Praise for Recapture Your Health

"Warning—if you follow the instructions in this book, you will forget what your doctor looks like."　　*—B.J. Vickers, Reiki Master, Lexington, Kentucky*

"*Recapture Your Health* is the ultimate survival manual that will show you how to look and feel better immediately. Everything Walt and Jan suggest works! I strongly recommend this book to anyone who has a strong wish for a better life than they're living now."

—Taylor Hay, author of Synergetics—Your Whole Life Fitness Plan

"*Recapture Your Health* is an excellent and energetic presentation of a common-sense approach to wellness. The book's pep-talk style is refreshing to read and its workbook layout is easy to follow. I recommend it!"

—Andrew W. Saul, contributing editor, Journal of Orthomolecular Medicine, *author of* Doctor Yourself: Natural Healing that Works

"This inspirational book about the 3LS Wellness Program will help transform lives by elucidating the steps necessary for a deeper and more personal healing."　　*—Bill Manahan, M.D., assistant professor of Family Practice and Community Health, past president of the American Holistic Medical Association*

"Walt Stoll has been a pioneer in the treatment and healing of people suffering from chronic illness. If you are committed to recapturing health, you'll find a wealth of information that will propel you down the path of healing."　　*—Banks Hudson, Marriage and Family Therapist*

"Based on sound principles, *Recapture Your Health* is an illuminating, cutting-edge health guide. It is a must for attaining and maintaining a sound, total health program."　　*—Aaron L. Mattes, Kinesiologist, author of* Active Isolated Stretching: The Mattes Method

"Dr. Walt Stoll's years of clinical practice and research pays off for the public in this volume. Nowhere have I found a better source for describing the foundation of diet, exercise, and relaxation for wellness and addressing chronic disorders."   —*Bob Sachs, Social Worker and Massage Therapist*

"True health comes about when our body, mind, and spirit are balanced. In *Recapture Your Health* Dr. Stoll and Jan DeCourtney have grasped this fundamental truth and present it in a way that is practical and understandable. It is a book which will be useful for both patient and physician."

> — *Gladys Taylor McGarey, M.D., M.D.(H.), past president of the American Holistic Medical Association, president of the Arizona Board of Homeopathic Medical Examiners"*

"If you want to improve your health, read this book. The time-tested, practical guidance for diet, relaxation, and exercise can help anyone feel better, have more energy, and reverse troublesome chronic symptoms. Highly recommended!"

> —*Beth Loiselle, R.D., L.D., author of* The Healing Power of Whole Foods

"Imagine a society devoid of most chronic illnesses or the need for revolving-door doctor appointments. The solution is inside this remarkable and comprehensive book!"   —*Kay Chambers, educator*

"What if you could find a healer that had more power than anyone to dramatically improve your health? Congratulations, that person is holding this book. This book describes a set of tools that you can use to create a wellness program that can change your life. It details a paradigm shift toward a view where causes, not symptoms, are treated on all levels."

> —*C. Meyer, Ph.D., scientist*

"This book is an absolute necessity for anyone interested in living a longer and healthier life. The authors of this book have compiled the most profound and comprehensive document on Holistic Medicine, and the connections among Nutrition-Relaxation-Exercise and Body-Mind-Spirit relationships to everyone's health."   —*Edward A. Wilbanks, M.S.*

"The 3LS Wellness Program is simple, so clear, and so effective."

> —*Terry Chappel, M.D., president of the International College of Integrative Medicine."*

Recapture
Your
Health

A Step-By-Step Program to
Reverse Chronic Symptoms
and Create Lasting Wellness

Walt Stoll, M.D. & Jan DeCourtney, C.M.T.

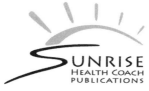

SUNRISE
HEALTH COACH
PUBLICATIONS

Boulder, Colorado

Grateful acknowledgment is made for permission to include the following: Target Heart Rate Charts from the International Fitness Association; an excerpt from "Holistic Health: What Is It?" and "The Holistic Health Practitioner: What Standards Set Him Apart?" by JoAnn Louk Axton, presented at the first conference of the Association for Holistic Health in 1975; an excerpt from the American Holistic Health Association website at www.ahha.org; and Appendix B, "Quick Reference Guides to the Perfect Whole Foods Diet" adapted from *The Healing Power of Whole Foods* by Beth Loiselle, R.D., L.D.

Publisher's Cataloging-in-Publication Data
    Stoll, Walt
    Recapture your health : a step-by-step program to reverse chronic symptoms and create lasting wellness / Walt Stoll and Jan DeCourtney
    p.   cm.
    Includes bibliographical references and index.
    ISBN-13: 978-0-9653171-2-2
    ISBN-10: 0-9653171-2-9 (alk. paper)
    1. Alternative Medicine – United States 2. Diet 3. Exercise
    4. Mind 5. Body 6. Self Care, Health
    I. DeCourtney, Jan   II. Title.
    RA776.5 S859 2005
    613 – dc20   2005907184 CIP

Contact: The authors welcome comments, additions, constructive criticism, or relevant experiences sent to the postal mailing address below. We'd be especially delighted to hear of your success with the 3LS Wellness Program. Give us feedback on what parts were particularly helpful and tell us how you put these ideas into action. Health care practitioners are invited to let us know of their success offering the 3LS in their practices.

For book orders, media inquiries, wholesale ordering (including health care practitioners who wish to resell our book), and serial rights information, please visit our website.

Sunrise Health Coach Publications
    PO Box 21132
    Boulder, CO 80308
    www.sunrisehealthcoach.com

*This book is dedicated to you, dear reader,
with best wishes for your health and happiness.*

*May this book provide stepping stones
for healing and self-development
of all aspects of your being.*

Acknowledgments

We would like to thank all who donated time and resources to help create this book. Each person's offering has been a beautiful gift of energy, love, support, and encouragement. It has touched our lives that so many have given so freely to help make this book available and serviceable to others.

People who have made a substantial contribution in terms of reviewing the manuscript, editing, concept evolution, and providing other significant support are Cathy Bauers, Psychotherapist; Joanne Catlin; Kay Chambers, Educator; Julien Coutellier, Graphic Artist; Noelle Coutellier, Artist; Linda Culp, Graphic Artist and Designer; Sandie Gorecki, M.A., O.T.R.; Holly Hayes; Mary Lilga, M.A., Scientist; Beth Loiselle, R.D., L.D.; Chris Meyer, Ph.D., Research Scientist; Barbara Munson, Editor; Walter Page, R.N., M.S.; Deborah Pageau; Bob Sachs, L.I.S.W., L.M.T.; Julia Schloesser, L.M.T.; Maggie Smith, C.M.T.; and Lou Zeman, C.M.T.

Volunteers who assisted by reading and commenting on the manuscript, assisting with sections of it, or providing other forms of support, are Carol Beline Keen; Maria Beaudoin; Abby Belasco; Sanford Coleman; Kathleen M. Diehl; Prue Dings, M.S.W.; Dave Fritts, Ph.D; Kim Glassburn; W. C. Green; Christie Hardin; Rebecca Herr; Linda Kelly, Physical Education Teacher; Bruce McCann; Nona Olivia; Brenda Orr; Michele Paiva; Corinne Rodriguez; Anita Rowe; Bill Stoll; Sunny Turner, M.A., Biofeedback Practitioner; Sharon L. Vadas-Arendt, Ph.D.; Betty J. Vickers, Reiki Master; Emily Walker; Ed Wilbanks, M.S.; and Doug Wray.

Special appreciation goes also to all individuals who contributed testimonials and endorsements to help inspire other people to begin their healing journey. Their names are with their writing. Thanks also to our families for their support and to the bulletin board participants at www .askwaltstollmd.com for their assistance.

I have been living all three aspects of the wellness lifestyle for some time now. The first month in about eight-and-a-half years that I did not get a migraine with my period, I was ecstatic! I can't explain to you how grateful I am to you for providing information on how to heal and become healthy. I feel I have the power in my hands and any health decision is mine, not a doctor's or anyone else's. I realize I still have a long way to go before I can say I am in a truly vibrant and healthy state. I went from 148 to my present 128 pounds. I can feel myself getting stronger every day. I was having four migraines per month and have gotten it down to a very mild one every once in a while. I can't tell you how much you have helped me and how much more I look forward to.

—*Donna El Hayek, Data Analyst, Diamond Bar, CA*

For six months I had been ill, with no relief in sight. I had symptoms of nausea, dizziness, constant fatigue, numbness, tremors in my hands, brain fog, and anxiety. I learned about Skilled Relaxation and the 3LS Wellness Program and started to incorporate these positive changes into my life. I learned about candida, leaky gut, and dysautonomia, and gained a better understanding of the cause of my problems. It was difficult at first, so I made changes gradually. After just one week of cutting sugar out of my diet, the brain fog disappeared. With each positive result, I was encouraged to make more changes. I started eating more whole foods and practicing Skilled Relaxation.

I had never even heard of bracing, but I was certainly guilty of it. Massages and stretching have helped with the bracing and my tremors are gone. I do feel like my body is starting to recuperate after six months on this program. I am now able to exercise in moderation, which is a big accomplishment considering that one year ago I could not even leave the house, I was so dizzy that I could not drive. I feel that my journey back to wellness will be a long one, there is no magic pill to fix all of my problems, but it is worth every sacrifice to once again enjoy good health.

—*Lauren, Registered Nurse, South FL*

Previous condition: symptoms related to fibromyalgia syndrome— insomnia, muscle strains and rigidity, foot pain, digestive problems (leaky gut syndrome), hypoglycemia, TMJ (jaw pain), dry eyes, constipation, food allergies, tingling in extremities, exhaustion. Present condition: Mild muscle stiffness, mild food allergies occasionally. Now I am not only able to stay well, but when symptoms rear their ugly head, I know why and how to turn my health around again. I'm still singing your praises and will be forever grateful for all the help you gave me when so many other "professionals" didn't have a clue what was going on with me. Your approach was most remarkable—you empowered me to do it myself. It's the path of survival.

—*Johnelle Donnell, Bible Study Teacher, Wichita Falls, TX*

My doctor doesn't think you can control Hashimoto's disease without medication, but my blood test came back today and proved her wrong. I have not treated my disease with meds but with diet and Skilled Relaxation. Lo and behold, my TSH levels are back to normal and so are my free T3 and T4's. I still show antibodies, but she said it is nothing to be concerned about. I told her I was going to continue to control my Hashimoto's with diet and Skilled Relaxation and see what happens. It felt so good to prove a doctor wrong and that going natural does work.

—*Lana Wilson, Bus Driver, Calgary, Alberta, Canada*

After turning 40 a few years ago I began to take stock of my fitness, or lack of it. I was overweight with borderline hypertension and couldn't walk up a flight of stairs without gasping for breath. While that was easy to blame on living in high altitude in Colorado, I was anxious to do something about my blood pressure. At the advice of a friend, I borrowed some relaxation and self-hypnosis tapes and began a daily half hour of skilled relaxation. I monitored my blood pressure daily, before and after each session. An immediate reduction occurred after each session, as I expected. But quite surprising to me was a longer-term reduction, over a period of several months, to a value well within the normal levels. Inspired by this improvement, I began a daily walking regimen and changed my diet. I walked four miles a day, ate more healthy foods, cut out late night snacks, and continued my skilled relaxation. A year later, I weigh 50 pounds less, feel great, and have recently started mountain climbing. Now it takes a climb to 13,000 feet and a wonderful view to take my breath away. Much of what I did was accomplished through trial and error, and I appreciate now the concept and practice of the "3LS Wellness Program" as discussed by Walt and Jan.   *—D.B., Ph.D., Boulder, CO*

After being plagued with herpes for years, and spending a fortune on every supplement/remedy under the sun, my relief came from effective Skilled Relaxation.   *—Anonymous*

I've had chronic pelvic pain for years. The key elements that have made a beneficial impact on my pain and severity of my symptoms are daily, effortless relaxation along with proper nutrition and moderate exercise. Giving my body what it naturally needs makes for a healthy mind and body. Calming my mind calms my body, which leads to less pain. Proper exercise and nutrition give my body what it needs to function properly, which also decreases pain.   *—Dayne Herren, Librarian, Topeka, KS*

By the time I connected with Dr. Stoll and his 3LS approach to wellness, I had been dismissed by my conventional doctor and 2 specialists, all of whom found nothing wrong with me. They condescendingly recommended I take Metamucil twice a day for the rest of my life and "just learn to live with it." I was chronically fatigued, bloated, constipated, lethargic, and was susceptible to yearly colds, sore throats, and sinus infections. My life drastically changed, however, when I began my holistic journey under Dr. Stoll's care. While being treated for Candida, I threw out soft drinks, processed foods (especially white flour and sugar) and began exploring the wonderland of whole foods. It was an incredible adventure and a blessing for my nutritionally starved body.

With the addition of aerobic exercise (regular hill-climbing walks), I am nearly free of all my symptoms and haven't been sick in years. I am finally beginning to embrace skilled relaxation, too (it's hard for me), and feel a greater sense of well-being just in the few months I've consistently practiced it. What a shame, all the years my insurance company foolishly reimbursed me for repeated appointments with conventional doctors and the drugs they prescribed. Discovering the nature/root of my illnesses and teaching me preventive methods like the 3LS Wellness Program is clearly the most effective therapy for a healthier existence!

—Kay Chambers, Educator, Louisville, KY

In October it will be four years since I was diagnosed with severe rheumatoid arthritis by multiple board-certified rheumatologists. I'd like to provide some longer-term perspective for those who may consider a wellness approach (diet modification/whole foods, relaxation techniques, light exercise) in dealing with this horrible problem and others like it. I started on this method about six weeks after diagnosis...I continue to be amazed at how my body continues to improve even after all this time... this past February I was able to start playing full-court basketball for 90 minutes once a week. My feet protested mightily the first time I did this, but this has also gradually improved. At age 44 and in good shape, I am one of the more mobile people on the floor, which includes people in their twenties. With the exception of some slight stiffness in my feet/ankles for a few minutes when I wake up in the morning, I feel better than I can ever recall. I feel like I have finally significantly backed away from Dr. Stoll's healthcare "cliff." It feels mighty good. It has been my experience that there is a definite pattern of improvement in the VAST majority of people who diligently try this type of approach.

—Joseph Hackett, IT Manager, Louisville, KY

For two years, I had gone from doctor to doctor trying to find a cure for my ills, wondering if I had some immune disease or HIV. These are the symptoms I was having: chronic post-nasal drip, chronic nasal allergies, stomach bloating and some reflux, hiatus hernia, and intermittent high blood pressure. I began doing progressive relaxation exercises, which is a form of the skilled relaxation Dr. Stoll is always raving about. I also tried his cure for hiatus hernia. It's been four months now, and all of the above, except for the bloating and reflux, are GONE! Even those are much less of a problem now (six months is recommended for optimal results on the progressive relaxation. I'm keeping at it). Also, I always used to get colds and the flu. Since I started the progressive relaxation I have not had one cold or flu. Trust me, Dr. Stoll's alternatives to Western medicine truly seem to be the key to a better quality of life. And the concept is so simple and ingenious that I didn't really believe in it at first. Just try it!

—Anonymous

Contents

Foreword by C. Norman Shealy, M.D., Ph.D. xix
Preface by Jan DeCourtney, C.M.T. xxi
List of Charts and Figures xxvi

PART I:
Introducing the 3LS Wellness Program

Introduction: What Can I Do to Improve My Health? 3
    How to Use This Book 4
    Key Phrases and Abbreviations in this Book 7

Chapter 1: How to be Healthy 9
    Practice Serious Wellness 9
        Are You Already Doing Some of These Practices? 9
        Two Key Ways to Use the Program 10
        How the 3LS Wellness Program Works 11
        Wellness Program Q & A 12
    About Healing Chronic Illness 21
        Focus on Resolving Your Condition 21
        Falling Off the Edge of a Cliff 21
        What You Think and Do Affects Your Health 22
        Ready to Start 24
    SUMMING IT UP 25
    Quick Start Guide 27
        Quick Start Skilled Relaxation 27
        Quick Start Perfect Whole Foods Diet 29
        Quick Start Right Exercise 31

Chapter 2: Skilled Relaxation 33

The Real Effects of Chronic Stress 33

    Bracing (Chronic Muscular Tension) 35

    Digestive Weakness (Leaky Gut Syndrome) 37

    Brain and Body Chemistry Imbalance 38

A Better Way to Relax: Skilled Relaxation (SR) 39

    Benefits of Skilled Relaxation 39

    How Skilled Relaxation Works 40

    Conditions Helped by Skilled Relaxation 42

    Anyone Can Do Skilled Relaxation 44

How to Do Skilled Relaxation 45

    First, Choose a Relaxation Technique 45

    Second, Begin to Practice 49

    Third, Evaluate Your SR Practice 53

Skilled Relaxation Q & A 59

For Immediate Relief 61

    A Quick Primer on Therapeutic Massage and Bodywork 62

Troubleshooting Guide for Skilled Relaxation 65

The Authors' Experiences 68

SUMMING IT UP 71

Skilled Relaxation—Steps to Take 72

Comments from Others About Practicing Skilled Relaxation 73

Chapter 3: The Whole Foods Diet 75

How do I Choose a Diet? 75

What is a Whole Foods Diet? 78

    Perfect Whole Foods Diet 78

    Liberal Whole Foods Diet 78

Benefits of the Perfect Whole Foods Diet 79

    Reverse Unusual Symptoms 79

    Weight Loss 80

    Increased Enjoyment of Food 80

    Self-Empowerment 81

    Increased Enjoyment of Life 81

Why a Whole Foods Diet Benefits Health 82

    The Krebs Cycle 83

    Refined Carbohydrates 84

How to Start the Perfect Whole Foods Diet 86

What is a Whole Food?..86

What is a Typical "Perfect" Menu? 87

Who can Benefit from the PWFD?..88

What to Eat and What Not to Eat 88

Where to Purchase Whole Foods 92

Whole Foods Diet Q & A..92

Getting Clear of Refined Carbohydrates 101

Should I Stop Eating Fruit?..104

The PWFD in Daily Life 106

Social Situations..106

Meal Preparation..108

Eating Out, Restaurants, and Travel 109

The Liberal Whole Foods Diet 111

Troubleshooting for the PWFD..112

The Authors' Experiences 118

SUMMING IT UP..121

PWFD—STEPS TO TAKE 123

Appreciation for the Whole Foods Diet..125

Chapter 4: The Right Exercise for You 129

Exercise—Love It or Hate It? 129

Choosing an Exercise..130

What's the Right Exercise? 131

Setting a Goal for Yourself 131

A Note to Athletes: The 3LS is for You, Too................................133

Aerobics! The Foundation of Any Wellness Program 134

Benefits of Aerobic Exercise 135

How to Do Aerobic Exercise 136

Aerobics: What You Should Know..140

Increase Your Metabolic Efficiency for Health 142

What is Metabolism?..143

Aerobics Q & A 144

Other Exercises and Their Effects 149

Non-Aerobic Exercise 150

Strengthening Exercise 150

Flexibility Exercise 150

Troubleshooting for Exercise 154

The Authors' Experiences 162

SUMMING IT UP 166
Aerobics Exercise Summary—STEPS TO TAKE 167
People Speak about Their Exercise Experiences 169

Chapter 5: The 3LS and Your Daily Life 173
Are You Procrastinating? 173
   Staying with the Program 174
   Maintaining Steady Progress 175
   How Long Should I Practice? 177
Troubleshooting Q & A for the 3LS 180
Relating to Family and Friends While Practicing 181
How Healing Progresses with the 3LS 187
   Exacerbations and Remissions 188
   The "Healing Crisis" 188
   Changing Techniques as You Heal 192
Two Essential Tools for Healing 193
   Tool #1: The Power of Your Awareness 194
   Tool #2: Constructive Use of Your Mind 200
The Authors' Experiences 202
SUMMING IT UP 205
Making Changes Step-By-Step 206
Comments on the 3LS Wellness Program 208
Charts Section 211

PART II
Getting the Most from the 3LS Wellness Program

Chapter 6: How Did This Happen?—Causes of Illness 217
What Are the Causes? 217
   1. Genetics and the Bell Curve 218
   2. The "Real" Stress 219
   3. Choice (Lifestyle Choices) 226
Genetics, Stress, and Choice Interact 228
The 3LS to the Rescue 229
   How the 3LS Practices Support Each Other 230
"Will I be Cured?" 231
Choosing Health 232
   Enhancing Your Opportunities for Choice 232
   Replacing Your Limiting Beliefs 234

How to "Choose" Health...236

SUMMING IT UP...238

People's Observations about the Causes of Illness 240

Chapter 7: Adjunct Approaches to the 3LS........................243

Steps to Healing...What Works for You?.........................243

Using Other Healing Methods Concurrently....................244

Self-Help..245

    Some Self-Help Methods.....................................245

    Eliminating and Decreasing Stressors.....................252

    Nutritional Supplementation 255

Using the Services of Physicians and Practitioners 261

    Allopathic Medicine...261

    Holistic Medicine..262

    Using the Allopathic Approach for Chronic Illness.........266

    Using the Holistic Approach for Chronic Illness.............269

Working with Practitioners Q & A................................272

Troubleshooting Checklist for Different Treatments
and Practitioners 274

The Authors' Experiences 275

SUMMING IT UP...278

People's Accounts of Using Additional Treatments............280

Chapter 8: Health for the Complete You:
    Mind, Emotions, and Spirit, Too 283

Wellness Is More than Just Physical Health 283

Body, Mind, and Spirit Are All Related 284

Healing Mind and Emotions....................................285

    Causes of Mental-Emotional Difficulty.....................285

    Conventional Treatments...................................287

    A Holistic Approach 287

    Understanding Brain and Body Chemistry 288

What You Can Do to Improve Mind and Emotions.............293

    Use the Pattern of the 3LS 293

    Employ Psychosocial Approaches to Healing.............295

    Use Holistic and Body-Mind-Spirit Therapies.............299

Healing Mind and Emotions Q & A 301

Troubleshooting Checklist for Improving Mind and Emotions.....302

The Spirit of Life and the 3LS...302
   Spirit is a Part of Life 302
The Authors' Experiences 304
SUMMING IT UP 305
Real Life Experiences Told 307

Conclusion...311
Defining Wellness 311

Afterword by Walt Stoll, M.D........................................315
Thoughts on the Issues of Modern-Day Medicine.................315

Appendix A: For Health Care Practitioners 323
Why a Section for Practitioners?......................................323
Practitioner Q & A...324
Ways to Empower a Patient..330
Working with the 3LS..334
3LS Q & A..335
Working with Patients to Improve Mind and Emotions 343
Including the 3LS in Your Practice....................................344
   Practitioner Resources..344
Comments from Practitioners 347

Appendix B: Quick References for the Perfect Whole Foods Diet.............351
Quick Reference for Food...352
Quick Reference for Additives 359

Notes..363

Glossary 369

Resources...381

Index..401

For 100 years the American Medical Association has dominated medical care in the United States, often squelching common sense. Over the past 40 years the AMA and most physicians have appeared to become pawns of the PharmacoMafia, offering a drug, or many drugs, for every symptom. While it is true that there have been some miraculous innovations in medical care, the vast majority of medical interventions are not useful in a majority of chronic illnesses. More importantly, the American Medical System is now responsible for a minimum of 250,000 deaths each year, as reported in the Journal of the American Medical Association in 2000. Interestingly some say that the figure might be as high as 789,000! Any way you look at it, medicine does not usually produce health. Indeed, most people lose health because of an unhealthy lifestyle.

Dr. Thomas McKeown, author of *The Origins of Human Disease,* has stated that 92% of the increased longevity enjoyed in the past century is not the result of medical innovations but is the result of common sense sanitation—improved handling of sewage, milk and water. The editor of the *New England Journal of Medicine,* commenting on that book, analyzed American medicine and stated, "Thus, we wind up barely on the positive side of zero"—just maybe one percent better than doing nothing!

The failure of drugs is perhaps greatest when applied to managing stress. Indeed, a wonderful article, "The Emperor's New Drugs," captured the situation best. The best antidepressant drug is 7% better than a placebo with a 25% complication rate. Those are not odds I would take! Anti-anxiety drugs are even worse—they convert anxiety into depression. Horse estrogen, promoted for over 50 years, may be great for horses, but when used for humans it is dangerous. And so on it goes.

Dr. Edmond Jacobson proved 80 years ago that deep relaxation would cure 80% of stress illnesses. Sir William Osler, the father of American medicine, stated that stress is the greatest cause of disease. *Drugs are never the solution to stress.* And neither is surgery, plastic or otherwise. Yes, there are good indications for drugs and surgery, perhaps 15% of the time. But for 85% of Americans, the solution is a common sense approach to health. Unfortunately, most Americans do not value health until they lose it. Thus the key for those who have lost it is to *Recapture Your Health—relaxation, nutrition and exercise!* These are also the keys to keeping health.

Ideally, those with real common sense will heed the message in this book to *keep* health. If you follow these guidelines you probably won't need to recapture health. It is well worth the minimal effort required to maintain health. Either way, keeping or recapturing, I urge you to heed the wise advice herein.

—*C. Norman Shealy, M.D., Ph.D.*
President, Holos University Graduate Seminary
Founding President, American Holistic Medical Association
Author of 90 Days to Stress-Free Living *and*
Life Beyond 100—Secrets of the Fountain of Youth

Preface by Jan DeCourtney, C.M.T.

Imagine what it would be like for you to have great health, to feel really good, and to stay that way! I hope you believe this can happen for you. If right now you are facing any kind of chronic health condition (with or without a diagnosis), and especially if you have been unsuccessful using conventional or other treatments, you may well find the health care answers you've been searching for detailed in this book. If you already enjoy good health, use this book for your health maintenance and prevention of illness.

The basic method of health improvement described in our book is Dr. Stoll's 3LS Wellness Program. This approach to wellness is time-tested, safe—and it works. His specific version of the traditional wellness protocol of Relaxation, Diet, and Exercise has been refined over more than three decades of clinical and personal experience. While most people know that relaxation, diet, and exercise are good for health, few people are aware that applying them knowledgeably, according to their individual specific needs, can be curative. People are often astonished to experience reversal of long-time, adverse health conditions just from using these three practices, but such recovery is commonplace.

It's called the 3LS Wellness Program because of the three essential practices—relaxation, diet, and exercise. You will find that it is different from other approaches which offer temporary disappearance of symptoms. Rather than just working with symptoms, the 3LS Wellness Program works on the causes to promote true healing. Physical health benefits are only part of what you gain. Other areas of your life may be enhanced as well. Since holistic healing works on all levels of your being, most who use the 3LS get an added bonus—their emotions, mind, and spirit become healthier as their chronic symptoms subside.

In this self-help book, we provide the tools for you to successfully apply this wellness program to your life and carry you through the entire process of healing. Expect to learn concepts, ideas, and tips for integrating wellness habits into your current lifestyle. Reverse your condition by cutting through the confusion of the latest fad treatments by understanding the actual causes of chronic illness and how to alleviate them. We've provided as much information as we could for you to move forward on your path to health.

We encourage you to start using the simple and effective practices right away. Only through experiencing the benefits of profound health improvements will you realize the importance of these practices and learn how much they can help you.

Dr. Stoll and I have different backgrounds and formal training. However, we both individually reached a deep understanding of a holistic lifestyle's benefits through our own personal experiences. Throughout this book, we share some of our experiences with you, both from implementing the 3LS Wellness Program to improve our own health conditions and from our work as health care professionals. First, allow me to share a little about my background and experience, and how Dr. Stoll's Wellness Program helped me improve my own health condition.

During my lifetime, I spent many years searching for solutions to my chronic health problems: constant fatigue, difficulty concentrating, terrible insomnia, anxiety, physical tension, palpitations, poor memory, excessive emotion, and a variety of strange symptoms that came and went. There was no name for this condition, but a good term for it would be "misery." I later found out many of my symptoms could be labeled functional dysautonomia (improper regulation of the autonomic nervous system) plus I had many nutrition and digestive issues. Short on funds for visiting health care practitioners (since I am without health insurance), and finding that the visits I could afford were mostly unhelpful, I grew determined to learn how to improve my health through self-help methods. One thing became apparent to me: my problem was deep and encompassing, and it would take working on all aspects of my being—body, mind, emotions, and spirit—to resolve my often debilitating condition.

For over 20 years, I explored healing philosophies and modalities, psychotherapeutic approaches, and spiritual paths. I learned everything I could, primarily from reading, taking classes and workshops, and seeking out and spending time with wise elders, teachers, therapists, health care practitioners, spiritual leaders, and others who were willing to share life wisdom with me. During that time, I also earned a college degree in Latin American Studies and lived in or was influenced by four different cultures (Hispanic, French, Chinese, and Native American) in addition to the US culture. I worked over 10 years for a small publisher of alternative health books. Next I took up formal training in Therapeutic Massage[1] and Polarity Therapy and became a certified health care practitioner. I continued learning in other disciplines so I would have more tools for helping myself and others.

However, despite improvements in the mental, emotional, and spiritual aspects of my life, my deep physical problems continued, so I kept searching for answers. Several years ago, it was my great good fortune to find Dr. Stoll's website and read about the "3LS Wellness Program." I first tried the Skilled Relaxation segment of the program and was astonished that it immediately helped me feel better. Then I added the other two aspects of the program— the Whole Foods Diet and Right Exercise. By practicing all three legs of this wellness triad simultaneously, I experienced dramatic improvements, and now, several years later, I am getting better still. I am rarely fatigued, I'm sleeping better at night, and my health is so much better than before. The poor concentration, anxiety, memory problems, and strange and varied symptoms have all but disappeared. I am also much more optimistic and relaxed than ever. I am looking forward to still further improvement as I continue to follow Dr. Stoll's protocol and healing advice over the years to come. Even my self-image and self-esteem have taken a dramatic turn for the better: I now think of myself as a healthy, happy person!

I was very impressed by Dr. Stoll as the first health care practitioner (and truly, the only one I have found so far) who understood both cause *and resolution* of chronic full-body muscle tension, which is something I see everyday in my massage clients. So after discovering his website, I began a mission to learn as much as possible from him. In particular, I wanted to learn more about self-help, since I knew that self-help can be one of the most effective forms of healing. I now pass along this new healthcare improvement discovery to my clients, friends, and family, so they too can receive the benefits of the 3LS approach to health. It is a pleasure to see them restoring health and happiness to their lives!

■ ■ ■

Dr. Stoll was first trained formally in American universities as a medical doctor, and he practiced conventional medicine for many years as a family practitioner. He had all the appropriate credentials and was well respected as a conventional physician and educator. He had some chronic conditions, too, which medical school had taught him he would live with for the rest of his life. However, after about 13 years of practice, he was introduced to alternative healing techniques, and much to his surprise, these methods resolved many of his health problems.

This enlightening experience led him to expand his practice. Dr. Stoll then became a holistic physician and a founding member of the American Holistic Medical Association. His unique and caring approach to practicing medicine included both conventional and unconventional healing methods. By coordinating the assistance of a team of practitioners using a wide variety of healing approaches, Dr. Stoll achieved great success in treating patients, especially very difficult cases. His Holistic Medical Center in Lexington, Kentucky thrived because it helped people transform their lives, and patients came to him from around the world for treatment.

Thereafter, Dr. Stoll proceeded to share what he had learned with his colleagues. Much to his surprise, not only were his healing methods resisted by many of his colleagues and the local medical establishment, but he was personally rejected and often harassed by many of his fellow physicians. He continued practicing holistically for another 17 years, but obviously was disapproved by the local medical board. After a long period of indirect political and economic harassment from the state licensing board (under the policy of the American Medical Association [AMA]), Dr. Stoll chose to stop practicing medicine and retire early. His experience, unfortunately, was all too common among holistic physicians in the 1980s and even today the "medical establishment" is not fully accepting of the holistic way of practicing medicine pioneered by Dr. Stoll and his forward-thinking colleagues.

Fortunately Walt Stoll did not stop helping people. He used the new opportunity to write his first book, *Saving Yourself from the Disease Care Crisis,* which led to his website, www.askwaltstollmd.com. Through the powerful medium of the Internet, his books, and his health coaching service, he has continued to carry his message of the healing power of holistic medicine to people around the world. He is dedicated to educating people on how to go beyond the dictates of conventional medicine to find a better solution to their chronic problems. Read more about the issues of modern-day medicine in the Afterword.

■ ■ ■

In the spring of 2001, I contacted Dr. Stoll with the intention of preparing handouts for my clients. He gave me permission to compile information from his website to do so and graciously offered his assistance. After a few months of work, I had gathered so much helpful information about the Wellness Program that the handouts became too long. Together, Dr. Stoll and

I decided to create this book. In the course of our collaboration, we have both contributed to and worked on all parts of this writing.

We have aspired to make this a user-friendly, easy-to-read book, so don't be surprised about the use of ordinary conversational speech or our including some humor. We may call doctors "docs" and use abbreviations, in the style of written communication used on the bulletin board of the website. No irreverence is intended. Also, in the book, we refer to him as Walt, doc, or Dr. Stoll, since he feels that in a truly effective healing relationship, titles can sometimes get in the way.

I would like to express my appreciation to Dr. Walt Stoll, who is a great inspiration and mentor in my life and work. He has been so very supportive and has taught me so much during the entire time we have been working on this project together. He has transformed my life.

We have no expensive cure to sell you. We offer you our knowledge and experience with the 3LS Wellness Program to improve your health. It is our hope that you will try this program and experience its benefits for yourself. We wish that you enjoy abundant health and happiness in your life.

The door to your future wellness is open—we invite you to walk through.

List of Charts and Figures

Introduction: How the 3LS Got Its Name 4

Chapter 1: The Edge of the Cliff..23

Chapter 2: Hypothalamus..34

Chapter 3: Comparing the Perfect and Liberal Whole Foods Diet 86

Chapter 4: Target Heart Rate Chart..138

Chapter 5: Two-Week Calendar for Tracking the 3LS................................210
    Symptom Tracking Chart 211
    Chart for Recording Results of Therapeutic Trials 212
    Blank Monthly Chart 213

Chapter 6: Bell Curve..219

Key: Authors' Personal Comments

When you see [■■■ JAN:] the following text is her specific comment.

When you see [■■■ WALT:] the following text is his specific comment.

Each one's comments ends with ■■■.

Part 1

Introducing the 3LS Wellness Program

Introduction

"What can I do to improve my health?"

"There are many paths to the top of the mountain." This statement by the great sages of human history can be used to describe the various ways to reach the goal of vigorous health and wholeness. And while this is a true statement, in our more than 38 years of working with patients struggling with a wide variety of conditions, we have found one particular path to wellness that reliably and effectively helps the most people with the greatest success. We recommend this path to you as the best way to improve your health.

■■■ WALT: This path is called the 3LS Wellness Program, a thoroughly researched, step-by-step protocol of Relaxation, Diet, and Exercise. I have worked with dozens of practitioners, thousands of patients, and a variety of methods and plans. I have witnessed again and again how patients who follow the path of the 3LS Wellness Program make remarkable improvements in their health conditions. Now, through this book, Jan and I would like to give you the opportunity to achieve the same type of health improvement as our patients.

You don't have to have a chronic health condition to follow the 3LS program, but this wellness protocol is especially effective for helping to reverse chronic illnesses, whether diagnosed or not. If you are healthy, the 3LS is useful and beneficial for maintaining that good health, as well as for preventing countless health problems in the future.

I would not have believed the effect of doing the three practices that comprise the Program could be so positive and spectacular had I not first experienced it in my own mind, body, and spirit. The changes brought about by my adopting the 3LS Wellness Program were so dramatic that my patients began to ask me what I was doing for *my* health. Sharing that information was what started my career in Holistic Medicine. (I like to use a specific definition of what I term Holistic Medicine: a philosophy of medicine that is responsive to all aspects of a person and uses a wide range of therapeutic modalities.) My area of interest and expertise in practicing medicine is optimal health (wellness). My specialty is educating individuals about options for alleviating chronic conditions that conventional medicine ignores. ■■■

How to Use This Book

To most effectively accomplish the 3LS Wellness Program, it is helpful to fully understand how this self-care protocol works as a whole. The more you understand, the more benefit you will get from the practices. Therefore, we recommend that you read the entire book from beginning to end so you will be able to implement the practices accurately and get the promised results. Look for the Summaries to help you catch the important points and to make

How the 3LS Got Its Name

We call this Wellness Program "3LS." The name originates with the old-fashioned image of a 3-legged stool. Picture a solid wooden stool with three stable legs…perhaps in a dairy barn. (Walt grew up on a dairy farm in Ohio.) Such a stool is a useful tool for the one who uses it. A 3-legged stool offers stability, support, and rest. Although you could sometimes balance adequately on one or two legs, this wouldn't be as steady as three and would sometimes tip over. Of course, adding more legs provides even more stability, but three provides the basic foundation.

This useful wellness program best supports your health when you use all three of its aspects, or "legs." Thus it was nicknamed the 3-Legged Stool, which has now been simplified to 3LS. The idea to use this concept came about because we wanted to give you a solid, stable image that you could recall every time you think about your health and well-being.

Another way you can think about this Wellness Program is that it provides "3 Lasting Solutions" for your health.

understanding easier. If you are too ill or weak to read entire chapters, the Summaries will help you.

For those who are eager to start implementing the Wellness Program immediately, you will find Quick-Start Guides starting on page 27. These Quick-Start Guides will give you just enough information to get you going so you can begin your path to health today and, while you are reading the rest of the book. We encourage you to select and begin at least one of the three practices immediately, so you will start progressing on your path to health even while you are still learning the details.

The Quick-Start Guides, however, do not give all of the instructions, so you will benefit from reading the rest of the book to learn how to make each practice effective and ensure your success. Let's look at the different sections.

- **Part I** of this book explores each of the individual legs of the Wellness Program. For each of the three practices, we have included a Summary that you can photocopy or tear out for ready reference or use as a reminder (for example, tape it to your mirror or refrigerator). Reading the Summaries will give you the minimum information to start learning and practicing the 3LS Program. In Part I we also teach you how to integrate the 3LS into daily life and how the process of healing occurs.

- **Part II** discusses holistic healing in general and gives guidance for maximizing your use of the 3LS. It discusses the causes of chronic illness and how the 3LS addresses causes and not just symptoms. Part II also instructs how to use other healing methods together with the 3LS, both self-help and professionally assisted treatments. Finally, it looks at mental-emotional health, and how the growth of one's spirit and a deeper meaning to life can be a result of following this Wellness Program.

- **Appendix A:** For Health Care Practitioners appears at the end of the book. Everyone can benefit from reading it. Understanding the 3LS from the perspective of health care professionals will help you work more effectively with your own providers, should you feel the need to seek their assistance.

- **Appendix B:** Quick Reference Guides for the Perfect Whole Foods Diet follows. These special guides provide a comprehensive list of foods and additives allowed on the diet.

The appendices are followed by a Glossary of abbreviations and concepts that will enrich your understanding as you read. (It's helpful to read the entire Glossary just to learn more, too!) A large Resource section comes next. After these sections you will find Reference Notes and an Index.

Comments from individuals who have used the 3LS are located at the end of most chapters. Many were written by participants on the Bulletin Board at www.askwaltstollmd.com. Some of these quotes include people's full names, but others have given initials or wished to remain anonymous. We respect people's confidentiality. The comments give you the opportunity to read about a wide range of experiences and understand the potential for change made possible by deciding to alter your lifestyle for the better.

You may photocopy any of the pages marked "This page may be photocopied" for your own use or to give to family and friends. Health care practitioners may copy these pages for patients or clients, and teachers may do the same for their students.

■ ■ ■

In working together to compile this information for you, we have done our best to make this book as complete and user-friendly as possible, with as many tools as we could add to help you learn, study, and assimilate. Because we have different experiences and perspectives, each of us have sometimes given commentaries on a particular topic. You will know which one of us is speaking by our names next to the text, and by the small boxes that begin and end our comments.

This is a self-help book, not a technical or theoretical book. We have based it on actual experience and real results in daily life. Rather than including lots of statistics and figures, we wanted to keep the focus on practical information you can use immediately to help yourself. We feel that reading the numerous experiences of others who have used the Program and actually doing the Program yourself will be more likely to convince you than statistics will.

But we also have included many notes, references, and resources in this book to guide you to find figures and statistics, should you want them. From this information you will find that the 3LS consists of time-honored practices that never go out of date, unlike current fad medications and treatments that are proven effective one year and then later proven ineffective or even harmful. These time-tested practices more and more are "taking up the slack" where conventional medicine falters.

We want you to succeed at this. If you need additional help or have questions, you'll find many ways to obtain assistance. Extensive information

archives and a bulletin board for asking questions are available at www
.askwaltstollmd.com, a practitioner network is located at the American
Holistic Health Association's website at www.ahha.org, and other resources
may be found in the Resources section at the end of this book.

—Walt Stoll, M.D. and Jan DeCourtney, C.M.T

■ ■ ■

Key Phrases and Abbreviations in This Book

Because some terms in this book may be new to you, here are definitions
of some of the key phrases.

Allopathic: Conventional medical approaches to health care.

Bodymind: The term bodymind describes the reality of how closely the
functions of mind and body are interrelated.

Chronic illness: An illness or symptom that persists over a long period of
time, or recurs (repeats). Most chronic symptoms or conditions appear
suddenly but have been building over a length of time. The natural
progression of chronic conditions is to become more severe. The term
chronic relates to the duration of symptoms rather than their severity.

Edge of the Cliff: A phrase that describes the point at which symptoms
begin to appear. The limit for any functional body system to cope with
or tolerate stress.

Healing: The use of inner power and resources of our mind and body to
restore our own unique balance and harmony. It is this balance and
harmony that results in full health and gives us the ability to live lives
of vitality and joy.

Holistic Medicine: Emphasizes the necessity of looking at the whole person and the whole situation, including analysis of physical, nutritional,
environmental, emotional, spiritual, and lifestyle values. Holistic medicine particularly focuses upon patient education and patient responsibility for personal efforts to achieve balance.

Holistic medicine, in its broadest sense, could include practically
every type of medicine, including all of the healing philosophies and
modalities in the world. It encompasses all safe modalities of diagnosis
and treatment (including drugs and surgery) and searches for the root
cause of illness.

Practicing Serious Wellness: This means practicing the 3LS Wellness Program, plus doing whatever else it takes to become healthy, including
learning and study.

Self-help: Self-help is about observing yourself, your habits, thoughts, feelings, and actions. It is about examining those aspects of yourself (body, mind, emotions, spirit) that contribute to your health condition and finding ways to make lifestyle changes that will enhance and improve your health and well-being.

Stress: Anything that puts the body in fight-or-flight mode (activates the sympathetic nervous system) causing an increase in the heart, respiratory, and blood pressure rates, and moving blood away from your digestive organs and into large muscles in preparation for a fight or flight. Countless factors and events can activate the fight-or-flight response.

Website: Dr. Stoll's website: www.askwaltstollmd.com.

Abbreviations

3LS .... "3-Legged Stool" or "3 Lasting Solutions" Wellness Program
AE........... Aerobic Exercise
AHHA .... American Holistic Health Association
AHMA.... American Holistic Medical Association
AMA....... American Medical Association
CAM....... Complementary and Alternative Medicine
EEG........ Electro Encephalo Gram
EFA......... Essential Fatty Acids
FOF .... Fight or Flight
GERD ..... Gastro Esophageal Reflux Disorder (also called hiatal hernia or acid reflux)
GSR .... Galvanic Skin Response
PWFD .... Perfect Whole Foods Diet
RE........... Right Exercise
SR .... Skilled Relaxation
WFD....... Whole Foods Diet

How to
Be Healthy

PRACTICE SERIOUS WELLNESS

The best way to avoid and resolve many chronic health conditions is to be too healthy to have them!

That is easy to say, but if you are pretty far down the slippery slope of bodily or mental dysfunction or disease and have lots of undesirable symptoms, you need to *get serious* about practicing the steps to regain health, and dedicate yourself to getting well again. The dream is within your reach.

This can be done by using the 3LS Wellness Program, which we also refer to as Practicing Serious Wellness. 3LS entails:

- Practicing an effective form of Skilled Relaxation (SR).
- Following a Whole Foods Diet (WFD).
- Choosing the Right Exercise (RE) for you.

Careful practice of these three interconnected legs of the Wellness Program can greatly enhance your health overall, and many chronic conditions will clear up totally. The benefits come from helping your body heal itself, because that's the only way you can truly be healthy.

Are You Already Doing Some of These Practices?

■■■ JAN: If you already have a Relaxation practice, think you're eating enough Whole Foods, or are doing pretty well with Exercise—congratulations! You're already off to a good start. However, you're still not "practicing the 3LS" until you have read each of the chapters and learned exactly what you need to know to make your practices work effectively enough to heal your chronic condition or generally improve your health. You have not actually "been there, done that" until you have followed the detailed instructions in each chapter of our book.

Why am I saying this? Take it from one who knows: I practiced relaxation techniques for 20 years, thought I was eating a healthy diet, and exercised occasionally—but did not get any health benefits until I read and followed Dr. Stoll's instructions precisely! I read them first on the Internet at www .askwaltstollmd.com. Before then, I wasted a lot of time and could have been feeling better sooner. By learning and putting into daily practice this specific information, you will most likely experience what I did—a great improvement in the effectiveness and results of your existing Relaxation, Diet, and Exercise activities.

If you are not yet doing a Relaxation practice, not eating a Whole Foods Diet, not Exercising, and have yet to begin your path towards wellness, congratulations also! You are taking a great first step by reading this book. ■■■

Two Key Ways to Use the Program

For a long time, the greatest holistic practitioners and teachers in the world have promoted using rest, diet, and exercise for health. This version presented in our book offers more detail and instruction on these three critical areas of health improvement than you will find in your typical health self-help book or program. Moreover, we show you how to effectively integrate them, step by step.

Below are two main ways to apply the Wellness Program as part of your personal health program.

1. To heal a chronic condition: short-term program

If you have a specific health problem or chronic condition that you wish to heal, for fastest results, start the 3LS Wellness Program and stick to it for at least six months to a year. We recommend:

- Skilled Relaxation for 20 minutes twice a day

- A Perfect Whole Foods Diet

- Exercise of any kind sufficient to create a positive, sustained improvement in your metabolism, which may gradually lead to doing Aerobic Exercise 20 to 30 minutes, three or more times a week.

We have seen this basic regimen produce the quickest and most certain health results for the largest number of patients. However, since results are individual, some people will get better sooner while others will take longer.

2. For health maintenance

After your chronic condition has improved or healed by using the first regimen, continue to use the 3LS Wellness Program in a slightly different way for health maintenance. This protocol is also for people who are healthy and want to stay that way. For everyone in these categories, we recommend:

- Skilled Relaxation for 20 minutes *once or twice a day*
- A *liberal* Whole Foods Diet
- Aerobic Exercise for 20 minutes or longer, three or more times a week (or whatever type of exercise you can do that leads to a consistent, sustained increase in your metabolism).

Once you are well (or at least on your path to wellness so that you feel noticeably better), you will know what wellness feels like, and then you can determine how much time and energy you need to devote to continuing the practices. It would not hurt anyone to continue the full health benefit program forever, but some people can choose to spend less time on certain aspects of their Wellness Program later on than they did at the beginning.

Practicing wellness is somewhat like making a good investment. You receive a return from what you put into it. Whatever you spend in terms of time, especially at the beginning, is returned in greater productivity and efficiency due to better health. You will generally not have to put in as much time later as you did at the start. However, you may feel so much better and enjoy the whole process so much that you choose to spend more time, effort, and money to continue to improve your health even more. You'll also notice the process soon becomes routine.

How the 3LS Wellness Program Works

We as men, women, and children have inherent in our being a wondrous system called the human bodymind. The term bodymind describes the reality of how closely the function of mind and body are interrelated. The human bodymind is the most powerful tool that we have for healing and preventing illness. Anything that helps part of the bodymind helps the whole, because everything works together and is interconnected like a spider's web.

The human species has yet to find a better way to rebalance a dysfunctional body system than utilizing the power of nature inherent in one's own bodymind. Sometimes, trying to hurry up the healing or rebalancing using certain medical approaches (for example, drugs or surgery) can actually cause damage instead of healing. Our position is that natural approaches to healing that use your own inner healing power, like the 3LS, are almost always safe and may be even more effective than the tools of current medical science.

The 3LS Wellness Program aims at enhancing the function of the bodymind. The 3LS improves the web of a person's total function, which allows the bodymind to do the job of rebalancing itself. The three aspects of Practicing Serious Wellness are most effective at this rebalancing when done comprehensively and simultaneously. Each aspect of this health triad enhances the others in an exponential way, creating a synergistic effect.

It works like this: let's say you get three points for doing one leg of the Wellness Program. When you add a second, you get nine points rather than six. If you add the third activity, you get 27! Our normal thinking is if we get three for each part, we end up with a total of nine. But the way in which the body, mind, and spirit respond to our efforts is not 3 + 3 + 3, but 3 x 3 x 3. Everything in the body affects everything else in the body.

Practicing only one or two aspects of the Program will still bring you health benefits, but not to the degree that all three do. This synergy explains why eating Whole Foods won't address or resolve *all* the problems without also adding Skilled Relaxation. And Exercise won't solve *everything* by itself. Moreover, the quickest results are obtained by using all three practices at the same time. However, you do not have to *start* all three simultaneously. If you suffer from a chronic condition and you are just beginning the 3LS, you may be better off choosing one leg and then using the benefits and energy gained from that part to start the next.

Wellness Program Q & A

Q: What conditions can be helped with the 3LS?

A: It is interesting that people want to see a list of diseases or symptoms that can improve from resolving the basic causes of illness with the 3LS. One could fill a book of 1,000 pages or more just listing the symptoms that could possibly be alleviated. Here we can only mention a few general categories of health problems that the Wellness Program can help. From decades of practicing medicine and as evidenced in the lives of thousands of people who have written in to the website bulletin board at www.askwaltstollmd.com, the 3LS Wellness Program has been proven effective with most chronic functional diseases, mental-emotional problems, musculo-skeletal disorders, and systemic problems. It is also proven helpful for patients who have unusual symptoms that are not nameable or identifiable as any specific condition, syndrome, or disease. The 3LS even helps conditions you might not expect it to address. One example is dental problems. Even conditions like TMJ (jaw pain), bruxism (night grinding), and tooth decay (caused by dietary issues) can be helped by practicing Wellness. The 3LS Program also helps most chronic conditions resulting from injury or accident.

Chapter 2 (Relaxation), Chapter 3 (Diet), and Chapter 4 (Exercise) have short lists of conditions that each practice helps most. But keep in mind the three aspects will work in some way (sometimes dramatically) for nearly everyone who uses them correctly. If this seems too miraculous, we don't blame you for your skepticism, since doubtlessly you've been bombarded by advertisements that claim unrealistic results that do not deliver. Thus, practicing the 3LS Program merits your careful consideration. You deserve to know everything possible about the 3LS for your evaluation, so we have included as much information as we could.

It is our experience that regardless of the condition or symptom that you have, if you do not practice Wellness, as time goes on you will end up with poorer health, fewer resources, and fewer options.

Q: Does the 3LS Program actually cure everything completely?

A: The term "reversing" may be a more accurate description of what happens with the 3LS rather than "curing." Yet besides just reversing a condition, practicing the Wellness Program can actually change a person's genetic potential by improving molecular, cellular, and atomic mechanisms. Thus holistic approaches such as Wellness and the synergy that results are many times more likely to actually cure something than conventional approaches.

Since most chronic conditions are progressive (meaning they keep getting worse), many people would be doing well just to see their health problem progress no further, and be very happy about that. By using the 3LS, they may become ecstatic to see their condition regress, and unbelieving when it actually disappears, which often happens.

In some cases, even if the Program does not totally resolve a problem in six to twelve months, the individual practicing it would be so much healthier by then, that anything else that needs to be done with the help of practitioners could work much quicker and more effectively, since the patient or client has done most of the groundwork already.

Keep in mind that some chronic conditions are structural in nature or origin, or have gone past the point of being curable, depending upon how much damage was done before starting the Program. An example of this is a structural condition one was born with or a condition that has produced so much scarring that only an act of God could reverse it. Although a wellness program would help those individuals get the most out of what remains of their health, these conditions would not likely be reversed.

The 3LS can even be used in death, dying, and hospice situations. We've had patients who, before they died, improved the quality of their lives and saw a reduction in debilitating, painful symptoms through use of these practices. Even though death will eventually come to all of us, until that day finally comes, we can significantly enjoy our lives more and for a longer lifespan through better health practices.

Q: What are the benefits you keep talking about that come from doing the practices?

A: The most obvious one is that some or all symptoms disappear. You may experience dramatic changes in how you feel. Strength and energy increase. You feel happier and more coordinated. Your mind becomes clearer and you make better decisions.

There are other payoffs, depending upon what symptoms or conditions you have had, and how long you have had them. Since benefits and improvements are individual depending upon the symptoms, they cannot be easily described. We encourage you to read the comments after each chapter to better understand the wide variety of benefits that people have received from practicing different parts of Wellness and from doing all of them in combination.

From our experience, we have seen notable improvement in many people who start even one part of the Program. Seeing their positive results, they become convinced of the validity of this wellness approach and are willing to expend the effort to start the second and then the third aspect.

One of the constants of holistic medicine is that when a person begins to do whatever their bodymind really needs (Skilled Relaxation, Exercise, Dietary changes, supplements, etc.) many unexpected benefits show up. So don't be too surprised if you experience improvements that you were not expecting.

Q: How long does it take to see results from practice?

A: The length of time it takes to see significant results or even total reversal of symptoms depends on how diligent you are in practicing, how many of the practices you do, and how deeply rooted your condition is. Many people experience significant improvement in three to six months if they are using all three legs of the 3LS.

We can also answer this question in terms of each of the three practices. Although most people see some short-term benefits almost immediately from doing Skilled Relaxation, you will not really see the more wonderful benefits for a few months. Skilled Relaxation needs to be done correctly for at least three months to begin to see the full potential for that person. In the case of the Perfect Whole Foods Diet, initial results can be seen in three and one-half days to a week, and maximum benefits in about six months. Any type of Exercise makes most people feel better almost right away. However, for aerobics, you will need to exercise for at least six weeks to begin to see the true benefits.

All of these estimates of results are based on many years of clinical practice using the 3LS with patients. Part II (which is about using the 3LS in daily life) has more information about combining the three aspects of the Wellness Program and how the healing process occurs.

Q: How do I know if what I have is a chronic condition or if I need to go see a doctor right away?
A: If you feel for any reason that you need to be seen by a doctor, make an appointment and see one. Chronic means something that is persisting over a long period of time, or recurring (repeating). Most chronic conditions first show themselves suddenly, and then the symptoms linger for a long time.

Many people wish to consult a physician or practitioner about their symptoms before beginning this Wellness Program just to be sure they don't have an acute or urgent problem. They are encouraged to do so.

Q: Do I need to see a health care practitioner while I'm practicing this Wellness Program, or can I use the 3LS on my own?
A: Practicing Wellness as we discuss it in this book is the safest, most commonly effective, and least expensive approach to reversing symptoms and conditions. Thus, the 3LS can be used by many, if not most, people as a self-help or self-care program. However, self-help has limitations, and some people will need to seek professional help. Some need encouragement and support while going through this process, and this support may be provided by practitioners. Individuals who have issues that cannot be resolved by the 3LS or who do not understand exactly what to do will also benefit from consulting a professional.

About 10% to 15% of conditions are best approached and treated allopathically (with medications or surgery).[1] Other conditions may be helped by using

When to Seek Medical Advice

Always seek appropriate medical advice, regardless of whether or not your condition is chronic, if you have the following:

- Fever, *with no other symptoms,* that lasts more than a day
- Any recurrent symptom you cannot definitely tie to a specific cause
- Urinary symptoms of any kind
- Swelling anywhere, unless you are certain of its cause (such as from an injury)
- Any unexplained alteration of function of any part of the body
- Exposure to poisons
- A foreign body, anywhere
- Any injury that remains painful more than seven days
- Chest pain associated with exertion or in any other way not clearly explained
- Any of the seven danger signs of cancer:
  —A change in bowel habits or bladder function
  —Sores that do not heal
  —Unusual bleeding or discharge
  —A thickening or lump in the breast or other parts of the body
  —Indigestion or difficulty swallowing
  —A recent change in a wart or mole
  —A nagging cough or hoarseness
- Any problem of living that begins to affect your ability to concentrate, sleep, or enjoy life

other healing methods. However, since improving health and well-being will help any treatment work better, unless your situation is urgent, you might practice the 3LS with determination and dedication before or while using other treatments for your chronic condition. This will bring more strength and resources to those treatments.

If your diagnosis is something your doctor says can only be treated, and not cured, Practicing Serious Wellness might be the best solution for you. However, if you tell your physician what you are doing, don't be discouraged if he or she says, "I've never heard of the 3LS, so it probably won't help." Just keep doing the practices on your own.

Keep in mind—healing does not necessarily require a medical license, and there are many practitioners who may be able to assist you. Chapter 7 (about working with health care practitioners) has more information about selecting and working with health care practitioners.

The holistic approach to healing empowers individuals to take charge of their own health, but it is also wise to seek help when it is needed. This is why we added a chapter about seeking additional care, and also why we added the claimer/disclaimer on our copyright page. The claimer/disclaimer says: "In the Holistic Healing model, each person is responsible for his own health and makes his own choices in healing. The information in this book is provided for your information and education. Any application of the information is at your own discretion. If you feel you need to do so, consult with your physician or knowledgeable practitioner before or while making use of this information or beginning any wellness program." Self-help requires intelligence, common sense, and the ability to take full responsibility for your own actions. We encourage you to make your own health care decisions based upon your research, or in partnership with a qualified health care professional, when available. If you suspect you have a disease or health-related condition of any kind, please do some research to understand your condition. Learn from more than one source.

Q: I've had my health problem for a long time. It seems pretty serious. My symptoms are really weird. Do you think it is still possible to help my condition using the 3LS?

A: Actually, the best way we know of to help a difficult, chronic condition, especially those with unusual symptoms, is the 3LS. Without even knowing your diagnosis, we can confidently say: your very best option is most likely Practicing Serious Wellness, beginning at once and continuing for the next year or longer. There is no harm in following this wellness program correctly, although it takes discipline and learning. At the very least, it will make you healthier for the rest of your life. Simply put, you have nothing to lose and so much to gain. If your illness seems severe, you need to put your health above everything else if you want to get better. We have yet to see this Wellness Program fail when properly and faithfully applied. Seek additional help at the same time if necessary.

Q: Why do you call it, "Practicing Serious Wellness"?

A: Practicing Serious Wellness means using the 3LS and doing whatever else it takes to get well. If you have symptoms, you must seriously dedicate yourself to setting goals and working with determination and effort toward getting better. Integrating some or all of the practices that make up the 3LS is the most important thing you can do if you are serious about improving your health. Continued learning and study may help tremendously, and you may wish to add other approaches that enhance the Program's effects.

Many people need to get a totally different perspective of what it means to work on improving health! Just as you would seriously focus on working a full-time job or going to college full time, you must put time and energy into practicing wellness. The ultimate determinant in your achieving health is your desire to do what you have to do to get better and then doing it. Your willingness to make and stick to the necessary lifestyle changes will create health for you. With this amount of effort, chances are that you can graduate from illness to essential wellness in only one year.

Some people find it easy and fun to practice the 3LS, and others find it challenging. One way to turn your process of Practicing Serious Wellness into an enjoyable experience is by considering it as a new, *wonderful* lifestyle change that will bring profound and positive benefits to all aspects of your life.

Q: I have been taking a prescription drug, and it has helped a lot. Should I continue taking it while I am using the 3LS?

A: At the beginning, do not stop whatever has been working for you. As with all regimens, you should not discontinue or even change the dose or timing of a medication without close consultation with a qualified practitioner. If taking something is helping you, use it while learning about the causes of your symptoms and as you begin the Program.

Remember, however, that when medications or non-toxic remedies such as herbs cause symptoms to disappear, *this is not necessarily a sign that your problem is gone.* Reducing symptoms without working on the cause of your problem is akin to putting black tape over the dashboard warning light so you don't have to see it. Symptom suppression is never a permanent solution to a health problem. Unfortunately, this is just what most people do, but they do nothing to address *why* their symptoms are happening. Their medications, herbs, or surgery work (for a while), but the causes creating the health condition are continuing to accumulate. Then the bodymind has to shout even louder for help by creating worse symptoms.

Here is a story that illustrates this point. Once upon a time, there was a couch potato, doing his thing chilling out on the sofa, when the doorbell started ringing. He didn't want to get up, so he didn't. However, the bell continued to ring until it was driving him to distraction. So, he got up and cut the wires to the doorbell. It stopped ringing and he went back to watching TV and snacking on junk food. Unfortunately for him, the doorbell ringing was his neighbor trying to warn him that his house was on fire. This may or may not be a true story, but we hope it helps you understand that the symptoms are a warning that something is wrong.

Q: Are there any side effects or harm from using the 3LS?
A: The "side effects" are gratifyingly positive. For example, if you have high blood pressure and are taking medication, you had better keep a close watch on your condition, since before the end of a year of practicing the 3LS, you will probably have to reduce your dosage due to the positive changes.

Appropriate implementation of the 3LS is without any known permanent or irreversible negative harm or side effects. With the 3LS, you may experience some temporary healing effects. Some examples include sore muscles for a few days when you start exercising or various gastrointestinal adjustments when you clean up your diet. For this and related reasons, we encourage you to carefully read the book so you know what you are doing when you implement the 3LS.

If you stick reasonably close to the instructions, you can only do yourself good. If you have any doubt about whether you are following the instructions correctly, or if something does not feel right about what you are doing, consult a qualified health care practitioner. Of course, anyone can create a problem for himself or herself by abusing or misusing any thing or any instruction. For example, if you do Skilled Relaxation for 12 hours each day for months instead of 20 minutes twice a day, it may not be an optimum choice with good results in your life.

Please note that for many people, success with the practices makes them more aware of other ongoing health problems they haven't noticed previously. For example, if your main symptomatic complaint gets better from using the 3LS, perhaps now you begin noticing a different health problem. Most likely this other problem is not new, but you were simply unaware of it because your main symptom was getting all your attention.

One of the tasks of self-healing is to pay attention, make appropriate adjustments to your healing program, and keep moving forward. So, it is true that when you go through a healing process, you may feel worse for part of the time along the way. Changes, even sometimes those that do not feel well, are often signals that you are getting better. This is called a healing crisis and is described fully in Chapter 5.

The increased sensitivity that comes with better health is a great asset. You will most likely become aware of increased energy and creativity, enhanced attention span and mental focus, elevated emotions, improved self-esteem, and a positive outlook. Your fit body and glowing appearance, plus your confidence and upbeat attitude, will be noticed by others, too. These are the typical "side-effects" of this program.

Q: How much does it cost to follow the 3LS Wellness Program?

A: One of the best things about this Program is that almost everything you need costs only your time and effort. Some people may want to refer to a few other books to learn some of these practices (see the individual chapters), which may be obtained through libraries. Some supplemental information is already so well written in other resources, and not everyone needs it, that it did not make sense to add it here. If you choose to purchase those books, you will find they are easy to obtain and inexpensive.

Moreover, the practices are best done at home, so the Wellness Program is convenient as well as inexpensive.

Q: Which aspect of Practicing Serious Wellness is the most important one, and which one should I start first?

A: The first and most important aspect of the 3LS for you to do is the one you *will* do. In other words, any of the three practices that you implement as recommended is almost certain to help improve your health and well-being, and subsequently move you towards practicing the whole program.

Getting started is the most important step to take. The trick to beginning the 3LS is to find one thing you are willing to do and practice it long enough to let it work. Once started, the healthy feeling (and increased horsepower) generated from doing that initial practice gives you the strength to take the next step.

However, here is a bit of insight for you. One of the truisms of holistic medicine is: the very thing a person needs the most, the less likely he or she is to do until the very last.

Q: I really want to get better, but I'm only going to do one aspect of the 3LS right now, and it really doesn't matter to me which one it is. I'm sure I will do all of them but have to make a choice. Which one would you recommend I start first?

A: If you have no preference, do Skilled Relaxation first.

ABOUT HEALING CHRONIC ILLNESS

Focus on Resolving Your Condition

Healing a chronic illness is not likely to be accomplished by continually going from doctor to doctor and test to test to try and come up with a name or a diagnosis. The search for wellness must still be done, but repeating a fruitless, time-consuming search is counterproductive and may even be harmful to your health and well-being. Symptoms often form a complex equation. Sometimes a distinct name can be given to that equation, but many times not. You could waste your money, time, energy, and health in a futile search for a name, a label or the "all-important" diagnosis that may not even exist for your condition. And, in the meantime, your health may still be getting worse.

The way to see chronic symptoms (including unusual, mysterious, or varied symptoms) melt away is to give your body what it needs to resolve its own issues. The 3LS is an integrated program that does just that. Thus if you suspend your focus on the question of "what to call it," you will free up a tremendous amount of energy that you can devote to making yourself better. Practice Wellness for a while, then see if your body is still sending you signs of a health problem. If you still have signs of illness, those issues will now be much clearer to read, diagnose, and treat.

People often wish they were healthier, but then in the next breath say they don't have enough time or money for improvement. Some of these people then spend lots of time and money visiting doctors, popping pills, and eating junk food. How is it that spending their time and money on those things is more important than practicing Wellness? It is important to set priorities straight.

Falling Off the Edge of a Cliff...

Our bodyminds are designed to compensate and adapt, and often they keep on compensating over time, and it seems we are doing just fine. Finally, however, the bodymind tries to compensate one time too many and symptoms suddenly appear. This is the way practically every serious chronic condition occurs.

We often refer to reaching the place where symptoms appear as "being on the edge of the cliff." This is an important metaphor that describes the edge or limit of one's functional capacity. Having a disease is called "falling off the cliff." Moving far enough away from the edge of the cliff to not have symptoms is called "being in the middle of the field."

To increase your distance from the edge of your cliff, and to restore better function, you have two basic options. You can either:

1.   Move the cliff edge away from you by improving your horsepower (your health) so you are stronger and healthier. This can be accomplished by practicing the 3LS.
2.   Move away from the cliff edge by removing or reducing stressors from your life.

Combining both approaches (moving away from the cliff and moving the cliff edge away from you) is the most effective and prudent thing to do and is why we have included both in our book. However, since modern society has so many stressors, and it is difficult to eliminate many of them, you will usually get the very best result by focusing most or all of your energy into increasing your body's horsepower by adopting the 3LS Wellness Program.

Once you have fallen off your cliff and experience symptoms or disease, just climbing back up onto the edge frequently is not always enough to re-establish normal function. Many people must move away from the edge, and back to the middle of the field, in order to achieve wellness.

Some individuals spend their entire lives walking right at the edge of the cliff with the foot closest to the edge slipping a little with each tiny stressor. Just think how much better they would feel if they were living even one yard away from the edge. Of course, the ideal place to be is far away from the edge, in the middle of the field.

By the way, symptoms are warning messages from your bodymind that something has to change because there is too much stress to one or more functional body systems. If you do not get the message, your bodymind will eventually send you a stronger message, i.e., a stronger disease or symptom. Chapter 6 has more information about how disease occurs.

What You Think and Do Affects Your Health

One last point before we start the 3LS. Let's look at how beliefs and choices influence health. The research being done in the Human Genome Project (a study undertaken to identify all the genes in the human body) indicates that only 20% of the cause of chronic illness is limited to genetic inheritance, and 80% is what we choose to do with that inheritance.[2] In other words, our choices determine the state of our health.

People make choices based on what they believe. There are basically two viewpoints that describe what people believe about the causes of health and illness. One viewpoint is called the internal locus of control (locus means

The Edge of the Cliff

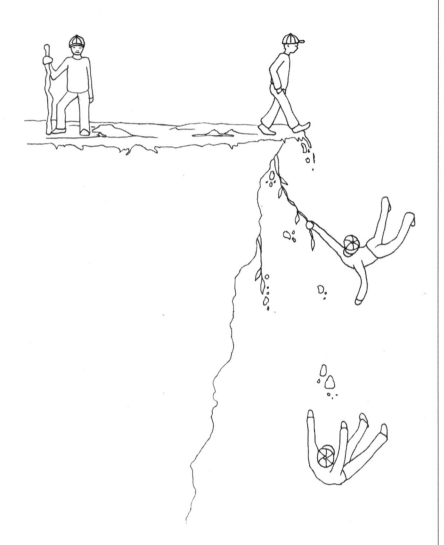

| Middle of the field (Wellness) | Edge of the cliff (Symptoms appear) | Falling off the cliff (Disease) |

▶ ▶ ▶ Increase your burden of stressors, move towards symptoms and disease ▶ ▶ ▶

◀ ◀ ◀ Decrease your burden of stressors, move toward wellness ◀ ◀ ◀

center). This is the belief that health originates inside the body, and the ability to improve health comes from deciding and taking effective action. If you have this belief, you will probably be very interested in learning and practicing Serious Wellness, and you will achieve good results with it.

The second viewpoint is called the external locus of control. This is the belief that outside influences determine your health and destiny, and you are helpless to do anything about your fate. If you have this belief, you might feel your life is determined by factors that you cannot control or you are a victim of some kind of attack that just sort of happens. This is not true! If you have this second viewpoint and are skeptical, just implement our recommendations as an experiment. It is through personal experience that you will find out these practices truly work. We hope you will try the 3LS before your suffering becomes extreme, and before you have spent a lot of time and money visiting a large number of professionals who are unable to help. If you still doubt that the 3LS can help resolve illness, skip ahead to read Chapter 6 (about the causes of illness).

By believing you can help your health, and by Practicing Serious Wellness, you can turn on your body's own solution to your health problems.

Ready to Start

We recommend beginning one or more of the practices right away by using the Quick Start Guide on page 27 while reading through this entire book. Starting immediately means you will get better sooner.

When selecting which practice to start, choose something that you will actually do. As we've mentioned, it matters less which aspect you try first. What matters most is that you start one of the practices. If whichever part you choose is done right, you will become healthier and eventually have the energy and interest to start another. The momentum will carry you.

We know this book contains a lot of information to digest. It is crucial that you avoid biting off more than you can chew and risk becoming overwhelmed. The key to working with the advice in this book and adopting any positive change in your life is to implement the steps in manageable amounts. Trying to do too much frequently leads to failure. Thus, starting with just one practice, but doing it correctly, is good enough.

That being said, all three practices can also be started simultaneously, *if wellness is the primary focus of your life.* But without sufficient time, attention, and energy to start all three aspects of the Program at the same time, most people starting all parts simultaneously soon quit. Most who succeed begin by choosing only one aspect of the program and doing it well before starting a second.

Chapter 1, How to Be Healthy—SUMMING IT UP

What is the most important thing you can do to help your health? The answer to this question is individual, but one path to Wellness that reliably and effectively helps the largest number of people with the greatest success is Dr. Stoll's 3LS Wellness Program.

The 3LS Wellness Program consists of three self-help practices:

1. Skilled Relaxation
2. A Whole Foods Diet
3. The Right Exercise for you

There are two main ways to use this Wellness Program with slightly different protocols.

1. As a short-term health benefit program for healing a chronic illness or condition
2. For health maintenance

The 3LS Wellness Program can improve most chronic health conditions, whether you have a diagnosis or not. This Wellness Program reverses many conditions and is more likely to cure chronic diseases or illnesses than conventional approaches. It can help other treatments work better. Even if a condition cannot be helped, practicing the 3LS will enable you to make the most out of what remains of your health. After you are healthy, if you want to use the 3LS Wellness Program for health maintenance, you can usually decrease the amount of time you spend.

The practices that comprise the Program are time-tested and have been thoroughly researched. In general, the only cost of this wellness program is your time and effort. Most people can use the 3LS as a self-help program, but some will need to see a practitioner for support. If you're already doing similar practices, you're off to a good start, but you will most likely experience more effective progress in reversing your chronic symptoms by reading and following the specifics in this book.

Getting started is the most important step in practicing the 3LS Wellness Program. Symptoms of poor health are signs of stress from one or more functional body systems. To distance from symptoms, you can either become stronger and healthier, or reduce your stress. Since there are so many stressors in modern times, becoming stronger is usually the most effective option, and this can be done by practicing the 3LS Wellness Program. The 3LS works by increasing the total function of your bodymind. Holding the belief that you can improve your health can propel you towards health and wellness.

You may begin practicing the 3LS Wellness Program using the Quick-Start Guide at the end of Chapter 1, but be sure to read the entire book to learn all the important details that make a difference in the effectiveness of the practices.

Quick-Start SKILLED RELAXATION
Practice Skilled Relaxation 20 minutes, 2 times a day

To begin, choose a relaxation practice. You may use a relaxation technique that you already know, or learn a new one.

If you've never just tried relaxing, here are a few suggestions for how to do it. Find a place where you won't be disturbed for about 20 minutes. Sit in a comfortable chair. It's okay to sit in a recliner or lay down, but do not fall asleep. You can either close your eyes or leave them open. Allow your thoughts to fade away and just relax and enjoy your time with no distractions or preocupations.

Some simple methods to help you get started relaxing in a 20-minute session include:

- listening to soft, soothing music
- focusing on different parts of the body starting with your feet and going up to your head, suggesting relaxation to each part
- breathing normally, and keeping your attention on your breathing. You may count your breaths to help keep your mind quiet.
- visualizing relaxing scenes or images
- meditation, done by sitting (usually with eyes closed) and being mindful of the sounds of your environment and being aware of your own body

Other suggestions for relaxation practices may be found in Chapter 2 and in *The Relaxation and Stress Reduction Workbook* by Davis, Eshelman, and McKay.

Practice your relaxation for 20 minutes, two times a day. The best times for most people are in the morning after waking or rising, and in the evening after returning home from work.

From the very beginning, start building the habit of regularly doing your practice twice a day. Your goal in each session is to reach a deeply relaxed state of body and mind, and stay in that state for at least a few of the 20 minutes. It takes some practice to reach this depth of relaxation, so it might take a several times to learn how to do it. Do not worry if you don't feel relaxed right away in the first few sessions, because such experience may be new for you. Here is a hint: *reaching deep relaxation is not something that you can make yourself do, but you fall into it* similar to the experience of falling asleep. You have to let it happen rather than make it happen. You will learn over time by just continuing to practice.

NOTE: If you have any kind of severe psychopathology or seizure disorder, using any kind of biofeedback machines, training devices (such as sound and light machines), or other mechanical devices, we advise you to seek professional help before beginning Skilled Relaxation.

This is just enough information for you to get started doing the practice of Skilled Relaxation. To know if you are reaching the relaxed state, and to learn further specifics about doing the practice correctly and successfully, read Chapter 2.

Quick-Start the PERFECT WHOLE FOODS DIET
Follow a Perfect Whole Foods Diet for two weeks
to begin to feel the benefits

To begin a Perfect Whole Foods Diet, eliminate all refined foods from your diet and eat only whole foods. A whole food is one that has had no parts removed. A refined food has had something taken out. For example, whole wheat flour is whole, but white flour is refined. The Perfect Whole Foods Diet focuses on eating all whole foods, but especially whole carbohydrates because refined carbohydrates cause many health issues.

One way to do a two-week trial is to follow a very simple, easy-to-prepare diet of whole foods for two weeks as outlined in the list below. For your meals, you might eat a basic menu of whole grains with vegetables and protein foods. Snacks can be nuts and seeds. Beverages can be spring water or herbal teas. Some spices or seasonings may be used. A variety of ingredients will keep the menu interesting.

Grains: brown rice, quinoa, 100% whole rye or other whole grain crackers, rolled oats, oat bran, 100% whole wheat flour.

Vegetables, all types: fresh or frozen, raw or cooked. Eat the peels if edible (be sure to wash carefully before eating), and avoid canned products.

Protein foods: meat, fish, poultry, beans, legumes, tofu, farm eggs, whole milk, cheese.

Spices or seasonings: Bragg's liquid amino acids, sea or mineral salt, black pepper, any individual spices (avoid pre-mixed), vinegars, olive or other whole (unrefined) oils.

Snacks: macadamia nuts, peanuts, cashews, pecans, sunflower seeds, popcorn, pumpkin seeds, walnuts; pure nut butters on 100% whole grain crackers.

Beverages: mint tea, chamomile tea, spring water.

These are just a few of the items on the complete diet, but the above will give you a very simple two-week trial. Refer to Appendix B for a more complete list or to know if what you are eating is allowable. Do not eat anything that is not on the list, even if it seems whole. Make sure that what you eat does not have anything added to it. All forms of sugars, starches, and alcohol must be totally avoided. If you eat no other than the items listed above or in Appendix B for two weeks, you will be following the Perfect Diet and will most likely experience significant health benefits. Thus, you will find out how much better you can feel and what the diet can do for you.

Another aid for doing a two-week trial is *The Healing Power of Whole Foods* by Beth Loiselle. This resource has many delicious recipes for the Perfect Diet. Ordering information is in the Resources for Chapter 3 (located at the end of the book).

There is one thing you must be aware of when doing your two-week trial. Some people go through a period of withdrawal when stopping consumption of refined foods. The withdrawal may last from one day to one week (average three-and-a-half days. This is described fully in Chapter 3). If you have this reaction, take it easy for those few days until you start to feel the health benefits of the new diet.

NOTE: if you are diabetic and are taking any oral hypoglycemic agents or insulin, you will need to be under a doctor's supervision during this two-week trial as your requirements for insulin may drop dramatically.

This is just a start. Be sure to read Chapter 3 as it explains the specifics of how to select foods, how the Perfect Diet works, and easiest ways to socialize and eat in restaurants.

Quick-Start RIGHT EXERCISE
Do enjoyable exercise of any kind, three times a week

To begin exercising, choose one or more activities that you like, and just begin. One of the keys to success in an exercise program is to have fun and enjoy it!

If you have not exercised for a long time or have been very ill and are weak, you can start with five or ten minutes of simple exercises like walking or rebounding (gentle bouncing on a mini-trampoline). Doing any these exercises once or several times a day will slowly start to build up your strength.

People who are stronger can choose any enjoyable activity that is reasonably comfortable. If you wish to begin aerobics, a general guideline is 20 minutes, three times a week (not including warm-up and cool-down time).

Exercising on a regular schedule is most beneficial. Remember it will take some time for your body to become used to this, so do not overdo it at the beginning. If you feel pain or discomfort during or after exercise, see a sports medicine practitioner or general physician.

NOTE: if you are over age twenty and wish to start aerobics or any type of exercise that affects the heart rate, check with your doctor to see if you need a stress test before beginning your exercise program.

Most people start to feel better almost immediately when they begin to exercise regularly. Some people may experience sore muscles, depending upon the exercise chosen.

Information to help you choose the kind of exercise that will benefit your specific health condition and other helpful tips are in Chapter 4. The more you know, the more your exercise can be effective in bringing the health benefits you desire.

Chapter 2

Skilled Relaxation

In this chapter:

1. How Skilled Relaxation (SR) reverses the effects of stress
2. Instructions for Skilled Relaxation
3. How to know if your practice is effective
4. Getting immediate relief from symptoms until the relaxation takes effect

THE REAL EFFECTS OF CHRONIC STRESS

Have you noticed how pervasive stress is in our culture? The average person today is exposed to more than 1,000 times as many stressors every day than people were just 100 years ago, more than 386,000 per day per person.[1] Stress of *any kind* can cause the fight or flight response (FOF).

No doubt you've experienced FOF and know what it feels like: your heart, respiratory, and blood pressure rates increase, and blood moves away from your digestive organs and into large muscles in preparation for a "fight or flight." Tension also occurs in different parts of your body. (This varies by individual, depending upon the person's genetic and lifestyle background.) In FOF, your body is in a state of red alert or readiness, as you get ready to run from that big ol' tiger or ready to fight for your life. The technical terms for FOF are "activation of the sympathetic nervous system" or "autonomic arousal."

If a person under stress who is in FOF does not discharge the arousal by actually fleeing or fighting in response to that stress (and many modern stresses cannot be run from or fought), the readiness to act is stored chronically in the hypothalamus. The hypothalamus is a part of the brain that functions as the connection between the mind and the rest of the body. It is like a switchboard that ultimately controls all parts and functions of the bodymind.

When stress occurs and a person goes into FOF, the *effect* of the stressor (called stress-effect) that is not discharged by fleeing or fighting accumulates in the hypothalamus as stored stress-effect. Over the years, the stored stress-effect increases, creating a heavier and heaver burden of readiness in the hypothalamus, until it completely changes how the hypothalamus runs your entire bodymind. The result is your bodymind stays in a continual state of FOF, which in turn influences how you respond to every stressor that arises.

The hypothalamus was designed, over millions of years, to function primarily and most efficiently in the rest mode, interspersed with short periods of total and abject terror in the FOF mode (when the saber-toothed tiger appeared, for example). It was not designed to cope with low levels of chronic stress and high levels of stored stress-effect persisting unceasingly for a lifetime.

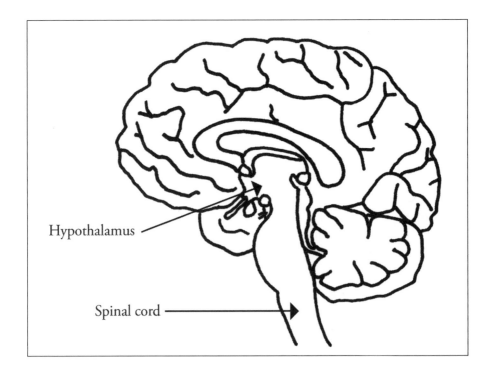

Hypothalamus

Spinal cord

Stored stress-effect directly affects function, and dysfunction, of body and mind, and is the root of many chronic (long-term) health conditions. Stored stress-effect does not actually cause illness by itself, but at least greatly aggravates and contributes to every illness to which humans are heir. No one yet knows exactly how the stress-effect is stored,[2] but chronic autonomic arousal is measurable in many ways, including blood pressure, pulse, perspiration, cholesterol levels, clotting speed, muscle tension, breathing rate, and cortisol levels. Chronic stress-effect and its subsequent storage also change the function and output of hypothalamic hormones (and thus the stimulus of other hormones), which discombobulates the rest of the bodymind's function.[3] More discussion of stressors and stress-effect is in Chapter 6 (about causes of illness).

At the present time, stress-related chronic conditions make up at least 90% of all office visits to physicians.[4] Functional diseases (meaning some part of the body is not working as well as it should, but may not show measurable structural changes such as distortions or differences on a blood test) can be traced back to FOF and stored stress-effect. To make a complete list of the conditions or diseases affected by hypothalamic overload would take a book all by itself! A partial list of conditions caused by stored-stress effect is on page 42.

If you are a typical human in the twenty-first century and especially if you experience chronic health symptoms, it is likely that you suffer from stress-effect. Three of the most significant results of having a hypothalamus overloaded with stored stress-effect are:

1. Bracing (chronic muscular tension)
2. Digestive weakness (leaky gut syndrome)
3. Brain and body chemistry imbalance (fatigue, or mental or emotional difficulties)

Each of these conditions in turn causes secondary conditions, such as stress and tension disorders, gastrointestinal and cardiovascular disorders, immune system disorders, and musculoskeletal disorders. Therefore, these three are actually the root of numerous other health problems. Let us briefly look at these common results of stored-stress effect.

Bracing (Chronic Muscular Tension)

Bracing is a curiously appropriate word. It is just like someone trying to "brace for impact," in the event of a crash or collision. Too many people are constantly braced for impact, in a state of constant tightness and tension.

Interestingly, bracing is usually below people's conscious awareness, which means that bracing typically cannot be felt by the person who is doing it. *The majority of people in this country brace for 24 hours a day without even knowing it.* Did you ever wake up in the morning feeling stiff and sore? You were even bracing in your sleep, so pronounced is your pattern of carrying chronic stress and muscular tension in your body.

Bracing is usually a full-body phenomenon that occurs in layers. Most people only become aware of the outermost layer (external skeletal muscles) when the area braced starts to manifest physical pain. Common areas where bracing is typically felt include shoulders (raised up towards ears), jaw (which causes the grinding of teeth), head (which causes headaches), and back and hips (creating stiffness and pain). However, any muscle in any part of the body can be chronically tense due to bracing. Bracing also occurs in deeper areas of the body (internal muscles, including some organs). Pain is not usually felt in these areas, but serious health conditions can arise.

The reason it is so important to understand bracing is because although you do not feel it, this tension can affect any part of your body and eventually cause serious health problems. Bracing, like any long-term factor causing illness, takes years to finally show symptoms and even longer to show damage that physicians can detect with current instruments.

The technical description of bracing is "chronic electrochemical discharge of myoneural junctions due to excessive sympathetic activation in the hypothalamus."[5]

What bracing is... and isn't

■■■ JAN: It's been my experience that it takes a while for most people to understand what bracing is and know if they are doing it.

What bracing isn't:

- Your headache (or backache, etc.)—that's only a *small* part of your bracing.
- Raising your shoulders (for example) when you're under stress—that's tension or clenching, which can be a *part* of your bracing, but is only the tip of the iceberg.
- Gone when your neck or other painful area stops hurting (for example) after a massage—that is only *part of your tension, and your full-body bracing still remains!*

What bracing is: constant, full-body tension, most of which you cannot feel.

Some people think if they feel themselves tense up, and have *some* muscle tension or pain, they are bracing. They are right, but that is only a small, external sign of bracing. I believe most individuals are only aware of about 1% to 5% of the total-body bracing that is going on.

It's true that most people brace. I don't think I've seen a single person yet in my massage office who doesn't brace. You may have to take a leap of faith to believe that you are bracing and begin the practice of Skilled Relaxation. If you are not sure if you are bracing, here is a hint: healthy muscles do not feel hard like rocks or bones, feel sore or tender to touch, nor are they flabby. Healthy muscles are soft, pliable, and firm and feel comfortable when touched or massaged.

In my massage practice, seeing people brace is an everyday event. It is true that most people are not aware they are bracing—*especially* those who are the biggest bracers! A person who is a strong bracer can be very active physically and feel fine most of the time. One of my challenges as a massage therapist is helping the big bracers understand why, after I have gotten their necks, shoulders, or backs out of pain, it is important that they begin self-care (Skilled Relaxation) for eliminating the bracing in the rest of their body.

Although massage often greatly helps muscular problems, for a person who is bracing, massage may not be enough. For example, you might temporarily alleviate the pain of a recurrent backache by getting massage, and this is a good thing. However, it does not mean that your bracing has gone away. What has happened is a few tight muscles on the outermost layer of your bracing have relaxed, and all the other muscles and layers continue to be tense even though you cannot feel this tension. Another painful episode could easily be triggered because your body is still very tight.

Bracing can begin as early as infancy. Besides being the root of many health problems, bracing may eventually lead to atrophy (weakness) as muscles become exhausted.■■■

Digestive Weakness (Leaky Gut Syndrome)

Stored stress-effect in the hypothalamus and chronic FOF cause blood flow to be constantly directed away from the intestines, weakening the digestive lining. This lack of support to the gastrointestinal tract is the cause of leaky gut syndrome (LGS), a condition in which incompletely digested proteins (peptides) pass through a weakened digestive lining and enter the blood stream causing an immune response. The symptoms of an immune response can differ among individuals, depending upon what part of their body is closest to the edge of their symptomatic cliff. For many people, the immune response is experienced as their usual chronic symptoms. For others, LGS manifests as fatigue, weakness, nervousness, anxiety, trembling, headache, sweating, hunger, dizziness, visual disturbances, mental confusion, and similar experiences.

Typically, LGS is the first of a series of digestive problems. A weakened digestive system with LGS easily becomes host to imbalance in the bacterial ecology. This imbalance, called dysbiosis, may then lead to hypersensitivities to foods (sometimes called food allergies or food intolerances). Dysbiosis also creates an environment favorable to parasites and the overgrowth of the yeast candida albicans. Some of the more serious digestive disorders that can occur later, after the onset of LGS, include GERD (Gastro Esophageal Reflux Disorder, also called hiatal hernia or acid reflux), Crohn's disease, ulcerative colitis, diverticulitis, and colon cancer. The effects of LGS are not limited to digestive difficulties, but also cause systemic problems in other areas of physical and mental function.

People who discover they have food allergies, candida, GERD, concentration difficulties, or the other health problems mentioned above first need to resolve the underlying LGS to effectively resolve their secondary symptoms. Most people are not aware that they have LGS. It has been proposed that approximately 75% of the US population has LGS.[6]

The technical term for leaky gut syndrome is "intestinal hyperpermeability." Chapter 3 has more information about LGS and digestive issues.

Brain and Body Chemistry Imbalance (Mental-Emotional Difficulties)

Stress, including stored stress-effect in the hypothalamus, can deplete the bodymind of specific nutrients such as vitamins and minerals. This depletion can result in chemistry imbalance, including hormonal imbalances, anywhere in the bodymind, but especially in the brain and endocrine system. Chemical imbalances are a direct cause of, or are a factor that increases susceptibility to, mental-emotional problems such as agoraphobia, alcoholism, anxiety, attention deficit disorder (ADD), depression, manic-depression, nervousness, panic attacks, phobias, and post-traumatic stress disorder (PTSD). Chemistry imbalances also contribute to fatigue, endocrine system disorders, and other health conditions. Chapter 8 (about mind, emotions, and spirit) has more information on chemical imbalance.

■ ■ ■

These short descriptions of bracing, digestive weakness, and chemistry imbalance demonstrate how stress and stored stress-effect can play havoc with the entire bodymind, from the most superficial layers to the deepest ones. The good news is that reversal of stored stress-effect may occur through the practice of Skilled Relaxation, and health can be restored.

A BETTER WAY TO RELAX: SKILLED RELAXATION

If you have health problems originating from accumulated stress, rather than focusing on relieving individual symptoms, often the best thing to do is to get rid of the mechanism causing the symptoms—hypothalamic overload of stored stress-effect. To get rid of the overload, stress-effect must be discharged faster than it is being accumulated. In modern times, there are too many stressors causing FOF to discharge that much readiness in the usual eight hours (or less) of sleep. The discharge of accumulated stress, however, can be accomplished through the practice of Skilled Relaxation (SR), in which you are actually changing your brainwaves.

Benefits of Skilled Relaxation

Whether you are trying to reverse a chronic condition or are using the full 3LS Program for health maintenance, SR supports your well-being.

SR is easy to do and brings two kinds of benefits. Short-term benefits relieve and lessen your immediate symptoms. Long-term benefits reflect an actual positive change in your health problem. By far, the greatest result from the consistent long-term practice of SR is the long-term benefit of moving far away from the edge of your symptomatic cliff.

Here is a partial list of the proven benefits of practicing Skilled Relaxation 20 minutes twice a day.

Skilled Relaxation…

- lowers bad cholesterol and elevates good cholesterol, increasing the type of blood fats that prevent heart attacks.
- increases energy, resistance to disease, physical capacity to handle stress, mind-body coordination, and physical agility.
- lowers resting pulse and breath rates.
- reduces anxiety, nervousness, depression, neuroticism and inhibition, feelings of mental and/or physical inadequacy, and irritability.
- improves self-esteem, self-regard, ego strength, problem-solving ability, organization of thinking, creativity, and productivity.

Here are some of the non-physical benefits of Skilled Relaxation...

- promotes self-actualization and fosters trust and capacity for intimate contact
- enhances the ability to love and express affection
- develops inner wholeness, increases autonomy, self-reliance, and satisfaction at home and at work
- moves one towards a more positive and mature personal expression
- reduces feelings of alienation and meaninglessness.[7]

> Note that the short-term benefits of symptomatic relief are *not* enough to sustain a health *change*. It takes the long-term benefits of reversing the condition to actually create health, about six to twelve months into a Skilled Relaxation program.

How Skilled Relaxation Works

Skilled Relaxation, along with its other benefits, automatically reverses the buildup of chronic stress-effect and does so at a rate 24 times as fast as normal sleep.[8] SR is an activity that produces a physical relaxation response that occurs when you slow down your brainwaves. When you practice SR, you consciously change the activity of your brainwaves from ordinary waking consciousness (beta brainwave) to *relaxed* (alpha or theta brainwave). This is not to be confused with sleep (delta brainwave) though. These brainwaves are nothing mysterious, unusual, or new. You experience all of them constantly and also sequentially every night when you fall asleep.

You can expect to experience health benefits fairly soon after correctly reaching alpha or theta brainwaves consistently in your sessions.

The brainwaves

Beta is the state of usual, wakeful consciousness with ordinary or fast thinking. As we are working, driving, talking, etc., we are most likely in beta. On the higher extremes, beta is sometimes associated with anxiety, panic, or stress. Beta's brainwaves range from approximately 14 to 20 Hertz.

Alpha is a state of light relaxation. It is not a sleep state, but is usually reflective of a calm, alert, focused mind. Alpha is sometimes called the "super-learning state" because the brain seems to be more receptive and open to new information. Alpha is also considered ideal for creative brainstorming. True meditation occurs in this state. (Note that many people meditate regularly, however, not all of them reach alpha regularly.) Alpha's brainwaves range from approximately 8 to 13 Hertz.

Alpha is simple to achieve and practice. Anyone who has become absorbed while actively and creatively doing something and has lost track of time has experienced this mode. Alpha is a clear mind with very soft, gentle thoughts or no thoughts at all.

Theta is a state of deep relaxation. Sometimes a sleep state, sometimes not, theta reflects a state of dreamlike awareness. Dreams and a deep, meditative state of consciousness are common characteristics of theta. Theta's brainwaves range from approximately 4 to 8 Hertz. Theta is almost a dream state, or a semi-aware state with deep, dreamy thoughts. It is usually experienced just before falling asleep.

Delta, the deepest of the brainwave patterns, is a state of deep sleep, or trance-like consciousness. Maintaining awareness into delta can result in opening access to the unconscious portion of our consciousness. Delta's brainwaves range from approximately 2 to 4 Hertz. Most people are asleep and are not conscious in a delta state, except for, perhaps, Zen masters!

All of the brainwaves are experienced by each person daily, and they are not unusual. For example, everyone goes through the alpha/theta rhythm on the way to sleep, like this:

$$beta \rightarrow alpha \rightarrow theta \rightarrow delta.$$

Relaxation feels good and supports your health

Alpha is the brainwave you wish to attain for at least several minutes during your SR session. Theta may also be reached. Alpha and theta indicate a relaxed *mental* state. The alpha state produces deep relaxation while still being alert, conscious, and focused. The relaxation of the theta state can feel somewhat like drifting.

Skilled Relaxation is a skill that you learn and develop. The trick to doing SR successfully is to learn how it feels to relax and reach alpha (or theta) brainwave, then reliably reproduce that relaxation response twice a day. This relaxation feels good both during and after your practice session.

This level of relaxation allows the bodymind to heal itself. Even discharging just a little of the stress-effect storage in your SR session helps. Over time, as you discharge enough of the stress-effect storage, your system eventually returns to normal, and your symptoms will improve or disappear.

Many people will notice almost immediate short-term results from reaching the alpha state or relaxation response for 20 minutes twice a day. Significant changes can usually be experienced in three months, but on the average, reversing the causes of an illness takes six to twelve months. When we say six to twelve months of faithful SR practice, for some people this means becoming totally free of symptoms and having permanent reversal of many chronic disorders. Until then, you will most likely continue to have occasional symptoms.

Conditions Helped by Skilled Relaxation

The following is a partial list of problems and conditions SR has been shown to help.[9]

Acne
Adrenal fatigue/
  exhaustion
Agoraphobia
Airflow (breathing)
  restriction
Alcoholism
Allergic skin reactions
Allergies
Angina pectoris
Anxiety
Arm pain
Arthritis
Asthma
Atonic (weak) bowel
Attention deficit
  disorder (ADD)
Autoimmune
  conditions
Back pain
Baker's cyst
Baldness
Bipolar disorder
Blepharospasm (eye
  twitching)
Bracing

Brain chemistry
  imbalance
Bruxism (grinding or
  clenching teeth)
Bursitis
Candida related
  syndrome (C-RS)
Canker sores
Cardiac arrythmias
Cardiac dysrhythmias
Carpal tunnel
  syndrome
Celiac disease
Charlie horse (leg
  cramps)
Chondromalacia
  (softened kneecap)
Chronic fatigue
  syndrome
Chronic pain
Cold hands and feet
Colds
Colon problems
Constipation (chronic)
Coronary heart disease
Costochondritis (pain
  in the ribs)

Cough
Cramps
Cranio-mandibular
  dysfunction
Crohn's disease
Depression
Diverticulitis
Dizziness
Dysautonomia
  (nervous system
  dysregulation)
Dysbiosis
Eczema
Endocrine imbalance
  or dysregulation
Epstein barr virus
  (chronic)
Fasculations
  (twitching)
Fatigue
Fibromyaliga (chronic
  pain in muscles)
Fibromyositis (chronic
  muscle inflam-
  mation)
Flu
Food allergies

Gall bladder disease
Gastritis
Headaches (all kinds)
Hemorrhoids
Herpes
Herpes simplex
Hiatal hernia (GERD or
  acid reflux)
Hives
Hypertension (high
  blood pressure)
Hypoglycemia
Hyperthyroidism
Incontinence
Injuries
Insomnia
Interstitial cystitis
Irritable bowel
  syndrome
Joint aches
Leaky brain syndrome
Leaky gut syndrome
  (LGS)
Leg pain
Lymph node swelling
Manic-depression
Menopause
Mononucleosis

Multiple chemical
  sensitivities
Musculo-skeletal
  conditions
Myofascial pain
  syndrome
Neck pain
Nervousness
Neuropathy problems
Osteoarthritis
Pain (chronic)
Panic attacks
Parasites
Pelvic congestion
  syndrome
Phobias
Plagiocephaly (skull
  malformance)
Plantar fasciitis
Post traumatic stress
  disorder (PTSD)
Pre-menstrual
  syndrome
Prostatitis
Psoriasis
Rectal problems
Renaud's syndrome
Restless leg syndrome

Rosacea
Scabies
Scoliosis (curvature of
  the spine)
Seborrhea
Shin splints
Sinusitis (chronic)
Sleep apnea
Spasms
Tendonitis
Thoracic outlet
  syndrome (pain in
  neck, shoulders, arms
  and hand)
Thrush (candida)
Tinnitis (ringing in the
  ears)
TMJ
Torticollis (twisting of
  the neck)
Ulcerative colitis
Ulcers
Unusual symptoms
Vaginismus
Vertigo (dizziness)
Vitiglio (loss of
  pigmentation)
Yeast infections

To get the permanent reversal of symptoms, however, you must get back far enough from the edge of your symptomatic cliff to allow your bodymind to heal itself. Thus, some people need to practice SR even longer than a year. No matter how long your healing takes, as you go along with your SR practice, if you keep a record of your symptoms and temporary exacerbations (times when your symptoms return for a while), you will likely discover that as time proceeds your exacerbations become less severe, last fewer days, and are farther apart.

Some people find it hard to believe that long-standing chronic conditions may disappear when approaching the problem at its source by sitting quietly in a chair for 20 minutes, twice a day. Yet literally hundreds of books and thousands of scientific articles certify the effectiveness of this technique. If you want to know if SR would be helpful for you, the simplest way is to see how you feel for a few minutes after your first *successful* SR session (meaning you have achieved an alpha or theta brainwave).

Anyone Can Do Skilled Relaxation

One of the nice things about SR, especially for chronically ill people, is that it takes very little energy to learn and practice. SR is very simple to practice without much effort. Even children can learn how to practice Skilled Relaxation. The Resources at the end of the book mention a book about teaching SR to children.

Older people also experience great benefits. Most individuals recognize a decline of function with advancing years, and usually believe it is due to the aging process. Actually, as mentioned earlier, a large percentage of health problems in older individuals are from the increasing stress-effect burden in the hypothalamus. As we age, the stress-effect burden continues to accumulate unless we practice SR twice a day. Therefore, older people who learn and practice SR diligently are often pleasantly surprised with improvements in their functional ability and how they feel overall. The main challenge for older people tends to be getting past old habits or ideas rather than the actual process of learning and using SR.

> Older people who learn and practice SR diligently are often pleasantly surprised with improvements in their functional ability and how they feel overall.

We would like to mention one precaution. If you have a history of psychiatric disorders or seizures, consult a professional before beginning SR. This includes individuals with severe psychopathology, including epilepsy, seizure disorders, acute psychosis, major affective disorders, history of dissociation experience, and borderline personality disorders. Under supervision of a qualified health professional, use active SR as described below and check your SR success using the written self-evaluation description. You may use passive SR or biofeedback methods (such as biofeedback machines or entrainment devices, see page 48) if they are under the supervision of professionals who are knowledgeable and experienced in these conditions *and* in using biofeedback. As far as we know, no harm has ever occurred to anyone practicing SR using machines, but the potential may exist.

For most people, practicing Skilled Relaxation is as relaxing and enjoyable as taking a short vacation twice a day!

HOW TO DO SKILLED RELAXATION

Generally, all it takes to be successful at Skilled Relaxation is a little instruction and some practice. To practice SR:

- First, select a relaxation technique (see pages 47–48) to effectively help you reach the alpha brainwave state.
- Then, practice whatever technique you choose two times a day for 20 minutes each time.
- Next, evaluate your SR practice. After two weeks to a month of regular twice-a-day sessions, evaluate your practice. Check your signs of relaxation with the list later in this chapter, or take a one-time test by a biofeedback professional to make certain you are reaching the alpha or theta brainwave. We describe each of these steps below.

Relaxation is actually a very simple and enjoyable thing to do. It can be as simple as just sitting in a chair.

Practicing SR is similar to falling asleep. When you go to sleep, you let sleep occur. You just ease into sleep. The same effortlessness applies to SR. In your SR session, you relax, almost as though you are going to sleep, but you don't actually sleep. You still maintain awareness.

More than 95% of people who start are able to learn SR easily. The 5% that need additional input to practice SR can facilitate their learning by using biofeedback for a while. For those few people, it is simple to use a biofeedback machine called a GSR at home to give you some clues about how to relax. We will discuss how to use biofeedback later in this chapter.

If you think you don't know how to relax, keep in mind that relaxation isn't something you do, it is something you fall into. There is no forcing or *making* relaxation happen. However, most of us are so used to being busy and tense that spending a little time doing nothing (just relaxing) may seem complicated. Once you get used to relaxing, you will see how good it feels and how simple it is. If relaxing seems to be a big challenge for you, just make a commitment to give it a try twice a day for at least a two-week trial, to see what changes occur for you.

First, Choose a Relaxation Technique

In general, to practice SR, choose any relaxation technique that you enjoy. If you already know a relaxation method, you may use it. A list of common practices or techniques is on pages 47–48. See if you already know how to do one or more of them. If you are new to relaxing, there are many ways to learn an effective method. Relaxation can truly be as simple as sitting comfortably in a chair.

To learn from a book, we recommend *The Relaxation and Stress Reduction Workbook* by Davis, Eshelman, and McKay. This book teaches a variety of relaxation techniques from which you may choose. You may buy the workbook or borrow it from a library. Your health care practitioner may also have a copy to loan or sell to you.

Key Resource:
The Relaxation and Stress Reduction Workbook,

by Davis, Eschelman and McKay

This is an effective self-help book for learning a variety of SR techniques. Earlier editions are also good. The workbook contains information on the following SR methods: breathing, progressive relaxation, meditation, visualization, applied relaxation training, self-hypnosis, autogenics, recording a relaxation tape, combination techniques, and thought stopping. The workbook also has a symptom effectiveness chart that may help you choose which one to try first. The fifth edition also includes useful information about body awareness, stress management, coping skills, time management, assertiveness training, and exercise. This is an excellent self-help book. (Fifth Edition, 2000, New Harbinger Publications, Inc.; published continuously since 1980.)

Besides the relaxation workbook, you can also learn Skilled Relaxation by taking a class in meditation, breathing, yoga, t'ai chi, or stress reduction. In addition, some SR methods do not require any learning; instead you use a device or CD to guide you into relaxation. These are called passive methods.

NOTE: Remember, if you come across unfamiliar terms, check the Glossary.

Examples of Skilled Relaxation methods

Since people enjoy relaxing in different ways, here is a list of different relaxation techniques. Choose any activity that would be comfortable and enjoyable for you. There are two main types of SR techniques: active and passive.

Active Techniques

Active Skilled Relaxation produces relaxation by a person training himself or herself to do it. It can be done as simply as sitting in a chair, yet most people find it helps to learn a technique or method. The activity helps you stay focused on relaxing. A well-known example of active SR is meditation. Since not everyone enjoys meditation, here are some other active relaxation methods from which you can choose:

Affirmations: Repeat positive phrases to oneself, via thoughts or words, to calm the mind.

Applied relaxation: Learn six different aspects of relaxation with the goal of relaxing in successively shorter periods of time. Also learn to transfer this state to everyday situations.

Autogenics: Repeat a series of phrases that suggest relaxation while focusing on different parts of the body.

Breathing techniques: Count breaths or hold the breath, learn to use breathing muscles correctly, and/or use awareness of breath to calm and relax the nervous system.

Centering or contemplative prayer: Focus on interior silence and quieting the faculties through prayer.

Chanting: Repeat names, words, or syllables in a rhythmic fashion to dissolve worries, soothe the nervous system, and still the mind.

Meditation (all forms): Still the body and mind. There are many ways to meditate, including sitting quietly, breathing deeply, and concentrating intently on some object or sound such as your own breathing, a word, or a candle.

Mindfulness: Be aware of the present moment without judging, reflecting, or thinking; simply observing.

Progressive relaxation: Follow a specific order and sequence for relaxing the muscles of the body. Sometimes muscle groups are tensed before relaxed.

Self-hypnosis: Use words to guide and create a state of relaxation. The wording must be precise to achieve the desired result.

Silva Mind Training: Use systematic mental processes, such as visualizations and affirmations, to achieve a relaxed mind.

Thought stopping: Slow and stop normal mental chatter for brief and then longer periods of time.

T'ai chi chuan: Follow a complex series of slow, dance-like movements that are intended to harmonize mental and physical functions and enhance energy flow. T'ai chi is a traditional Chinese meditative exercise and martial art.

Visualization: Invent or imagine your own relaxing images or scenes to create a peaceful mind and body.

Yoga (many kinds): Hold specific postures over a period of time while practicing slow breathing. Yoga originated in India and builds strength, endurance, and flexibility in addition to relaxing the bodymind.

Passive Techniques

Passive SR leads the brain to the correct brainwave by using a device providing electrical, magnetic, auditory, or visual input. Some people find that it helps to have something external to get started, and that is why there are so many passive devices on the market.

An example of passive SR is the use of machines (called mind machines or sound and light machines) that actually send a pulse of electricity, magnetism, sound, or light into the brain and depend upon entrainment (producing a similar vibration) to get the brain pulsing at the alpha or theta rhythm. Other machines that are less stimulating only give feedback about what is happening as you relax (as with a biofeedback machine).

Audio tapes or CDs: Listen to soothing music or music especially designed to induce alpha or theta brainwaves.

Biofeedback: Use a biofeedback machine that monitors physiological activity and displays the results via a dial or tone. This provides instant information about whether you are relaxed or tense and what changes will create relaxation.

Guided imagery: Visualize relaxing images or scenes by listening to a recorded cassette or CD that guides the process.

Isolation tank or float tank: Float in a dark soundproof tank in salty water at skin temperature and achieve a state of quiet through reduced sensory stimulation.

Light goggles, mind machines, or sound and light machines: Use a machine that sends a pulse of electricity, magnetism, sound, or light into the brain. This gets the brain pulsing at a similar, relaxed rhythm.

The reason there are so many choices is because people are different, and each form of SR works best for only a percentage of people. No single approach works for everyone. For example, meditation is one of the more well-known techniques that produces the relaxation response. However, less than half of those who try meditation enjoy it. You can even make up your own relaxation technique; the key to success is to find and "do what works for you."

We did not put exact instructions for doing just one or two of the techniques in this book, because by offering only one or two approaches, you might get the false impression that every person would enjoy and be successful with those few. This list gives you options for finding the right practice for your success at Skilled Relaxation.

■ ■ ■

You might explore several methods before you choose one to practice regularly. You will soon discover a way that fits with your personality, physiology, and lifestyle, is easy for you to do, and produces immediate benefits. When you find your way, you'll know it, because it will feel comfortable.

In our personal and professional experience, the most effective approaches to SR are the active ones that can be practiced at no cost. However, Skilled Relaxation can be experienced in any of these techniques since SR is about the goal, not the process. The techniques are just guidance to help you become relaxed. Whether you use a passive or an active method of relaxation, once you know how to reach the desired brainwave, the technique may eventually become unnecessary as your familiarity with the practice enables you to slip easily into a relaxed state.

Second, Begin to Practice

Here are some helpful tips for starting your SR practice:

Start by simply building the habit of practicing twice a day without being too concerned with results. Just do your practice and relax.

Tell family members what you are doing and why, and elicit their support for having enough uninterrupted time and space on a regular basis for your practice.

Take it one day at a time. If you miss a session, get back on track the next day. Consider scheduling your SR sessions into your day-timer or daily schedule.

Stay motivated by reminding yourself that doing the practice regularly will make feeling good an ongoing trend in your life rather than an infrequent event.

Think of SR as a habit or necessity like brushing your teeth—something automatically done twice a day. Isn't it as important to feel good all over as it is to have clean teeth?

Reward yourself appropriately and regularly for successfully completing a week or a month of doing twice-a-day sessions. Give yourself a healthy treat.

When to practice:

- SR can be practiced any time *except* within two hours before sleeping and two hours before the next SR session. No one knows for sure why doing it right before bed does not provide the long-term results needed to resolve chronic health issues. However, empirical evidence shows that one needs to be awake for about two hours after a session, and space the sessions two hours apart, for SR to produce long-term results.

- Do not do SR right *before* exercising. If you must practice SR before exercising, we would recommend waiting two hours. However, scheduling your SR session right *after* exercise magnifies the benefits of both. Exercise followed immediately by relaxation is a wonderful combination. It can be helpful to have a cool-down period of about 15 minutes before starting SR to give your heart rate a chance to slow down.

- Practicing SR right after meals is not recommended, but this may not be a very important consideration. Some people have difficulty relaxing if they are too hungry and might want to eat a light snack before relaxing.

For most people, the best times of day to accomplish the two SR sessions are upon arising and after work.

The above guidelines came from observing people who have been successful at reversing their chronic symptoms through the practice of SR.

Length and frequency of practice: Alpha (or theta) brainwaves need to be reached at least twice each day. It is all right for SR sessions to be more frequent than two a day, and actually fine to practice SR as many times a day as you wish. Don't forget that you need about two hours after one relaxation session before doing another one to get the most long-term, cumulative benefit.

Most people need a session lasting at least 20 minutes to reach alpha or theta brainwaves. Ultimately, the required length of your SR session depends on your success in reaching the alpha (or theta) rhythm with your chosen relaxation technique. Since most beginners cannot just switch into that rhythm at a snap of the fingers, it generally takes 20 minutes just to settle down and to reach the relaxation response. If it takes you longer than 20 minutes, plan to spend more time. For example, if you are reliably reaching alpha in 30 minutes, then twice a day for 30 minutes would be much better than for only 20 minutes. Once you get really good at SR, you can practice several times a day, spending only a few minutes each time.

You do not have to spend the entire 20 minutes in the desired relaxed brain state. All it takes is a few minutes of alpha (or theta) during each of the two sessions to obtain beneficial results. Also, nobody will reach the deeply relaxed state 100% of the time during their practice. Just becoming that relaxed in about 90% of your sessions is desirable.

Longer duration or more frequent sessions might create a short-term effect of bringing immediate relief from symptoms, but may not contribute much to the long-term effect of reversing your condition. Based on our extensive experience, 20 minutes twice a day has proven to be optimal for most people.

Staying awake during SR sessions: You want to get the most and best results possible from the time you spend working towards improving your health. Napping does not give the same results as SR, so do SR instead of taking a nap. Once you get into the habit of doing regular Skilled Relaxation, you will probably find that naps are unnecessary anyway.

Also, falling asleep during SR cancels out the benefit of doing the practice. If we cross over into sleep and into the delta state, we have gone past the window of opportunity where alpha reverses the buildup of stress at a rate 24 times faster than delta. Measurable parameters of stored stress-effect empirically and consistently show greater healing effects from alpha (or theta) brainwave than the delta (sleep) brainwave. If just going to sleep resolved health problems, people wouldn't have any problems!

People who do *not* fall asleep during their SR sessions do much better than those who drowse. If you find yourself falling asleep during your practice, here are a few suggestions for staying awake.

- Change locations or positions: If you are trying to accomplish your SR session in bed, move to a different location to avoid the association with sleep. Sit up during your practice or use a semi-recliner, but do not lie down.

- The big spoon trick: Hold a wooden or large serving spoon, or any object such as a paperback book, in your hand. If you slip past alpha and theta into delta (the point of sleep), muscular control is lost, and whatever you are holding in your hand will fall and wake you up. Pick it back up, and go on with your SR practice.

- A special approach to help beginners stay awake in sessions was contributed by a practitioner helping clients with SR. He remarked that people struggling to stay awake have found that taking a short nap before SR helps. Later, after doing SR routinely, they don't need the nap.

What you might experience during SR: In a successful SR session, lowered body temperature is very common. Try draping a warm blanket over yourself. Some people are sensitive to noise during SR, and insulating oneself from loud noises by practicing in a quiet place is a good idea.

Sometimes a person will get slightly jolted out of his or her practice of SR. This is normal. It's similar to being asleep and being jolted awake by your leg jerking. Some experience an eye twitch (same effect, different part of the body). This comes from being so tense all day that the body reacts to finally relaxing a little with this release. This typically happens to people who have been maximally tense for many years. As the total stress storage decreases, this will no longer happen. If this happens to you, it is a good sign, not a bad one. It proves that you are on the right track.

Some people may even feel sore for a few days. It takes a lot of effort (even unconsciously) to hold muscles tight, thus the letting go can cause a soreness that replaces the tension for a short period of time.

Individuals occasionally experience curious temporary phenomena as part of their healing process. Here are some examples:

- Patient A: "I have been doing SR everyday for over a week now. I have noticed two things: one is that the last few days I've had lots of anger and have been very moody. I can't pinpoint what I'm mad at, but I don't like it."

- Patient B: "Sometimes during SR I notice I have a rapid heartbeat while the rest of my body seems to be getting relaxed."

- Patient C: "In my long-time practice of SR, I am experiencing a completely new thing. After about five minutes, I start to involuntarily rock back and forth and during my last session, it got fairly intense."

If something like these examples happens to you (chances are that it will not), tell yourself, "This, too, shall pass," and persist in your practice. Such experiences are usually part of the "healing crisis" which is a normal aspect of healing (see Chapter 5). Unusual sensations usually subside with regular practice, or by switching to a different relaxation technique.

SR has so many benefits. Over time, as you practice SR, you will become more aware of your tendencies to brace, both during your SR sessions and in your daily life. You may begin to notice more subtle tautness in your lower back, hip joints, or hands. You might become aware of the tightness that has overcome your digestive system and your breathing. Then, you will observe the tension fade away. Overall, you will become more conscious of your entire body as you lose the numbness that comes from full-body bracing.

When you reach the relaxation response or the alpha (or theta) window of brainwaves, not only does your mind get a vacation, muscles everywhere in your body release their tension, your pulse rate drops, your breathing slows down, and you need a lot less energy for bodily maintenance. Meanwhile, anywhere in your body that there is disease, restoration and healing occur. If there was any one thing that could be considered a magic pill, SR is it. Even if SR alone does not totally resolve a problem in six to twelve months, you will be so much healthier by then that any other treatments that might be needed or that you are currently using will work much better.

Changing techniques: After you have been practicing SR for some time, do not be surprised if the method that worked so well for you in the beginning stops working effectively and you need to select a different technique. This often happens as a person moves closer to the goal of health. As the bodymind changes, the healing path needs to change too.

After you have learned what the relaxation response feels like for you, it is easy to tell when your technique no longer works and it is time to find the next method. Experiment with other relaxation methods until you find a new one that works for you. If you have tested your practice with biofeedback, you most likely will not need to go for biofeedback testing again, because you already know what the relaxation response feels like. It has been our experience that passive approaches have to be changed more frequently than active ones.

Third, Evaluate Your SR Practice

There are two ways to know if you are relaxing and getting the right brainwave.

1. Self-evaluation
2. Biofeedback

1. Self-evaluation

Some people can tell if they are achieving an alpha or theta brainwave (mental relaxation) just by reading a description of how it feels to experience a quiet mind. The brainwaves have been described on pages 40–41.

Here's another way to know. If you are achieving alpha or theta brainwaves, you will also experience relaxation in your body. Thus, knowing what *physical* relaxation feels like is also useful. If you are experiencing a physically relaxed state, this confirms that your SR practice is producing the desired effect.

The physical "relaxation response" is a term coined by Herbert Benson, M.D. It is a relaxed physical state that comes from having a relaxed mind. When you reach the relaxation response, you will feel sensations in your body indicating you are relaxing. Generally, in an SR session, a person will first reach the alpha or theta brainwave, then the body will make some kind of physical shift. The body itself shows the signs of relaxation.

Signs of Reaching the Relaxation Response

- Abdominal breathing
- Awareness of gas in intestines
- Blank spots (not knowing where the mind was the last few seconds)
- Exhalation less controlled
- Extremities warm, heavy, or tingling
- Eyelids stop fluttering with eyes closed
- Facial muscles soft and less defined
- Feel like floating on a cloud or sinking (melting) into the rug
- Feel the pull of gravity
- Fingernail beds consistently pink
- Forehead smooth
- Growling in stomach
- Heart rate slower
- Heartbeats less pronounced
- Increased awareness of bladder fullness
- Increased or decreased awareness of hunger or thirst
- Increased salivation
- Jaw slightly open, not clenched
- Legs separate slightly (if seated)

- Lengthened breathing cycle
- Lightness (a light feeling)
- Loss of sensory proprioceptive input (can't feel clothing, jewelry, or position of hand in contact with other surfaces)
- More frequent swallowing
- Neck muscles soft
- Neck pulse less visible and slower
- Palms consistently pink (not speckled or white)
- Shoulders drop
- Sighing
- Time perception altered (time expands or contracts)
- Toes point outward more (if lying on back)

You will not feel or be aware of all of these sensations, of course, but may experience one or several. Since every person has a different sensation when reaching the relaxation response, each person has to experience it for himself or herself. Descriptions can only help in a general way.

For most people, it is easier to know if you've reached a relaxed state through bodily awareness (physical sensation) than by the brainwaves.

Q: Is the relaxation response the same as relaxing when I take a break at work, get a massage, watch TV, or go fishing?
A: There are moments in ordinary activities such as receiving a massage, going fishing, swimming, doing artwork, or even drumming when deep relaxation can occur for many people. However, even if a person does achieve an alpha or theta brainwave during these activities, unless practiced two times a day (impractical for most people, although maybe not for a fisherman, swimmer, or artist) and reaches the relaxation response reliably, those activities cannot be considered SR. The relaxation in a Skilled Relaxation session is usually a bit deeper than what most people consider to be relaxing.

Brainwave changes don't always occur during ordinary relaxation activities. What many people think is relaxation doesn't usually include an alpha brainwave and physical relaxation response. SR goes beyond ordinary relaxation, although ordinary relaxation happens on the way there.

Skilled Relaxation cultivates the ability to reliably reach a deeply relaxed state in a short period of time. We call it "Skilled Relaxation" because it is a skill that needs to be learned and practiced.

If you are still unsure if you are relaxing, you may use biofeedback to obtain definite confirmation. Actually, it is a good idea to use biofeedback at least once to know if you're reaching the relaxation response. That way you won't waste months doing the practice incorrectly. You cannot count on getting benefits from SR unless you know for sure that your practice is effective and you are reaching the desired relaxed state.

2. Using biofeedback

We recommend that everyone go for biofeedback testing after practicing a form of SR for about two weeks (or after a month if practicing less often, but of course we hope you are doing this twice a day). If you get checked by biofeedback shortly after you have started using your SR technique, you won't risk finding out it isn't working after practicing for months. The worry about "am I doing this right?" can easily be put aside by checking your practice with a knowledgeable biofeedback trainer or using a biofeedback machine at home. The sooner you know for sure when you are reaching alpha (or theta), the easier it is to learn how to reliably reproduce that state each time you practice SR.

Biofeedback is the most reliable way we know of to scientifically establish whether your technique is producing the correct results. We do have to put in a disclaimer here about the term certify, since it actually is not 100% certain. It is, however, the best proof that we have and close enough.

A biofeedback practitioner can test you to see if your home procedure is working. If your method is working, one session is all it takes to verify that you are reaching the desired brainwave. Note that it is a little harder to have moving SR practices, like t'ai chi or yoga, checked by biofeedback than the other techniques. We would like to repeat the precaution for individuals with a history of seizures or psychiatric disorders. Individuals with those conditions may check their SR practice using the self-evaluation descriptions above, and need to be under the direction of professionals who are experts in those conditions and in using biofeedback.

What kind of biofeedback to use: When using biofeedback, either by being tested by a technician or using a machine at home, we are mostly concerned about what happens to your body's connection to the hypothalamus, which means making sure you are learning how to reach the physical relaxation response. Here are four biofeedback methods that you can use:

1.   Verification that you are reaching the physical relaxation response may be done by Galvanic Skin Response (GSR is sometimes also called EDA or Electro Dermal Activity), so that is what to ask for when you go for biofeedback. The GSR is the body measurement that most quickly changes with the relaxation response. A GSR monitor records

a change in electrical resistance of the skin by using a signal such as a light, tone, or dial. The smallest reduction in arousal will cause that tone (or signal) to drop, which indicates an increase in relaxation. The GSR is the preferred method for checking your SR practice.

2.   The machine that directly measures brainwaves is EEG (Electro-Encephalo Graph). The EEG machine can tell you if you're reaching alpha or theta. While the EEG doesn't tell you specifically if your body is becoming relaxed as the result of your practice, no one can produce pure alpha or theta over and over again for weeks on end without the body becoming more relaxed. Thus, if the person who helps you can only test your brainwave using an EEG, it is still okay.

3.   The muscle tension machine (Electro-Myo Graph or EMG) measures the electrical activity of each individual muscle cell monitored and the sum total of a targeted group of muscle cells. For example, since most people hold tension in their neck and shoulders, that is a good place for testing and reflects results in achieving the relaxation response.

4.   Skin temperature biofeedback indicates changes in autonomic nervous system activity (i.e., FOF or relaxation of the hypothalamus). As a person relaxes, the skin temperature of the extremities increases and warmth is felt. (Increased autonomic activity is why very nervous people frequently have cold hands and feet.)

If you can do only one of these four ways, we recommend using a GSR machine. The second choice for biofeedback is the EEG. Ideally, you would be tested using both a GSR and an EEG simultaneously, if available. Use the other two options, muscle tension and skin temperature, if GSR or EEG testing is not available. While muscle tension biofeedback and skin temperature biofeedback work, they take too long to respond, so we do not usually recommend them. However, if that is all that is available for you, they can still be somewhat useful.

When a biofeedback practitioner or technician hooks you up to any of the feedback monitors, focus on doing your relaxation practice. The feedback, by way of a tone or signal, lets you know whether or not you are moving into a relaxed state, if you are becoming more tense, or if you are not making any change. Pay attention to how you feel. Whatever you are doing that successfully helps you relax is what you need to continue in your practice. It is a very simple process to relax and listen to the tone telling you about your state of relaxation and tension.

It is not necessary to use all the forms of biofeedback, but if you could be hooked up simultaneously to all four biofeedback methods, you would experience how the response time differs for each method. The EEG (brainwave) reflects the relaxation first, followed very closely (seconds rather than minutes) by the GSR (skin response), then comes the muscle tension feedback a few minutes later, and finally the skin temperature registers. We mention this to help you understand how they work, because the response time of the biofeedback method you are using influences your learning process. The faster ones give you more immediate feedback so you can pay immediate attention to the subtle changes in your body.

What if you are not achieving relaxation? If during your biofeedback session, you have no decrease in GSR or an alpha brainwave is not reached, then are you not reaching the relaxation response. This means that your SR is not working. If this happens, the therapist should be able to tell you what to try next from the readings on the machine and the technique you are using. Use those recommendations to alter your future attempts. Go home and practice some more, and return a few weeks later to see if the new approach is working.

Most people are able to learn SR by this time, because it is really quite simple. However, if after that second time you are one of the few whose technique is still not working, you might obtain a machine for home use for a while to experiment and learn what works for you. Some biofeedback instructors will rent you a GSR to take home for a week or a month, usually at a reasonable cost. Machines can also be purchased. Use the biofeedback machine each time you practice your technique, and try different methods of SR if necessary until you find one that works for you. We have never known anyone who needed a machine more than a month. Most only need it for a week or so. It may seem like a lot of effort, but the end results will be worth it: improved health.

How to find a biofeedback practitioner: If you obtained or heard about this book from a health care practitioner, that person may offer biofeedback or be able to give you a referral to a biofeedback practitioner. Otherwise, try the Yellow Pages under pain management or biofeedback. If unsuccessful there, ask local psychologists or neurologists, or their office staff, for suggestions about where to go. Refer also to the Resources at the end of this book.

When you speak with a prospective biofeedback technician or therapist, simply say that you are practicing relaxation techniques and you want to be tested to see if you are reaching the relaxation response. If the technician doesn't know what you're talking about, or wants you to come in for a whole series of appointments, look around for another technician. One session is usually all it takes to verify if your practice is working.

Purchasing your own machine: ■■■ WALT: If there is no technician or biofeedback practitioner in your area, and no one else who knows enough to test you, you can purchase a machine for home use. The biofeedback machine I would recommend that you purchase is a GSR. For individual use, the GSR is more effective, less expensive, and easier to use than an EEG.

EEGs actually measure brainwaves, but tend to be expensive and difficult to use as biofeedback machines for self-monitoring of Skilled Relaxation. Thus most people would not get the best feedback from an EEG machine. Today this is all done by computer, and may be easier, but generally other biofeedback machines are more suitable.

GSRs typically use finger contacts or a bar that you hold in your hand. GSRs generally come in two types: more expensive ($300+) and less expensive (around $100). The more expensive machines are more sensitive and have more options for feedback, such as dials, volume control, or a flashing light. The less expensive machines are much less sensitive and have fewer options for feedback. Although I believe that it is much easier to learn with a more sensitive machine, the less sensitive machines are still probably sufficient to certify the effectiveness of your technique. For those bothered or distracted by a machine's response, such as dials, flashing lights, or tones, it helps to have a choice to be able to select the least distracting one. Some machines (the less expensive ones) only have a tone, so if you are better served by the lights or dials, and a tone is all there is, you may need to consider spending more money.

You may be able to find used machines on the Internet. If you buy one, after you are certain that you are producing the relaxation response, you can always resell it to someone else. ■■■

SKILLED RELAXATION Q & A

Q: How can I know if I am bracing?

A: Like most people, you are probably bracing and are not aware of it. The fact that you have chronic symptoms is a clue, but a massage therapist or other bodyworker can tell you if you are bracing.

You will also be able to know for sure if you have been bracing after you have started practicing Skilled Relaxation regularly and have managed to reduce the bracing somewhat. Your body will become more relaxed, and that feels very good! After a few months of regular practice, you will most likely start feeling better all of the time, and you will say, "My goodness, what was I doing before?"

Q: Since I can't tell that I'm bracing to begin with, how do I know when I'm no longer bracing?
A: Believe me, you will know. You will feel so much better and be very relaxed. Remember how good you felt right after one deep, total-body, therapeutic massage…or after a long, restful vacation? That is how you feel with just *some* of the bracing gone.

Q: When you say, don't exercise after doing SR, does that include mild exercise like rebounding and gentle walking, or do you mean vigorous exercise like aerobics?
A: This mainly refers to vigorous exercise. Doing such gentle exercise is probably not a concern, although doing it *before* the SR session is best.

Q: Patient A: Can I do my SR practice only *once a day* for 20 minutes? Patient B: Can I do it once a day for *40 minutes?*
A: It is the unusual person who resolves chronic tension or chronic illness with once-a-day SR practice. Practicing SR only once a day helps about 5% of people resolve their chronic problems. The other 95% need twice a day.

Even with the advantage of twice a day, it still takes the average person in our stressful culture six to twelve months to resolve most health conditions. Keep in mind that you probably continue to accumulate stress even as you are working to discharge it. It takes twice-a-day practice to discharge more stress from the system than is accumulated during the day. If you did SR only once a day, it could take you years to resolve your symptoms—if at all.

Q: Can I do SR to help me fall asleep or if I awaken in the middle of the night?
A: It is okay to use your new skill to get to sleep, but don't count that time as one of the twice-daily sessions needed for long-term accumulation of benefits.

Some relaxation techniques are specifically for falling asleep, but that is the only benefit derived from them. Some of these are in the form of a CD or audiotape that induces the delta or sleep brainwave. If you do SR before sleeping, you may get short-term benefits of temporary relief of symptoms, but since you go to sleep, you do not notice them.

Q: If I am interrupted while doing SR, do I need to start the 20 minutes over again or can I just continue as if nothing happened?

A: Just go on. However, it is best if you arrange things so you are not disturbed.

Q: I've been practicing SR for twelve months and have seen much improvement, but still have occasional times when my symptoms return. How long do I have to do SR twice a day to become totally symptom-free? Is there a time when I can do it only once a day?

A: There is a threshold you need to pass before your bodymind will take over for you so that you will not have to do the practice as frequently. If you still have some of your symptoms, you are not there yet.

After a year of being symptom-free, many people only need one session a day to maintain progress. However, you will continue to gain additional benefits for at least the first five years if you continue practicing relaxation at least two times a day. Some individuals would benefit from practicing twice a day for ten years.

Q: Is SR a religious or spiritual practice?

A: Skilled Relaxation is not spiritual or religious in nature. None of these techniques have any religious connotation. Many of the SR approaches have no basis in any ancient philosophy at all, such as autogenics, biofeedback, breathing, and self-hypnosis. Others date back many centuries.

One of the books recommended as containing many Skilled Relaxation techniques is *Awakening: Ways to Psycho-Spiritual Growth* (see Resources). This book makes the point that SR is not spiritual or religious. It does point out, however, that some of the great founders of the world's major religious and spiritual traditions discovered the relaxation response, or were taught it, and found it so profoundly moving that they created something around it. Thus, some of the techniques have a basis in ancient philosophies.

One can add a religious connotation to SR if desired, but that connotation is not necessary for the techniques to be effective. Prayer, for example, is also one way to reach this level of healing brain rhythms.

FOR IMMEDIATE RELIEF

Many people experience immediate benefits from their practice of Skilled Relaxation, but if you have long-term chronic pain or symptoms, you may wish to use additional treatments to provide greater immediate relief until the benefits of SR accrue. If you are in a lot of pain, visiting the health care professionals mentioned below can help, especially while you are learning SR to work on the cause.

Since so many symptoms are due to bracing, the paragraphs below discuss healing methods that can help alleviate the pain or discomfort caused by bracing.

A Quick Primer on Therapeutic Massage and Bodywork

Many people can obtain quick relief from bracing by getting a series of six therapeutic, deep-tissue massages in two weeks (90-minute sessions). Two other bodywork methods, Rolfing or Hellerwork, can give symptomatic relief for up to a year. Do a series of ten sessions over ten weeks if you choose the latter two modalities. Any kind of deep, total body, therapeutic bodywork done in a series over a short period of time will probably discharge enough of your chronic bracing so that you will be able to tell what it feels like to be without bracing.

Alexander Technique and Feldenkrais are practices that you can learn to do yourself that give similar results and offer even longer benefits. Like SR, you have to keep practicing these last two methods regularly.

With massage, Rolfing or Hellerwork, another person is grabbing you by the arm and "dragging you back from the metaphorical cliff edge" for a while. Alexander Technique or Feldenkrais are techniques you do on your own. None of these methods are harmful and will not have permanent effects without Skilled Relaxation. That is *not* to say that you shouldn't use them, just that you need to be realistic about what to expect from them. They will provide relief until your Skilled Relaxation accumulates the long-term effects and acts at a deeper level.

A massage therapist's perspective: relief until SR starts working

■■■ JAN: My experience alleviating bracing with massage is that the exact number and length of sessions is best determined individually depending upon the type of problem you have and the severity of your condition. Six 90-minute massages in two weeks is a good general guideline or average therapeutic trial. Some of my clients prefer to receive one deep tissue massage every week or every other week for their entire first year of doing SR. The number and frequency of sessions is very individual.

There are two basic ways massage relieves bracing. One way is focused work directly in areas of pain, and the other is full-body sessions for overall relaxation. Some people use a combination of these two approaches to obtain maximum relief. ■■■

If you are challenged by learning Skilled Relaxation practice because you have difficulty relaxing, a series of bodywork sessions may be especially helpful for you. Some people just have too much accumulated stress to do SR easily. They need to reduce their symptoms a bit and become more relaxed before SR becomes possible for them, and getting bodywork can help tremendously. Massage and Rolfing can help lessen or release your bracing a little, making it easier to start SR.

It would be unusual for anyone actually walking right at the edge of a cliff to truly relax! Our bodyminds really work this way, and getting some extra assistance from massage and other bodywork modalities when you are at the edge of your symptomatic cliff can be of great assistance.

The bodywork treatments mentioned above can also be beneficial if your symptoms are related to digestive issues or mental-emotional issues. Additional information about working with such conditions is provided in Chapter 3 (diet), Chapter 7 (additional treatments), and Chapter 8 (healing mind, emotions, and spirit). Also consider adding the other aspects of the Wellness Program—Diet and Exercise.

Symptom relief Q & A

Q: My chronic neck pain decreased after I received some massage. Since I feel better, why should I practice SR?

A: Localized conditions are often just the tip of the iceberg of total-body bracing. If you resolve the local condition with massage, the problem will often be back in a year or so, since the total-body bracing will still be present.

Q: I bruise easily when I get bodywork or just in general.

A: For many people, this is resolved by taking up to three grams of pure bioflavinoids every day. Within a few weeks you should see results, with complete clearing in a few months. Once you are clear for a month or so, cut the dose in half. If no more bruising occurs in a few months, cut the dose in half again. You will eventually find a dose that is not enough to prevent this bruising, and go back to the last dose that did. That is your maintenance dose.

Q: Can my back pain (or other musculo-skeletal problem) be resolved through massage and chiropractic alone, or through other physical techniques, without doing SR?

A: ■■■ WALT: Sometimes it can. However, if you are also bracing, those approaches alone will not usually give a permanent solution. At the Holistic Healing Center I had in Lexington, a chiropractor to whom we sent patients needing structural help would adjust them so that they would come out feeling better. However, a few days later the patients would come back and say, "It didn't last." The chiropractor would say, "The adjustment didn't hold." We finally began to catch on to the fact that the reason they were recurrently out of adjustment was because their tight musculature was pulling them out of alignment—bracing.

So then we brought in a massage therapist, who worked with the patients and was able to stretch out the times between adjustments significantly, but eventually the adjustments still didn't hold. At that point, we realized bracing can't be cured with massage alone; it was necessary to teach the person SR. Once we got an individual doing that (it might take a year of doing SR regularly and adequately twice a day), then the patient's goals could often be achieved with less massage and chiropractic. ■■■

A massage therapist's perspective: muscle pain

■■■ JAN: I had my clients in mind when I contacted Walt about writing this book. Many of my clients have made the rounds to many doctors, chiropractors, and physical therapists, and used many modalities, various drugs, vitamins, and supplements…some even attempted surgery. Yet they ended up in my office still looking for relief. Massage can help considerably; it resolves many muscular problems, and is the only relief available for some people.

However, if your pain continues to recur or move from one part of the body to another, and if you have underlying full-body bracing, then massage and other external treatments will likely not be enough to resolve your condition. In addition to working from the outside, you must also work from the inside using the 3LS. I have found that the combination of Skilled Relaxation and regular bodywork can bring fast progress for creating health. My clients who practice SR are delighted with the results. ■■■

Q: Why can't I just take a pill, such as muscle relaxants, to resolve my symptoms?

A: ■■■ WALT: I say the same thing about all things people can take for chronic conditions. My statement has been for years:

> *Chronic conditions will never be permanently resolved*
> *by something you take, but by something you do!*

I have no doubt that some products can give temporary benefits (even years) for many chronic conditions. I am talking about changing your health forever.

The regular practice of Skilled Relaxation at least twice a day for 20 minutes can reverse a multitude of chronic conditions. Taking things will, at best, provide temporary benefits. Even the effective treatments stop working eventually and you are right back where you started, only older, and whatever your symptoms are, they will probably be a little worse. ■ ■ ■

Points to Remember About Skilled Relaxation

- Relaxation is cumulative over time. If you are doing your SR practice correctly, it can take several months to feel the effects, although many people notice improvement immediately. Remember, it took a long time for your chronic condition to build up to the point of pain. It probably won't take as *much* time and effort to heal it.
- If you are in pain, you may try increasing the frequency or length of your SR sessions to obtain more short-term benefits.
- After you have learned what successful practice feels like, you may adjust the length of time of your sessions according to your awareness of your brainwaves and your body.
- If you become sleepy during the day, try a SR session instead of taking a nap. You will be more refreshed.
- Patience and persistence in doing the relaxation regularly are the passwords to success for SR.
- Relaxation is actually very simple to do. Just begin and you will get the hang of it.

TROUBLESHOOTING GUIDE FOR SKILLED RELAXATION

The following are answers to questions from patients and participants about SR that may be helpful to you down the road.

Q: I've been practicing SR for one month and haven't seen any results. What's going on?

A: Here you are after one month, wondering why you are not better? Remember, it takes three to six months of SR (done correctly) to start seeing results and six to twelve months for resolution. There is no real trick to doing SR, although at this time it would be wise for you to make sure your practice is effective by going for biofeedback. Success at SR does take the three D's— Diligence, Dedication, and Discipline.

Q: I've been practicing SR for one year and haven't seen any results. Why not?

A: This is very unusual. The first thing that comes to mind is that you are daily exposed to some kind of stressor that is exceeding your efforts at reversing the effects. Second, look at the checklist on page 67 to be sure you are doing your practice correctly. Third, have you tried adding the other parts of the Wellness Program in combination with your SR practice? Stress-effect storage is rarely the sole cause of a chronic condition, so it is wise to consider adding other healing approaches along with SR.

Q: I've been trying really hard to relax in my SR sessions, but I just get upset instead or my mind races. What am I doing wrong?

A: Like going to sleep, one cannot make relaxation happen, one has to *let* it happen. The harder you try, the less likely it will occur. Learning to do SR is like how you felt when you were a child trying to learn to ride a bicycle. If you think too much about keeping your balance, you fall. But when you let go and let your body make its own adjustments, you succeed. SR is actually a lot easier to learn than riding a bicycle!

Since SR is similar to going to sleep, for some people it works just to pretend to be falling asleep.

As mentioned earlier, some people who have too much accumulated stress to do SR easily would benefit from the massage or Rolfing series. These healing methods can help you relax enough to settle down during your SR session.

A few people find that moderate exercise before their SR sessions helps them fall into an alpha state easier.

Finally, if you can't seem to do SR, you may have chosen the wrong technique for you. Try a different technique. Experiment and keep practicing until you learn SR. You will be glad you did.

Q: I haven't been doing SR practice regularly lately—I don't have the time— but when I catch myself bracing in stressful situations, I do SR and it seems to help me relax.

A: Great! It sounds like you have become aware that SR can help you relax. However, we encourage you to re-read the information about bracing on pages 35–37 to be sure you understand the concept. The tensing up that you describe is most likely only a small part of your total bracing.

Also consider this: if you do enough SR to alleviate both the bracing you are aware of and the bracing you are not aware of, then you will most likely be feeling so much better, have increased energy, and be so much more relaxed on an ongoing basis, that you will end up feeling less tense in stressful situations any time they occur.

We encourage you to persist at finding a way to make regular SR a part of your day. No one yet has discovered how to discharge all the stored FOF response without an investment of time. Those who practice SR soon find that they are getting back more time than it is costing them.

Q: My health problems were really severe, but I'm doing much better since I've been practicing SR. However, if I miss the second SR session in a day, my symptoms come back slightly.

A: You are making progress. From your description of the severity of your condition, it sounds like it may take you two to three years to be finally rid of all your bracing. I would guess that you have been doing your SR practice for less than a year, so persist. Try your best to do your SR twice a day, as the long-term accumulation of benefits really only happens with that frequency. Also add the other two parts of the Wellness Program.

Troubleshooting checklist for SR practice

- ✓ Are you doing your SR practice twice a day for 20 minutes?
- ✓ Are you spacing your sessions two hours apart?
- ✓ Are you doing your SR at least two hours before sleeping?
- ✓ Are you doing your exercise before, not after, your Skilled Relaxation sessions?
- ✓ Have you tried several different techniques to find one that works for you, or a new technique if you've been doing SR for a while?
- ✓ Are you arranging your sessions so you are undisturbed?
- ✓ Are you trying too hard rather than allowing yourself to just fall into a relaxed state?
- ✓ Are you certain you're achieving the relaxation response by having your practice checked with biofeedback?
- ✓ Have you given your SR practice enough time to work (six to twelve months)?
- ✓ Have you gone for a massage or Rolfing series to help you get further away from the edge of the cliff?
- ✓ Are you falling asleep during your sessions?

If your activity does not seem to be working, consider beginning your wellness program with a different aspect of the 3LS, or adding one of the other two aspects of the program.

When to get professional help for skilled relaxation

Skilled Relaxation is very safe to practice. If your activity seems to be stimulating concerns, read the section in Chapter 5 about the healing crisis to understand the body's response to healing. Below are the few situations we have heard of that may require professional help.

- Decreased need for medications. Some people's health improves so much they need to decrease the medications they have been taking. If this is the case with you, talk to the health care professional managing your medications.

- SR may be a catalyst that opens up buried pre-existing emotional, spiritual, physical or historical issues needing to be addressed. If you have a history of psychiatric disorders, or you feel extremely anxious about practicing SR or experience strong emotions that you cannot handle alone, consult a mental health professional or psychotherapist before beginning any regular relaxation practice. If you experience disturbing ongoing energetic phenomena in your SR sessions or in your daily life (such as the examples on pages 52–53), consult a teacher of kundalini yoga, an energy practitioner, or transpersonal psychotherapist. If you experience physical symptoms that seem to be new, take care of them or consult an appropriate practitioner for assistance. Such symptoms are likely pre-existing and you have now just become aware of them.

- Seizures. As mentioned, the use of passive relaxation or biofeedback machines is said to have the potential to induce seizures in certain individuals. See page 44.

THE AUTHORS' EXPERIENCES

■■■ WALT: When I first started SR, I had so many serious, long-term problems that I regularly went to a neurologist, psychiatrist, orthopedic surgeon, internist, general surgeon, and chiropractor. All of the allopaths had me on at least one medication, and all said that I would have to take them for the rest of my life. This was how I had been trained to treat every one of these conditions, and this is how I actually treated my own patients until I learned about SR. Of course, the surgeons strongly recommended surgery.

Within six months of doing SR, I was off all my medications and became free of the following symptoms: hemorrhoids, chronic indigestion, sinusitis, high cholesterol, arthritis, hypertension, chronic depression, insomnia, pain, and muscular tension. I also no longer needed to wear a back brace for ruptured discs. I have not had those symptoms again since they went away (25 years already). I never had the surgery, either.

The SR method that worked best for me was Silva Mind Training. It was effective for a number of years and then I began to see that it was not working as well. Following that, I used autogenics for a few years, then tapes, then breathing; then I made up my own. I tried nearly every technique that is listed in this book, so I could say I had a personal experience with them. I discovered, when I first learned to do Skilled Relaxation, that I became so healthy I wanted to meditate for hours.[10]

I did not learn about SR until I was about 40, and I sincerely wish I had learned this relaxation at a younger age. ∎∎∎

∎∎∎ JAN: The practice of SR came easily to me since I had been a meditator for many years, and it did not take long for me to learn what alpha brainwaves and the relaxation response felt like. I had my practice checked with biofeedback, however, just to be sure. My deep healing started by adding the second SR session to my day. I got such good results from doing SR, I practiced it three times a day for over a year!

I would like to tell you how I experienced some of the changes in my body from SR. After practicing SR for about a month, one day my entire body suddenly relaxed. It was a huge shift and felt wonderful. Jubilantly, I thought I had stopped bracing. Then, after another month of serious SR practice, my entire body suddenly relaxed even more, and I thought, "What happened? I thought I had already stopped bracing last month! I guess I have *really* stopped bracing this time." However, about a month later, a third wave of relaxation melted tension in my lower body—abdomen, pelvis, thighs, and calves. At that point, I started to anticipate that there would be more changes to come from regular SR practice. And I was not disappointed. The next big relaxation surge included all the muscles of my upper body—the muscles between and over the ribs, and my neck, shoulders, and jaw. It was wonderful. I felt like I was being released from a straitjacket. Over the next months, the relaxation continued randomly in different spots in the body, including my limbs and deep within my torso, and even in my feet. At one point, my breathing eased, and I could suddenly feel the breath flowing deeply throughout my body. Then around eleven months of practice, some kind of critical mass was achieved and my energy increased tremendously, bringing about improvements in total body function. This whole process was amazing to me.

Since I knew so much about muscles from my training as a massage therapist, even at the beginning, I had no doubt that I was bracing, but I was ultimately surprised at the extent to which I was doing it. I only found out how uncomfortable I had previously been after practicing SR consistently for a year. Now, as I continue my SR practice, and the more I de-brace, the more surprised I become at how many places in my body have been tight without me even knowing it. Much of the tension was deeply internal.

For the first several years of SR practice, I found that 30-minute sessions were usually best for me. That extra 10 minutes seemed to relax my bodymind more. Later, after I had mastered achieving alpha states, I only needed about 10 minutes for each SR session. Four years into the program, after my health was so much better, I see the wisdom of always scheduling two SR sessions each day. As I continue doing the practice, the health benefits continue to accumulate. Skilled Relaxation is wonderful! ■■■

Chapter 2, SKILLED RELAXATION—SUMMING IT UP

Stress causes the Fight or Flight (FOF) response in the body, which is characterized by an increase in heart and respiratory rates, higher blood pressure, increased muscular tension, and reduced digestive activity. If not discharged from the body, the physiological effects of ongoing stress (stress-effect) are stored in the hypothalamus (brain), eventually causing a change in the function of the entire body. Some of the results of this stress-effect storage include bracing (chronic muscular tension), digestive weakness (also called leaky gut syndrome), and brain and body chemistry imbalance (mental or emotional difficulties). Each of these conditions, in turn, is like a foundation that results in secondary health conditions or complications.

The way to reverse the accumulation of stress in the hypothalamus is to practice Skilled Relaxation (SR). SR is a skill that you learn and develop to undo the effects of stress. Anyone can practice SR, and there are many benefits to doing so. The goal of the practice is to reach an alpha or theta brainwave at least twice a day, without falling asleep. Many different techniques can be used to practice SR and reach the desired brainwaves. The two main types of techniques are active (the person trains himself or herself to relax) and passive (a device is used to provide relaxing input). A few examples of practices are: applied relaxation, audiotapes or CDs, breathing techniques, guided imagery, meditation, mind machines, progressive relaxation, self-hypnosis, visualization, and yoga. SR is easy to do and feels good, too.

You can know if you are reaching the right brainwaves in two ways. One way is through self-evaluation by understanding the brainwaves and the physical relaxation response. The other way is by going for a biofeedback session, which is optimally done after you have been practicing SR two weeks to a month.

Most people notice immediate improvement from practicing SR, but it generally takes three to twelve months to experience significant change in a chronic condition. To get immediate relief from uncomfortable or painful symptoms, it can be helpful to go for a series of therapeutic massage or bodywork sessions.

For an abbreviated version of the steps to practice Skilled Relaxation, see the next page.

Skilled Relaxation—STEPS TO TAKE

- Choose and learn a relaxation technique. If you don't already know a suitable relaxation technique, obtain and read *The Relaxation and Stress Reduction Workbook* by Davis, Eshelman, and McKay; take a class; or see a practitioner. Examples of SR techniques include: applied relaxation, relaxation audiotapes, autogenics, breathing techniques, guided imagery, imagination, light goggles, meditation, progressive relaxation, self-hypnosis, Silva Mind Training, thought stopping, t'ai chi, visualization, and yoga. There are many others. If necessary, try several different techniques until you find one that feels comfortable.

- Practice two times a day, for 20 minutes each time. Remember, relaxation isn't something you do; it is something you fall into. Just like falling asleep, you have to let it happen.

- SR can be practiced beneficially any time except two hours before sleep and two hours before exercise. However, doing SR immediately after exercising magnifies the benefits of both. You also need to space your sessions about two hours apart to get the greatest benefits.

- After two weeks to a month of regular, twice-a-day practice, have your SR tested by a biofeedback professional. That way you can be certain you are reaching the relaxation response or alpha/theta brainwave, and you will avoid spending months doing the practice incorrectly. You only need to reach that state of deep relaxation for a few minutes each session. Your SR will not give you the results you desire without it!

- Done correctly, you will most likely start feeling better quickly. It takes an average of three to six months to start seeing *significant* results and six to twelve months for the *resolution* of chronic health problems. Continue practicing twice a day until your problems have been totally gone for a year or so. After that, you may only need one session a day to maintain progress. However, you will receive additional benefits during the next five years if you practice regularly twice a day.

- Skilled Relaxation is only one aspect of the 3LS Wellness Program. Do all three parts for fastest results, greatest health, and numerous benefits.

COMMENTS FROM OTHERS ABOUT PRACTICING SKILLED RELAXATION

I was having panic attacks, multiple chemical sensitivity, vertigo, and some other really "fun" things that I was experiencing on a regular basis. When nothing else helped, SR did and that is a miracle to me after over a decade of spending lots of $$$$$ and never finding an answer.

—Sharon R., IT Consultant, Denver, CO

At first, I thought I was one of those people that just wouldn't be able to do SR, but I could (after a few months). I had it verified with biofeedback, although I already knew I was doing it effectively...I now have no bracing-related symptoms (for instance, back problems, costochondritis, prostatitis), except when I don't do SR. SR is very effective in treating this. I had relief within a couple of months of starting SR. Even my holistic doc missed the bracing diagnosis.   *—R.L., IT Consultant, Mississauga, Ontario, Canada*

I wrote five months ago about my chronic hives, swelling, rosacea, and overall health. About a month after that I started SR, once I got the required info, books, etc., I have been doing SR (self-hypnosis) twice a day for 25–30 minutes and the results are amazing. Within ten days of doing SR, my outbreaks of hives decreased dramatically, and it's only gotten better. It's been four months without swelling, my rosacea has dramatically improved—almost gone—and my hives are almost non-existent. I may still get the occasional one here or there, but they don't increase in size or intensity, no itching, and they only last for a couple of hours. In fact, sometimes a session of SR will make them disappear. It's also been about two months without diarrhea and the cramping in my stomach. I am totally grateful to you for your advice. Thank you! I know I still have a ways to go and need to work on my diet and exercise, but funnily enough, incorporating SR into my daily routine has been really easy, and now I can't imagine not doing it.

—S. Willers, Communications, Toronto, Ontario, Canada

SR was the last thing I was willing to do. I didn't believe in it, and I didn't want to slow down ... I finally gave in because of desperation. It paid off. Until you are to that point, yes, other stuff [such as vitamins or medications —ed.] helps, but they are short-term helpers, not long-term reversal.

—Johnelle Donnell, Wichita Falls, TX

I have suffered greatly from fibromyalgia. I have only been practicing SR faithfully for about 5 weeks and my fibro symptoms have improved at least 75%.   —*Anonymous*

Had costochondritis off and on for a couple years. Never was completely off, could always feel it faintly, even if not painfully flared. Completely disappeared and has not returned since beginning SR (meditation) 2x/day. —*Anonymous*

I have been doing SR on a more regular basis for the last few weeks. Lately I have been noticing stressful things/situations that I previously didn't see as particularly stressful. For instance, I was driving today in heavy traffic on the freeway and started to notice that I was somewhat stressed. I immediately applied some breathing techniques to calm down. What I am finding is that as I do SR more regularly, I am becoming more relaxed and therefore noticing the stressful situations more. Prior to this, when I got in a stressful situation, I didn't notice because I was actually "living" in a state of stress most of the time. I was always stressed but didn't know it and was believing this state was normal. Now my eyes have been opened and I am very excited about where I am headed with this.   —*Mary Koehnen, Student/Homemaker, St. Paul, MN*

I was diagnosed eight years ago with interstitial cystitis. I was 40 and thought my life was over. I was in a vicious cycle of pain meds, bladder dilations and intra-bladder installations of chemicals. The pain was so bad that a pre-malignant ovarian tumor was almost overlooked. My doctors thought the pain was from the interstitial cystitis. DR. STOLL'S SKILLED RELAXATION WORKS!!! It took a little while, but if you stay with it, you WILL get relief. After six months of twice a day SR, I no longer suffer constant IC symptoms. As a matter of fact, for a year and a half, I rarely have had any symptoms at all. It takes a lot of stress and no skilled relaxation time for the IC to flare up and it is never very bad.   —*Anonymous*

I began feeling more positive, hopeful, and peaceful, and I looked forward to my SR time every day. Since I started doing SR on a daily basis, many doors and opportunities for healing and personal growth have opened for me. SR brought a synergy to my healing process and helped me understand that true healing comes from the inside out.

—*Mary Lilga, Environmental Scientist, Richland, WA*

Chapter 3

The Whole Foods Diet

When it comes to eating whole foods, the phrase "nutrition plan," or nutritional approach, better depicts what is being accomplished than the word "diet." Many people associate the word diet with weight loss programs—attempts to lose weight by temporarily changing eating habits. The Whole Foods Diet is meant to support your health and well-being through good nutrition as a lifestyle change rather than a temporary expedient to weight loss. It is very true that many people lose weight easily by switching to eating exclusively whole foods. Regardless, in this book, when you see the word "diet," think "nutrition plan" rather than "weight loss program."

In this chapter, you will learn:

1. About finding the correct foods for you
2. Why modern food weakens the body by creating poor health and chronic illness
3. How to follow a Perfect Whole Foods Diet

HOW DO I CHOOSE A DIET?

Q: How do I choose which foods to eat and what kind of diet to follow? I don't know what to think! A few years ago the general consensus was that one diet was correct and that a different diet was rubbish. Since then I have read about four other diets and they all say different things about what

the body should be getting. Could it possibly be that they are all wrong, because they can't all be right? All I want is to eat the right food for me.

A. ■■■ WALT: The subject of diet is a bit complex. There are so many nutritional theories around that it is hard to know which one to try. People would like to find just one dietary formula that solves everybody's problems, but no one way of eating is right for everyone, despite the claims of many books. Nearly all the different diets are beneficial for a small but specific percent of the population, but even so, chances are that any pre-determined nutrition plan you try will still require adjustment to meet your body's needs. ■■■

Let's look at several factors involved in choosing what to eat.

First, each person has different nutritional needs

Some people need more of particular nutrients than others. Genetics is one reason why some must eat more or less of certain foods (for example, meat) than others and why nutritional supplements can help (see pages 255–261). Genetics determines the way a person's metabolism (chemistry) works, and therefore what type of nutrition is optimal for any person. Since everybody has different nutritional needs, selecting foods to eat is an individual matter.

Second, each diet does something different

All dietary systems are just approaches that have worked for some people, and many are meant to resolve a specific problem rather than be used as a lifetime plan. For example, the Perfect Whole Foods Diet is different from the "elimination diet" and both are used for different purposes (the former is for resolving the health problems caused by eating refined carbohydrates, the latter is for relieving symptoms of food hypersensitivity—more about both shortly). A "metabolic diet" may help someone's general health considerably because it works according to a person's body chemistry, but it is not going to do much (directly) for resolving candida overgrowth, which requires a different eating strategy.

Third, the human body is complex

Often the best diet for any particular person will be a combination of several different dietary approaches. For example, a person who feels best eating only vegetarian food might wish to add the non-meat aspects of the Whole Food Diet to create a nourishing dietary program. Another person who has food allergies might combine the Whole Foods Diet with an elimination diet for the most supportive nutrition plan.

Fourth, dietary needs change

Dietary requirements change according to factors such as age, activity, and livelihood. For example, babies and young children have distinct dietary needs, and the nutritional requirements of older adults varies from that of young adults and middle-age individuals. Also, fashion models need a different diet than construction workers!

Dietary requirements may also change according to your health condition. This is especially true if you practice all three parts of the 3LS Wellness Program. After a few months of Skilled Relaxation, combined with exercise and nutritional improvements, you may stop being in the chronic fight-or-flight (FOF) mode. Consequently, your physiology will most likely become radically different and your body's dietary needs will probably change as well. **Thus the diet that was ideal for you at the beginning of your healing journey may not be your ideal diet later when you are healthier. Thus, any specific diet that helped you at the beginning *may* even make you sick after your health has improved.**

Fifth, certain dietary changes may only have temporary effects

For example, going from the junk many Americans call nutrition to any slightly healthier diet will help many people feel better for a while. However, any continued departure from a truly nutritious diet will eventually catch up with you, and you will likely go back to feeling poorly again. Therefore, small dietary improvements are ideally only beginning steps towards a truly nutritious diet.

Sixth, having some knowledge makes a difference

The more you learn and know, the better you will become at choosing for yourself. Sometimes it takes a pretty big commitment in learning about food, nutrition, and cooking, and practicing what you have learned, to find out which foods are best for you.

Since everyone is different, each individual benefits most by finding his or her own way. Thus, the most reliable way we know of for selecting an optimum diet is for you to become a real student of diet and use trial and error to find out which foods benefit you most. This means learning about any dietary approach you are interested in, trying it accurately, and then listening to your bodymind to see how much good or harm it does. Putting forth this effort can be life-enriching and literally life-saving for many people. When the human genome is much better understood, we will hopefully have practical, affordable laboratory tests that accurately predict which person will do best with certain diets, but such tests are not yet available.

■■■

Recognizing that each diet must be adjusted to suit each individual, there *is* still one nutritional approach that will likely be an improvement to the dietary habits of most people. This diet *may even provide full recovery* for the chronic conditions of many of those who try it precisely. This dietary approach is the Whole Foods Diet (WFD). All of the widely recommended diets on the market agree on this point—the fewer refined or processed foods eaten, the better. That's exactly what the Whole Foods Diet emphasizes. We promote the Whole Foods Diet because, in our experience, it helps most people improve their health greatly with minimal effort and expense.

WHAT IS A WHOLE FOODS DIET?

Following a Whole Foods Diet basically means you eat foods that are whole and avoid refined foods. A whole food is one that has had no parts removed. In contrast to a whole food, a refined food is one that has had something taken out. For example, a potato with the skin on is whole, but if you remove the skin before eating it, the potato is refined. A Whole Foods Diet focuses especially on eating whole carbohydrates, because refined carbohydrates cause so much trouble (read more about this on pages 83–86).

In this chapter, we present two ways to follow a Whole Foods Diet.

Perfect Whole Foods Diet

The first way, called the Perfect Whole Foods Diet (PWFD), is total avoidance of refined carbohydrates. If you are looking for maximum results in curing your chronic symptoms, or wish to feel better quickly, use the Perfect Whole Foods Diet. This nutrition plan will not hurt anyone (people in centuries past used to live just fine before foods were refined) and will help almost everyone who uses it accurately. In fact, we believe nearly 100% of people in this country would see significant benefits from following the PWFD, even after just two weeks.

Liberal Whole Foods Diet

The second way, called the Liberal Whole Foods Diet, is exactly the same as the perfect diet, but you occasionally eat small quantities of refined carbohydrates. The liberal WFD is a great standard wellness diet that helps promote general health.

The PWFD is considered the most curative of the two ways to eat whole foods, and is the approach recommended in this book as the starting place for making this dietary change. You may decide to choose the more liberal WFD for health maintenance after first using the Perfect Whole Foods Diet to resolve a chronic condition. If necessary, at any point after the first few weeks, either the PWFD or the Liberal Whole Foods Diet can be modified with other dietary approaches (examples are described on page 114–116) to create an optimal nutrition plan for your health.

BENEFITS OF THE PERFECT WHOLE FOODS DIET

Eating a Perfect Whole Foods Diet brings a number of benefits. We describe some of them below.

1. Reverse Unusual Symptoms or Conditions

The Perfect Whole Foods Diet can help correct or prevent a variety of diseases or symptoms. If you have health problems that are puzzling your doctor, or if you have gone from one doctor to another in search of help, to no avail, then following this diet perfectly may well prove very useful to you. Some of the most dramatic reversals of poor health to good health we have seen have been in those people who have followed a perfect diet even just for a week or so. After following the PWFD, most people are *amazed at how well they feel and how much their health has improved.*

Just some of the conditions that are helped by the Perfect Whole Foods Diet include:

Agoraphobia	Cravings for sweets	Low blood sugar
Allergies	Depression	Manic-depression
Anxiety	Diabetes (caution	(bipolar disorder)
Arthritis	– must be under a	Nervousness
Attention deficit	doctor's supervision)	Overweight
disorder (ADD)	Digestive disorders	Panic attacks
Behavior problems in	Elevated triglycerides	Phobias
children	Elevated cholesterol	Poor health in general
Candida albicans	Environmental illness	Post-traumatic stress
overgrowth	Fatigue	disorder (PTSD)
Chronic muscle aches	Headaches	Pre-menstrual
Chronic fatigue	Hypertension	syndrome
syndrome	Hypoglycemia	Weakened immune
Constipation	Learning disabilities	system

The PWFD also helps many symptoms with no names and many undiagnosable health conditions.[1]

2. Weight Loss

In addition to healing chronic illness, one effective way for most people to lose weight is to follow the PWFD strictly until reaching a normal weight (the level at which you feel best) and then continuing the diet for at least six months. Most people automatically lose weight when they follow the PWFD. How does this happen? The body's appetite center responds to the need for micronutrients, not just calories. People with continuous hunger usually have deficiencies in dozens of micronutrients and tend to eat large quantities of refined foods to try and satisfy (unsuccessfully) the hunger for those micronutrients, causing them to gain weight. The perfect diet provides those micronutrients and satisfies cravings.

Healthy people are neither fat nor skinny. Eating whole foods always brings a person to a healthy level, thus people who are overweight will most likely experience weight loss. People who are underweight will gain weight, although at first, during a transition period, they may lose a little. Any weight loss will most likely be temporary for those who are of low weight and permanent for those who are overweight.

3. Increased Enjoyment of Food and Enhanced Taste Sensitivity

Another benefit of this diet is how great the food tastes! Not only is the food delicious, but the ability to taste—and the range of taste—also increases after being on the PWFD for some time. This increase occurs because most people's taste buds are numb from eating the sweet/fat/salty diet promoted by manufacturers. You see, the manufacturing process removes much of the natural flavor from food and adds copious quantities of salt and sugar. To the manufacturers, what matters is that the food blasts the taste buds more. Anything sweet (that has been extracted from its source) especially tends to numb the taste buds to other tastes. Eventually, from continually eating overly sweet foods, our taste buds lose their sensitivity. So we have been trading the few good tastes being peddled to us by the manufacturers for the thousands of wonderful tastes available in natural foods (these tastes, by the way, can often tell us which foods our bodies happen to need at that time).

Thus, a universal experience is enjoyed among those who follow the PWFD. Within one week of avoiding any sweeteners, people's taste buds start to wake up and recover their natural sensitivity. People become amazed at how many whole foods have their own natural flavor and sweetness. Within about three months, their taste buds are completely restored and they immensely enjoy the wonderful tastes of whole foods. Anyone who has done the Perfect Whole Foods Diet can tell you of this experience. Those of us who have stuck with it for more than a few months know how the old junk food no longer tastes good and how much more we enjoy our food than before.

Spices, herbs, and condiments are the secret to making whole foods very tasty until the taste buds stop being numb from the mischief of the food processing companies. To learn how to use flavor foods, check at your health food store for a simple booklet on the use of herbs and spices in cooking and diet. Also, be sure to read the label of whatever spices you use, because some may contain refined carbohydrates or additives.

4. Self-Empowerment

Another benefit of the WFD for many is the satisfaction that comes from having controlled and conquered a challenge by doing something so well. People who are sick have often lost self-esteem. The accomplishment of following the diet and reclaiming your health can restore your sense of worth and confidence. Caring about what you eat is also a fulfilling act of caring about yourself, which can enhance your feelings of worth and value.

5. Increased Enjoyment of Life

Many people find that eating whole foods nurtures them on more than just the physical level of the food. This means more than just having extra health and energy. Shopping, cooking, meal preparation, and eating may all become wonderful activities that nourish you on emotional levels as well as physical. Besides the increased nutrition making you feel better, the simple act of preparing wholesome meals can enhance your enjoyment of eating, without adding extra calories. Meals become more like feasts as the "junk" quality of eating is put aside.

Learning about new foods and how to cook them can be a delightfully fun hobby and pastime. Improving your cooking skills and knowledge can give you an interest, talent, and ability for pleasant interaction with other people. You may share with others what you are learning about nutrition and healthy eating. This diet can be really fun and adventurous to follow if you explore new stores, new foods, new tastes, new cookbooks, new restaurants, and new cooking methods.

WHY A WHOLE FOODS DIET BENEFITS HEALTH

You might have noticed that new essential micronutrients are being discovered regularly. Bioflavinoids, phytochemicals, and arabino-galactans are examples. It was less than 100 years ago that vitamins were discovered. In the future, how many more micronutrients will be found?

In the human body, all of the essential nutrients and micronutrients (trace nutrients) are known to work in concert with each other for health. To receive the benefits of the synergy or teamwork that occurs among all nutrients, both trace and essential, by far the best source for obtaining them is the whole foods in which they are found naturally. In those whole foods, the nutrients exist in the exact proportions needed for that synergy to occur. Whole foods also contain all those other nutritional substances we have yet to discover and name.

If a food has been refined, part of the food has been removed, making it no longer whole. Generally at that point, only the macronutrients are left: carbohydrates, proteins and fats. In order to metabolize those macronutrients, our bodies are forced to provide from bodily storage all of the micronutrients that have been stripped from the food. Eventually, after eating refined food over an extended period of time, we no longer have enough micronutrients left to provide for metabolism, and the body no longer has access to the functions of those micronutrients. Consequently, the body becomes a little less efficient.

After years of eating refined carbohydrates, so many micronutrients are missing that our bodies become more and more inefficient, and we start experiencing symptoms of a chronic condition. The type of symptoms depends upon our genetic uniqueness, since genetic individuality always determines which part of the bodymind will falter first.

> To summarize: since eating refined foods causes a deficiency in our bodies of essential substances, even if we eat *more* refined foods, we have *less* nutrition available to nurture our bodies.

■ ■ ■

The only place where micronutrients can be found is in whole foods. The basic reason for refining foods has been to prolong their shelf life (No self-respecting fungus or bug will eat them. They know better). Refined foods have a certain appeal to the palate, but refinement destroys a food's nutritional value.

Actually, refined carbohydrates cause more stress to our systems than all the other nutritional stressors combined. Each stress to which we subject ourselves decreases the reserves we have to cope with other stressors. Eventually, from the long-term or chronic stress of eating a poor diet, our reserves become depleted, increasing our susceptibility to disease.

■■■ WALT: The reason humans survive eating refined foods is that we are the most complex organisms on the planet. We may not die from eating refined foods, however we do become chronically ill and end up paying the medical system a lot of money just to treat the symptoms of our "incurable conditions." Since the standard American diet is now about 75% refined foods (and this percentage is increasing every year),[2] is it any wonder that the current medical establishment makes so much money?

Please note that the National Research Council's recommended daily allowance of refined carbohydrates is *zero*.[3] The fact that any refined carbohydrate in the diet reduces health has been known by the government since it was first studied—more than 100 years ago.[4]

In the United States, where refined foods are so prevalent, eliminating refined carbohydrates from the diet is a very correctable cause of chronic poor health. In my practice, I have regularly seen wonderful health improvements occur in patients when they started eating whole foods. You may be amazed at how much refined carbohydrates decrease your health and quality of life; this is something you can only know after you have lived without them for a while. I hope you will discover for yourself how your quality of life can be extraordinarily improved by eating whole, nutritious foods. ■■■

The Krebs Cycle

To understand the importance of eating the micronutrients that are missing from refined carbohydrates and why eating whole foods is so healing, first it is helpful to know a little bit about the Krebs cycle. In the wondrous, complex system that is our body, the Krebs cycle is a series of chemical reactions that take place within almost every cell. The Krebs cycle produces and provides the energy for you to live and be active. Cells produce energy for every function of the body by means of the Krebs cycle, and it is vital that this metabolic process functions well.

The Krebs cycle requires nearly 100 different minerals, vitamins, enzymes (made up of trace nutrients), and catalysts to perfectly accomplish the production of energy (ATP) from carbohydrates. But every time the bodymind runs out of one of those nutrients, the process of creating energy

(ATP) becomes a little less efficient. After a lifetime of eating refined carbohydrates, most of these trace necessities are absent, and the cycle is nearly nonfunctional.

■■■ WALT: Impairment of the Krebs cycle is, in part, how disease or illness happens. When the cycle loses its function or becomes impaired in a particular part of the body, symptoms are expressed in that body part or in a related part. Which symptoms manifest depend upon genetic uniqueness and upon what body system is the closest to the edge of its symptomatic cliff. There are different levels of impairment of the Krebs cycle. There is also probably a different symptomatic reaction for each tissue in the body, although the Krebs cycle is the same for all. We could give many examples of what kinds of symptoms manifest due to an impaired Krebs cycle. Here are just a few: when and where the Krebs cycle is not working correctly in the brain, a person would experience symptoms like poor concentration, heightened emotional reactions, or what is commonly considered mental illness. In the muscles, an impaired Krebs cycle might show up as fibromyalgia; in the liver, detoxification processes might be impaired; in the lymph tissue, immunity breaks down; with the skin, infections, eczema, or psoriasis occur.

The Krebs cycle is just one of the many chemical reactions (such as lipolysis, protein synthesis, immune globulin production, and hormone production) occurring in a person's metabolism that is dependent upon good nutrition. To improve your nutrition, the PWFD is a good place to start because it provides the micronutrients needed for the Krebs cycle. ■■■

Refined Carbohydrates—Addiction or Allergy?

In addition to Krebs cycle problems, refined carbohydrates can cause other dysfunctions in the body. We would like to point out one health problem that becomes apparent to many people upon following the Whole Foods Diet perfectly: they discover, with amazement, that they have an addiction to refined carbohydrates and/or an immune reaction from eating them. This is revealed by physical reactions that occur when they discontinue eating the refined foods.

Addiction? When starting on the PWFD and stopping the consumption of refined carbohydrates, a person may experience symptoms of withdrawal and cravings, usually for an average of three and a half days. The withdrawal response is similar to discontinuing the use of any addictive substance such as tobacco, drugs, or alcohol. Addiction is defined medically as occurring "when withdrawal of a substance causes symptoms." Thus, the withdrawal symptoms that occur when stopping consumption of refined carbohydrates provide evidence that some kind of addiction has been occurring. The mechanism causing addiction is still not well understood. However, it is known that certain genetic hormonal patterns make an individual more or less susceptible to addictions of any type. Typical withdrawal symptoms are described on page 101.

Allergy/Immune response? In addition to the addictive response, another phenomenon may be observed when one stops eating refined carbohydrates. A very basic immunological mechanism may be noticed that is similar to an allergic (hypersensitivity) reaction.[5] This is how it appears: after stopping consumption of refined foods, if a person then eats some refined carbohydrates during the next six months, an immune response will often be restimulated.

Many people who eat a lot of refined carbohydrates have an allergic response every time they eat refined foods, but are unaware that they even have this response. Since their consumption is so frequent, the reaction is constant, and they have lost the ability to feel their bodily response. The body becomes numb to the feeling, but it is still happening even if they are unaware of it. Your body is by far the most sensitive laboratory ever developed. You just have to get it clear enough of refined carbohydrates to hear the message.

Most immune (hypersensitivity or allergic) responses disappear, if not restimulated, after about six months. Remember the tetanus booster shots you were given when young? The booster is given within six months after the first shot to restimulate the immune system memory. Similarly, eating any refined carbohydrates within six months of starting the PWFD will restimulate the immune trigger for refined carbohydrates.

Some experience the immune system restimulation as a symptomatic reaction (described on page 101–102). We do not know exactly why the symptomatic reaction can become so intense from about a week to a few months after the bodymind is totally free of refined carbohydrates. However, it is a consistent observation made during decades of clinical practice working with the PWFD.

■ ■ ■

One or both of these two health factors, apparent addiction and apparent immune response, may be noticed when starting the PWFD. Since the symptoms of each are so similar, it is unclear whether two different mechanisms occur or if it is just one.[6] Even though we don't know all the answers, we do know that reactions occur for many people. The point is, whatever mechanism is at work, the Perfect Whole Foods Diet ends it and thus can be wonderful for helping your health. After six months, most people's health will likely have improved considerably and reactions are unlikely to occur.

HOW TO START THE PERFECT WHOLE FOODS DIET

Now that you know some of the superb health and other benefits of eating whole foods, we will focus on starting and following the Perfect Whole Foods Diet.

We recommend that people seeking health improvement begin with the Perfect Diet rather than the Liberal. After six months or longer, after they are feeling better, they can switch to the liberal diet. The PWFD and the Liberal Whole Foods Diet are compared in this chart. Information about how to liberalize the Perfect Diet is described on pages 111–112.

COMPARING THE PERFECT AND LIBERAL WHOLE FOODS DIETS

	Perfect Whole Foods Diet	Liberal Whole Foods Diet
Foods	Totally eliminates *all* refined carbohydrates, *all* alcohol, *all* caffeine, and for some people, fruit.	The same as the perfect diet, but allows occasional small quantities of refined foods.
Benefits	Brings the fastest improvements to your health. For those wanting to cure a chronic condition and are willing to put forth some effort to do so. Expect dramatic results in your health. No risk of triggering responses if you are perfect with the diet.	Your health should still improve, but over a longer period of time. You will run the risk of experiencing triggering responses for a long time.
Success Rate	A much higher percentage of people succeed. Eliminating the addiction to refined carbohydrates quickly and totally brings fast results.	Most people drop out if they start with a liberal diet. The longer it takes for benefits to appear, and if triggering responses appear, people tend to give up and say this nutrition plan is too hard.

What Is a Whole Food?

What's the difference between whole and refined food? Here are some examples. An unpeeled wheat grain is whole, (i.e., whole wheat), while refined wheat (white flour) has had the peeling and germ removed. Brown rice is whole, but not white rice. An unpeeled potato is whole and a peeled potato refined. Most of the essential nutrients in a potato are in the peel, and nearly all the calories are in the white stuff inside. Basically, a peeled potato has had its micronutrients removed and so it is refined. People throw away the peel at their peril! This distribution and concentration of nutrients in the peel or skin is, however, not true of citrus and vegetables that have very hard skins. Therefore, for example, you don't need to eat the peels of oranges or spaghetti squash.

What is a Typical "Perfect" Menu?

■■■ JAN: The menu will differ for each person, since dietary needs are individual. However, just to give you an idea how delicious the PWFD can be, here are some of the meals that I enjoy.

This morning for breakfast I ate oatmeal cooked with chopped pecans in a bowl with milk, topped with chopped sweet potato (or sliced fruit), sprinkled with cinnamon and a little stevia (a natural sweetener). I also ate a few slices of bacon (an additive-free type called side pork), lightly salted, and I had a half grapefruit on the side.

For lunch I had fresh grilled salmon, tossed salad with oil and vinegar dressing, stir-fried asparagus with garlic, and steamed wild and brown rice blend. I had a few raw cashews for dessert. Yum!

For dinner I ate a lamb steak, a baked potato (with skin on) topped with olive oil, mineral salt, and fresh ground pepper, and stir-fried red cabbage with balsamic vinegar and caraway seeds. It was delicious.

Last night for dinner I savored a pan-fried pork chop with Italian seasonings, steamed broccoli, and a really delicious, expensive but healthy whole-grain spelt bread with a little olive oil on top (instead of butter). Then I had a few macadamia nuts for dessert.

Another favorite meal consists of brown rice spaghetti, tomato sauce with ground beef and mushrooms, a vegetable, and a salad.

Everybody eats differently, so the PWFD can be adapted to meet your tastes, preferences, and habits. These are just the types of meals I especially enjoy.

Here are a few more: pork and sauerkraut with potatoes and carrots; tofu and vegetable stir-fry with brown rice; baked chicken breast with fresh green beans and quinoa-olive salad (quinoa is a grain substitute); split pea soup, chili, or lentil stew with a sandwich made from whole grain bread, turkey, lettuce, and tomato; curried meat and vegetables with brown rice; beef, pork, or turkey burgers with chips and pickles; Brazilian black beans and brown rice with a salad. There are so many delicious things to eat. Ummm, now I'm getting hungry. Later in this chapter, you'll find suggestions for delicious whole foods snacks.

This list is just to give you an idea of the kind of menus you can create. You can be creative and prepare foods you enjoy eating. The food on this diet *can* be very enticing. People who quit eating refined carbohydrates generally find that they can eat very well, and the only real sacrifice made is their former poor health. ■■■

Who Can Benefit from the PWFD?

Would you benefit? If you are even looking for a dietary approach to feeling better, you may assume that you might benefit from a two-week trial of the PWFD. In any case, we have seen the Perfect Whole Foods Diet help nearly everyone who follows it. Moreover, nearly 100% of them should see significant benefits in just two weeks. Even many people who feel pretty good are totally amazed at how much better they feel after starting this diet.

Please note one situation in which the PWFD can be a risk. If you are diabetic, you are advised to be under a doctor's supervision while following this nutrition plan. Diabetics taking insulin or oral hypoglycemics may find that their diabetic condition improves so rapidly that they will most likely have to dramatically reduce their dosage (frequently even to the point of stopping completely).

However, other special populations, such as children, older people, people who are constantly physically active (such as athletes), and pregnant women need have no concerns about following a Perfect Whole Foods Diet.

What to Eat and What Not to Eat

Below is a basic summary of the PWFD, both foods allowed and foods disallowed. Typical foods to eat on the Perfect Whole Foods diet include all kinds of vegetables, whole grains, beans, nuts and seeds, fruit, and eggs; meats, poultry, dairy products and some fats/oils; and select condiments and seasonings. Any food that is whole is generally allowed.

Typical Foods to Eat on the Perfect Whole Foods Diet

Vegetables: all kinds of fresh or frozen, raw or cooked vegetables (like broccoli, carrots, celery, mushrooms, parsley, spinach, tomatoes, lettuce, cauliflower, and potatoes (that includes the skins)

Whole grains: brown rice, rolled oats, oat bran, millet, hulled barley, popcorn, whole corn grits, whole corn or whole cornmeal, whole wheat flour, and unsweetened 100% whole grain bread and crackers

Beans: dried beans and peas (like pintos, navy beans, split peas, lentils, black beans, tofu, and tempeh)

Nuts and seeds: natural peanut butter, almond butter, cashew butter, tahini, raw or plain roasted nuts and seeds like almonds, walnuts, pecans, pumpkin seeds, sesame seeds, and sunflower seeds

Beverages: spring water, peppermint tea, chamomile tea, ginger tea, herbal teas without additives (but not decaffeinated teas)

Meat, fish, and poultry: unbreaded fish, canned tuna in spring water, unbreaded and skinned chicken, turkey, beef, lamb, and buffalo

Dairy products: plain yogurt, milk, natural cheese, and dry milk

Eggs: farm eggs

Fats: unrefined oils and butter

Condiments and seasonings: fresh and dried herbs and spices, apple cider vinegar, mineral or unrefined sea salt, stevia, unsweetened canned tomato products, carob powder, baking yeast, and baking soda for leavening (if made without starches)

Foods Not to Eat on the Perfect Whole Foods Diet

All sugars: including honey, syrup, molasses, corn syrup, sorbitol, and mannitol. Any word that ends with −ose is a sugar: sucrose, dextrose, lactose, fructose, etc. Also, eliminate any sweetener added to foods (occasional use of saccharine may be okay, and stevia is fine). Some people may even have to avoid fruit for a few weeks, months, or longer because of its high sugar content. Some people will be able to eat whole fruit, fresh or frozen, without added sugar.

Foods that have parts omitted (and are not whole)—for example:

- refined grains, such as white flour (eliminate any flour that doesn't specify 100% whole grain), white rice (brown rice is okay), refined cornmeal (whole grain cornmeal is okay), etc.
- peeled vegetables, such as potatoes, carrots, cucumbers, tomatoes, etc. (i.e., whole potatoes are okay if the skin is eaten; the smaller the potato, the better).
- Any kind of starch added to foods, such as cornstarch, potato starch, etc.

Caffeine: *completely* eliminate caffeine. Discontinue even decaffeinated coffee and tea, because they are not totally caffeine-free. Caffeine is a contributing cause to the addiction, because one of its effects is releasing very significant amounts of pure sugar (glycogen, which is two linked glucose molecules) from the liver into the blood without any of the trace nutrients needed for metabolizing it. This counteracts the diet.

All alcoholic beverages: and all ingredients ending in −ol such as sorbitol, alcohol, etc.) and any use of nicotine. Alcohol is one of the most refined carbohydrates and will cause an immune system triggering response to occur. Nicotine will cause an elevation of blood sugar, which also tends to defeat the purpose of the diet.

To avoid eating excluded foods, read every food package label (including the label of any nutritional supplement, vitamins, etc., that you take). As an example of how sugar is found everywhere in packaged foods, note that even many brands of common table salt now have sugar added to them.

Even eating a *trace* of refined carbohydrates will defeat the purpose of this diet. A trace of refined carbohydrates may cause the immune system triggering response that we described earlier in this chapter.

An additional resource

To learn the specifics of following the PWFD and adapting this nutrition plan to fit your own dietary needs, we would like to refer you to a book written about this special diet called *The Healing Power of Whole Foods,* by Beth Loiselle, R.D. You may buy it or borrow it from a library. Your health care practitioner may also have a copy to loan or sell to you. This book is the best reference we know of to tell the difference between whole foods and refined foods, along with the specifics and details of the PWFD. It is much easier to be perfect on the diet with Beth's book than without it.

Until you can obtain a copy, there is a ready reference adapted from Loiselle's book in Appendix B: Quick References for the Perfect Whole Foods Diet. The reference lets you know what foods are allowed and what to look for on the labels of the products you buy.

Key Resource:
The Healing Power of Whole Foods

by Beth Loiselle, R.D.

Loiselle's easy-to-understand and inspirational book is an invaluable resource for those wanting to learn every aspect of eating and healing through whole foods. It contains information about the PWFD, the Liberal WFD, and adapting your nutrition plan to address candida, food allergies/sensitivities, digestive problems, and weight loss. It also has references for determining if specific foods, additives, and brand name products are appropriate for the PWFD. The book is full of delicious recipes and has a foreword by Walt Stoll, M.D. (Healthways Nutrition, 1993). Order from Healthways Nutrition, 93 Summertree Drive, Nicholasville, Kentucky 40356-9190, (859) 223-2270 or (800) 870-5378, or online at *www.wholefoodsforlife.com*. It is also available through Amazon. com and major booksellers.

■■■ WALT: People wonder if other books about whole foods would work just as well. I would like to explain why I recommend this particular book. I have had many years of clinical practice promoting the PWFD, and at the beginning, patients came back complaining that they felt worse after starting the PWFD. Even if I explained the concept of immune reactions, they were unable to follow the diet successfully without using this book as a resource. So I finally had to recommend that no one even try the diet without *The Healing Power of Whole Foods.*

Beth Loiselle is a former patient of mine. She is a registered dietitian. When she came to me, she was eating what her formal education trained her to believe was a good diet, but she had many symptoms. She was quite surprised to discover that her extreme fatigue was not due to having two young children, but rather caused by what she had been eating. Through our experience together, she became exuberantly healthy and then proceeded to write her book.

Her book is the best I have yet seen. The difference between Beth's book and all other books about whole foods is that hers includes the exact information needed to break a refined carbohydrate addiction. Other books on the topic do not teach the perfect diet and do not have this information. Beth's book will guide you to follow the diet perfectly and avoid exacerbations of your symptoms. ■■■

Where to Purchase Whole Foods

Health food stores carry a wide variety of whole foods. Some communities also have good natural food co-ops. Regular grocery stores are increasing their shelf space for whole foods or may special-order items for you. Whole foods may also be mail-ordered from some health food stores. Search the Internet to locate some.

Several of these options have not yet reached many small towns, but it certainly is much easier today than it was 20 years ago. Customer requests make a difference in what items the stores will carry, so ask your store manager to order or carry the whole foods products you wish to purchase or to include a natural or whole foods section in your local store.

WHOLE FOODS DIET Q & A

Q: How can I know if a food is whole?

A: One simple guideline to help you understand the concept is to consider whether that food will grow. Whole foods will grow and refined foods will not. Try, for example, placing both white rice and brown rice in separate sprouting containers and watering them. The white rice will not grow, but the brown rice will, so you know the brown rice is whole. Some whole foods do have parts that you remove, but it does not affect the integrity of that food. An example is an egg. You eat the inside of the egg and throw away the shell. Following our guideline of whether something will grow: an eggshell is not part of what grows into a baby chick, so if you remove it you are not making the food less whole. Similarly, you throw away the nutshell when you eat a nut. A growing nut sprouts through the shell, but does not need the shell to grow. This is just a general guideline, to help you understand. If in doubt, consult Appendix B.

Q: Is pasta a refined food? Can it be eaten on the diet? Can we eat processed foods that are whole foods on the PWFD?
A: You may eat any prepared or processed food you wish, as long as it is made of all whole foods and is not refined. If you read the ingredients on the labels of processed foods, you will know which ones contain all whole foods. Read every label, every time, because sometimes ingredients or recipes change. Refined carbohydrates are found in almost everything, even products from the health food store, although a few "safe" brands exist. Most ordinary grocery-store pastas are not whole foods. However, most health food stores sell at least some whole grain pastas.

Q: Why are vinegar, oils, nut milks, dairy (cheese, yogurt), cuts of meat, and tofu included in the PWFD? They do not seem like whole foods. Vinegar is made from fruit juice; oils, tofu and nut milks throw away the pulp; cheese and yogurt aren't made from whole milk; and certainly I cannot eat a whole cow. Would removal of the outer layer of an onion make it a refined food?
A: Refined carbohydrates are really the main foods that need to be avoided, and none of the foods you mention have refined carbohydrates in them. Oils and proteins are not carbohydrates. Onion skins are just dried layers of the onion, and each layer is whole within itself.

Whole milk has lactose in it (remember –ose words indicate the presence of sugar), but contains enough protein and fat, in relationship to the lactose, that it is much more slowly absorbed, and has sufficient micronutrients to run the lactose through the Krebs cycle. This ratio of nutrients prevents any reaction from occurring in nearly all people (unless they are lactose intolerant or have a food hypersensitivity to dairy).

Evaluation of whether a food can be eaten on the diet is related to the nutritional ratio within that food. Yet, what a person can ultimately eat depends upon the condition of his or her Krebs cycle. People without Krebs cycle problems or whose health condition allows them to follow a liberal diet may do all right just following the general guidelines given in this book.

For those wishing to overcome severe chronic health problems or Krebs cycle problems, who need to be absolutely certain whether a food is allowed on the PWFD, consult the lists in Appendix B. We also recommend you read

The Healing Power of Whole Foods. If you have a doubt about a food, it is best to avoid that food—especially during the two-week trial period.

Q: Does the food eaten on this diet have to be organic?

A: The concept and application of the Whole Foods Diet works differently from avoiding pesticide residue, so eating organic food is not the primary concern. Avoiding refined carbohydrates is the most important principle.

However, organic food has a higher nutritional content, so it's more nutritious for you if you can eat organic whole food. We recommend you eat it as much as you are able according to local availability and cost, but eating organic is not required to be successful on the Whole Foods Diet.

Q: Is the PWFD expensive to follow?

A: Some people find buying whole foods to be more expensive and others find it less expensive. Water costs a lot less than soda pop, for example. You pay less for unprepared foods than prepared ones. Grains, beans, spices, etc., are the most dramatic examples of how doing your own cooking costs much less. Until you learn what to do in terms of shopping and cooking, however, you will probably spend more for whole foods than you did for refined foods. Keep learning, and you will become more and more efficient and economical in following this nutrition plan.

■■■ WALT: I continued to learn about food selection, preparation, and cooking while I followed the diet, and soon I found my grocery bill was less than when I just ate typical meals. Within a year, my grocery bill was half what it had been the year before. Then I read a telling statistic: for every extra penny one spends for wholesome food, one saves a dollar in medical costs and lost wages (the smallest cost of illness). ■■■

■■■ JAN: Most of my expense when starting the diet came from restocking my kitchen with the new whole foods. With time, I spent less money as I became a better cook and made more meals from scratch. Eating at home more also meant spending less in restaurants.

However, not long after starting the PWFD, I made a conscious decision to increase my food budget and buy higher quality ingredients and a wider variety of foods. This decision came after feeling so much better from using the whole foods nutrition plan. I came to understand the importance of having the best nutrition I could possibly afford. I do economize by cutting coupons, timing purchases around sales, etc. ■■■

Q: Is there anything else I can do together with this nutrition plan that will help me get better faster?

A: Yes. Below we describe two food products that are typically refined or altered, and their whole food counterparts. Switching to these products will be of assistance to your health.

PWFD TIP #1

Nutritional Supplements: Most multi-vitamins are not made from whole foods and most likely lack micronutrients. To boost your recovery after years of eating refined carbohydrates and to help restore missing micronutrients, take concentrated whole food supplements for a few months. Select a supplement that is made from a wide selection of whole foods. Several brands of whole food supplements are now available on the market (see the Resources). These supplements will help fill in the gaps left by a lifetime of less-careful diet.

Also note that most or many other kinds of nutritional supplements contain starches or sugars, so remember to read their labels. See pages 255–261 of Chapter 7 for further information about nutritional supplements.

Salt: Ordinary table salt (refined salt) is refined to be 99.6% sodium chloride with all the other minerals removed. Some common brands of salt also have sugar added to them. To eat a healthier salt, you can purchase unrefined salt called mineral salt. Mineral or unrefined salt (mined from ancient evaporated seas thousands of feet underground) contains all of the original trace minerals in salt and actually tastes better than refined salt. It is very light tan in color and has little colored flecks in it. Mineral salt can generally be found at health food stores. The negative effects medically reported for salt are mostly (Walt believes all) due to the imbalance caused by eating pure sodium chloride while avoiding all of the trace minerals. Unrefined sea salt is okay as long as it has the little colored flecks in it.

Q: What kind of snacks can I eat on the PWFD?
A: ■■■ JAN: I'm a voracious snacker, so here I have listed a few ideas for you to get started giving up donuts and cream puffs and switching to healthy whole food snacks. This is the "no fruit" version of my snack list since I don't eat fruit. If eating fruit is a possibility for you, then you can surely include eating fresh fruit as a snack, too.

- Whole rye crackers, Triscuits, brown rice cakes, or whole grain bagels with peanut butter, almond butter, cashew butter, sesame tahini, or cheese.
- Popcorn with mineral salt and nutritional yeast.
- Whole grain cereal and milk (or nut, soy, or rice milk).
- Whole corn tortilla chips or whole grain bagel chips with salsa, guacamole, baba ganoush (eggplant dip), or bean dip.
- Raw veggies (zucchini, cucumber and sweet potato rounds, carrot and celery sticks) with homemade hummus (bean dip) or dipped in mineral salt.
- Whole sweet or baked potato. You can also bake yams whole and eat the pulp separately. On the skins, spread butter or oil, salt and pepper (parmesan cheese optional) and broil until crispy.
- Deviled egg halves (be sure to read the label of the mayo or use unsweetened yogurt).
- Chickpeas coated with olive oil and mineral salt, and roasted in the oven at 400 degrees until slightly crunchy.
- Leftovers from breakfast or dinner.
- Turkey hot dogs (remember to read labels).
- Homemade beef, fish, or turkey jerky.
- Canned tuna mixed with chopped green olives (yogurt or mayo optional), whole grain bread.
- Black olives, green olives, pickles (don't forget to read the labels).
- Hot or iced herbal tea.
- Canned smoked oysters, shrimp, or scallops.
- Whole grain pasta salad.
- Homemade ice cream.
- Homemade soft potato chips—slice a whole potato (or a sweet potato) and coat with olive oil, sprinkle with mineral salt, then bake until cooked through.
- Hot beverage using milk (or nut, soy, or rice milk), liquid stevia and roasted carob powder (instead of chocolate) with some alcohol-free vanilla and nutmeg (optional). Substitute pumpkin or apple pie spice for the carob powder for a different taste.
- Pistachios, almonds, cashews, macadamia nuts, sunflower seeds and peanuts. These can be seasoned with Bragg's Liquid Aminos (instead of soy sauce), curry, or cayenne, and roasted.
- Eggplant sliced thinly and dipped in a beaten egg and then in homemade whole grain bread crumbs combined with some herbs

(parmesan cheese optional). Spray with a bit of olive oil and put it in a very hot oven (450°–500° F) until brown and crisp.

Umm—now I'm *really* getting hungry! Enjoy! ■■■

Q: I'm having trouble starting the PWFD. Do you have any suggestions?

A: Most people tell us that they are willing to do anything to get rid of their vexing symptoms. If they knew that hanging from their thumbs for a

TIP #2 Starting the PWFD

- If you have previously eaten a poor diet, really don't know how to cook, and don't feel well either, in the beginning just take it slow. Relax and maintain a positive attitude, and keep learning. Just start and gradually keep adding more whole foods and removing more refined foods from your nutrition plan. In several weeks, you'll get the hang of it and accomplish the changes necessary to follow the perfect diet.

- In your day-timer, schedule "time in the kitchen" for meal planning and preparation. This will be especially true for those who are used to fast foods and take out, but less so for those who usually cook meals.

- View the diet as an adventure in eating, and use it as an opportunity to explore new foods and create new dishes.

- Find an appropriate healthy way to reward yourself for starting the diet, and periodically, for doing well with it.

- Remember that the need to eliminate *all* refined carbohydrates from your diet will not be forever. Take it one day at a time.

- Substitute customary comfort foods with new, interesting, or exotic comfort foods. For example, instead of eating chocolate or candy, try eating macadamia nuts, cashews, fruit, or pistachios. Instead of having coffee, have a blended herbal tea or some warm milk (of any kind) with some spices and stevia. Instead of wine, have an exotic vegetable juice blend.

- Vary your menu so you do not become bored with your food and feel tempted to eat refined carbohydrates. Try previously unexplored produce foods, visit new grocery stores to hunt for items, etc.

- Avoid stressful and social situations during the withdrawal period. There is no sense in putting undue pressure on yourself.

week would do the trick, they would seriously consider it. Being totally free of refined carbohydrates for a two-week trial is considerably easier than that!

■■■ WALT: The only people who I have seen become believers in the PWFD are those who have actually tried it and experienced the truth with their own bodies. Personally, I have seen magnificent changes occur when people have stuck to the PWFD 100%. I hope you choose this program and give your body a chance to find out how good you can feel. It is a matter of making up your mind that you are going to do it, and then figuring out the easiest way to accomplish it. ■■■

Q: After months of denial, I now must admit that I am without doubt addicted to sugar. I know I have to break this sugar addiction. Most people say if you can do without sugar for several days, the cravings subside, but I have not found that to work for me. What can I do?

A: We think the easiest and quickest way to break a sugar, alcohol, or refined carbohydrate addiction is to follow the Perfect Diet and accomplish the change quickly.

The problem with sugar addiction has to do with the missing micronutrients rather than with the actual glucose (simple sugar). Sugar is no different from any other refined carbohydrate, and cravings may be strong, especially during withdrawal. If you have an addiction to sugar, taking in any form of glucose can trigger the addiction/allergic response and keep the cycle of addiction going.

You may simply have to go through a longer withdrawal period than other people (more than three and a half days), and we encourage you to hold fast to your plan to do without sugar until the cravings subside. If this is impossible for you, here are some suggestions from a bulletin board participant on the website (www.askwaltstollmd.com) about how you might cut down gradually on sugar over a short period of time in preparation for what you really need to do—follow the PWFD.

> "I have been addicted to sugar, too, several times in my life. I've also unaddicted myself. One way is to start small. Quit drinking soda pop. Just that one thing—and you know you can do that much—will make a huge difference. So, start thinking about what you can substitute instead of soda pop. You've got to have a substitute! Of course, water would be ideal, but if you can't do that, pick something else: iced tea (even if you put sugar in it), lemonade, watered down fruit juices, SOMETHING else. Don't drink diet drinks either. Once you see that life as you know it is

still worth living, you can make better substitutions. Hey, if all you can do is quit drinking soda pop, you've made a huge and positive change in your diet. From little changes, big things happen. And if soda pop would be too hard to give up, pick something else. Quit eating baked goods, or quit eating cookies. Continue with the rest of your typical diet. Just pick something you can be successful at eliminating. *Just one thing.* From little changes, big things happen. Do not despair. Do the best you can. That's all any of us can do."

Another participant, who was once addicted to sugar, had this to say about ceasing to eat it:

> "The only way for me has been to stay away from anything with even a little sugar. All it takes is one little bite and WHAM! The cravings are back. I try to treat my sugar addiction as an alcoholic would alcohol: total abstinence. I've just accepted that there are some things I cannot handle a little of."

Some people's genetic make-up makes them more susceptible than others to addiction. Sugar addiction is the hardest addiction of them all to break. Alcohol is similar. Alcohol is the most refined carbohydrate (even more refined than sugar), which is one of the reasons that it is so hard to break that addiction.

Q: I've been struggling to quit smoking (or insert your particular habit: stop drinking coffee, stop drinking alcohol, etc.) for 20 years. I really want to improve my health, and I want to eat better. Won't going on the PWFD (except for that one thing that I have struggled with and haven't yet been successful at changing) still help my health anyway?

A: *If* you want to see the dramatic changes in your health promised by the PWFD, then the nicotine, coffee, or alcohol have to go. Some people can continue smoking and still break the addiction to refined carbohydrates, but there is a risk that doing so might not be successful. If your goal is wellness, why risk it?

Q: This diet is too strict. Isn't there any other way to do this?

A: Some friends who read this book while we were writing it felt we are too firm with this diet by stipulating that people follow it perfectly. If the diet does not always work when a person is less than perfect, would you expect us to tell you to do otherwise? We want to ensure your success and your health.

However, people and personalities are different, and since diet is not "one size fits all," you *can* adapt this program to meet your needs. Do what works for you, but also still remember that we aren't making up the need for perfection! We want to be sure that you get where you want to go—to good health. Unfortunately, we—especially Walt—have seen too many people drop out of the program because they failed to get results due to lack of accuracy with the PWFD. This is why we promote perfection with the diet.

If you are making dietary changes haphazardly rather than making a complete break from refined foods, chances are that your bodymind is telling you about it by giving you reactions. Hopefully such uncomfortable feelings will motivate you to achieve perfection on the diet as soon as possible.

As you make improvements in your habits, pat yourself on the back for making whatever positive changes you can make. Do not be harsh with yourself and keep moving forward with your plan. Any way you can move forward in a positive direction will still be good for your health.

Ultimately, continuing to eat foods that harm your health will not be beneficial for you. However, to allow for differences in people's personalities, you can certainly do whatever works for you if it brings you beneficial results.

TIP #3 Take It Slow

People who need to make many big changes to follow the PWFD may find making them all the changes at once to be too challenging. Therefore, if you are making many major changes (for example, if you need to quit smoking, go off caffeine, stop a sugar addiction, *and* change your entire way of eating) to follow this nutritional plan, and you are feeling overwhelmed, slow down. Make one change at a time, in a way that works for you. Go forward with whatever part of the diet you *can* do well until you are able to add more improvements and follow the Perfect Diet. Make your goal to be achieving the Perfect Diet in as short a time as possible.

■■■ WALT: This question brings up the real reason why it is so helpful and necessary to be perfect with eating only whole foods. The human body cannot heal itself if it continues to be aggravated by substances that are toxic to it. Therefore, if you are less than perfect on the PWFD, your healing will not likely happen. You body indicates this by the reactions you will probably experience whenever you eat refined foods. Completely eliminating refined foods from your diet, and not having reactions, is ultimately easier and more effective for reversing chronic symptoms than doing this any other way. We describe these reactions below so you will understand the importance of being so careful with what you eat. ■■■

GETTING CLEAR OF REFINED CARBOHYDRATES

This section describes the common withdrawal/immune system responses that may occur, which were mentioned on pages 84–85. Some people do not experience them at all, but since some people do, we have included this description. The withdrawal symptoms are an indication that an addiction to refined foods is present.

Withdrawal: When you begin following the nutritional guidelines of the PWFD, for a few days you may experience one or more of the following withdrawal symptoms: fatigue, weakness, nervousness, anxiety, trembling, headache, sweating, hunger, dizziness, visual disturbances, cravings, tingling of lips or tongue, chilliness, unsteadiness, drowsiness, flu-like symptoms such as nausea and vomiting, coughing up mucous, runny nose and sore throat, and mental confusion. You may also experience the withdrawal as strong cravings for certain foods.

Some people will have a mild experience, but others may experience a fairly dramatic withdrawal. Withdrawal tends to average three and a half days (for some, it is as short as one day, and for others as long as a week). Having more withdrawal symptoms is generally a signal that you have chronic symptoms that will be improved by following this nutrition plan. Thus if you feel exceptionally poor during the withdrawal, be profoundly grateful, because it means that your efforts will be greatly rewarded just by sticking to the PWFD. Having a withdrawal response proves that you are on the right track.

By going off refined foods totally and completely, you will minimize the withdrawal response. Slowly tapering down your use of refined foods causes the withdrawal to last longer, sometimes for a very long time.

Immune system responses (triggering responses): During the first six months of this nutrition plan, *if you eat any refined food in any quantity,* an allergic or immune system triggering response can occur. The symptoms can differ among individuals, depending upon what part of their body is closest to the edge of their symptomatic cliff. For many people, the symptoms seem like an exacerbation of their usual long-standing health problem, and for others, the symptoms are similar to the withdrawal symptoms listed above.

Most people have to experience the immune system response to actually believe it happens. Here is a description of one patient's experience:

> "I have been on the PWFD for about one and a half to two months now. Yesterday, I had to go to a seminar for work, and they had sandwiches and cookies. I was so hungry because I didn't have food with me, so I indulged. I had one sandwich on pure white bread and four cookies!! Oh, my God—once I ate one cookie I didn't stop myself. I could have, but I didn't want to. The symptoms started shortly after that, with that low headache just above the eyes. Well, I tried walking last night and did it, but felt horrible during and afterwards. I could only make it for 20 minutes. I went home and crashed into bed and slept for 11 hours straight.
>
> This morning I woke up with two huge, swollen bags under my eyes, and I am dizzy, grouchy, and tired. Besides that, my legs are aching like crazy! It's not because I overdid it walking. I have been exercising since February a lot harder than I did last night. I am not touching sugar or refined carbohydrates for a long, long time. By the time I am well, I probably won't want it anyway. I have heard that after you are really over that sugar thing, it tastes terrible anyway. I am glad I did that yesterday. It made me realize what I have been doing to my body for so long."

■■■ WALT: I experienced a similar type of reaction when I was first learning about this. After following the diet perfectly for about three to four months, I was invited to a friend's house for a fancy dinner party. She was a good enough friend that I could say to her, "Now, you know how fanatic I have been about my diet. How can I be sure that there will be no traces of refined carbohydrates in the dinner?" She assured me that she was a student of my work and knew how to do that. So I attended the dinner party. During my entire lifetime, I used to be constantly hungry (24/7) until about a month after starting the perfect diet. But about halfway through the dinner, I started getting hungry again. Then after dinner, I fell asleep in the middle of the living room floor in the midst of all those guests, another trait that had been a lifelong problem until I started the perfect diet. The next morning I had to drag myself out of bed—something else I did not experience since I had been on the perfect diet for about six weeks. So, I called my friend and said, "I know you did your best to be perfect with this meal, but there was something in the meal that was refined."

She insisted that there could not have been. However, when I described what I had experienced (one aspect of which she had witnessed—my falling asleep on her living room floor) she said she would check everything she had done once again. A few hours later she called back, upset. It seems that her husband had come home from work early to help her with the dinner. During the preparation, he ran out of mineral salt. In rummaging for more, he came across some Morton's Iodized Salt in the back of the cupboard. From that point on, that was the salt used. That product contains dextrose (sugar). So far as any of us could determine, that tiny trace of refined carbohydrate was the only refined food in that meal. ■■■

Not all salt contains sugar. Check the label of your salt package to find out exactly what is inside. After you get in the habit of reading every label, you may be surprised to find out what the food manufacturers include in different products and what you've been eating all these years.

Most people have a period of sensitivity during which they experience triggering responses like this. However, it is also important to understand that these are just general principles or guidelines, and everyone is different. Some people don't have reactions at all.

If you are having food reactions after starting the PWFD, look at what you are eating with a magnifying glass, and be sure you are avoiding all refined foods. Consult the guides in Appendix B to make sure you are not eating any disallowed foods (also see the troubleshooting section below). If your diet is not perfect, you may continue to experience triggering responses. Rest assured, if you are doing the diet perfectly, you will not experience withdrawal reactions after the average three and a half days.

Generally the immune system needs to remain clear for six months to stop reacting to triggering substances. Therefore, any time you have a reaction, you must start the six months over again.

The longer you go without triggering the immune response, your bodymind resets itself at a healthier homeodynamic, and then you will be unlikely to get sick or have reactions to traces or even large amounts of refined food. By that time (six months or longer of being totally clear), your system will have enough reserves that you would just feel bad for a few hours or days if you stumbled or had a holiday splurge, and you would do all right as long as you got right back on track with the nutrition plan. The real risk of any splurge is becoming addicted to refined carbohydrates once more, leading to the compulsion to eat refined foods regularly again. If you do become re-addicted, however, at least this time you will know what you need to do to get well.

It is also a good idea to stay with the Perfect Diet for as long as possible. Walt remained flawless for three years at the time he first tried the diet. Also be aware that people who go in and out of a perfect diet may experience withdrawal each time they move to perfection again.

Should I Stop Eating Fruit?

■■■ WALT: In her book, *The Healing Power of Whole Foods,* Beth Loiselle presents eating fruit (fresh or frozen) as all right for the perfect diet. Eating fruit is the only place I differ with Beth about the Perfect Whole Foods Diet. When starting the PWFD, I believe it is prudent for most people to do without fruit during a two-week trial period. Some people (especially those trying to break a refined carbohydrate addiction) may have to avoid fruit for a few weeks or even for six months. A certain percentage would succeed on the diet by eating some fruit, but in my experience, it is not worth the risk. However, if you are following a liberal WFD, a judicious inclusion of fruit is okay.

The problem with eating fruit while following the PWFD is that today's fruit, which is primarily grown for its sweet taste, is basically the same as sugar. Remember, fruit has fructose (fruit sugar) in it. When a person already has a problem metabolizing refined carbohydrates, currently available fruit (even the very best and most organic fruit) affects the body like pure sugar does. This tendency for fruit to cause trouble is especially true for those with candida overgrowth and those whose Krebs cycles are impaired. It is the ratio of calories (short-chain carbohydrates) to the micronutrients in fruit that impairs the already damaged Krebs cycle and continues the symptoms a person experiences.[7]

Everyone who eats sugar is damaged by doing so, because like all other refined carbohydrates, sugar depletes the body's micronutrients, causing the Krebs cycle function to decline. Some people have more reserves of micronutrients (or more efficient genes) than others, and this is the only reason some people can eat fruit and others cannot. If anything is worse than sugar for damaging the Krebs cycle, it is alcohol, because alcohol is the most refined carbohydrate that exists.

The Krebs cycle is so important that a few people who have very damaged Krebs cycles will not even be able to eat starchy vegetables like potatoes without experiencing reactions. These individuals have to start repairing their Krebs cycles by eating very small meals every half hour. I think that all

TIP #4 Going Off Fruit, Caffeine, and Nicotine

Fruit: Choosing the beginning of autumn to make this change may be easier than other times of the year. In autumn, there are still many fresh fruits on the market, but the most delicious fruit is less readily available, so there is less temptation.

Caffeine: To avoid withdrawal headaches, decrease consumption slowly rather than stop suddenly. For the first week, reduce your consumption of caffeine by half. For the second week, reduce it by half again. Then discontinue caffeine altogether for the third week. Also if you do end up with a caffeine-withdrawal headache despite tapering off gradually, you can drink a thimble-full of coffee to abate that response. Don't forget that decaffeinated products still contain traces of caffeine.

Nicotine: Starting aerobic exercise may make this process easier. Also see the Resources section for a book to help with breaking a nicotine addiction.

Some people struggling to quit sugar, caffeine, and alcohol may find that if they normally eat a lot of red meat, shellfish, hard cheese, and eggs, switching to white fish and chicken may help dampen their cravings.

high-carbohydrate foods are a little risky for such individuals because they will most likely have a reaction to eating those foods.

After starting the PWFD, some of my patients had withdrawal symptoms that persisted much longer than two weeks, so they believed that the diet was not working. The most common thing that solved the problem of continued symptoms was totally eliminating fruit. However, a few individuals had trouble understanding how the avoidance of fruit applied to a whole foods diet, since they saw fresh fruit as a whole food. I told them fruit is certainly whole if it is not refined, but the amount of fruit sugar in it creates the same effect as if it were a refined food. ■■■

We recommend that you test eating no fruit on your own body to see how you respond. Go on the PWFD for two weeks without fruit, then eat a piece of fruit, and see if it triggers a response. If no negative symptoms occur (such as those listed as being a withdrawal response on page 101, or your usual symptoms), you could probably stand to eat some fruit while you follow the PWFD. If you do have a reaction to the fruit, it is a good idea to stay away from it. The longer you go without fruit, the more likely you will eventually be able to have small amounts of fruit without risking your progress. Several months later, after you are feeling great, you can try some fruit. If you experience symptoms, you will understand that it is not a good idea for you to eat fruit, and then you also will have to restart the six months needed to clear the immune system all over again.

Each person must decide for himself or herself if fruit can be tolerated or not. People just have to know that if they eat fruit, they may not get rid of the withdrawal/immune system responses.

THE PWFD IN DAILY LIFE

Social Situations—Will My Friends and Family Understand?

When you are following the PWFD, share the process with your friends. You might have to spend some time teaching your friends why you are following this nutrition plan and how it works. They may try to influence you in your eating choices. Some will not understand why you're being so strict, even if you explain it to them. They might not intentionally try to get you off your diet, but they won't understand that it is important. Others will really try to get you to go off. Be firm with them, but polite, about your diet. It is better to hurt their feelings rather than hurt yourself by eating something that will cause a reaction and set you back. This is a good test to find out who your real friends are. Those who care about you will help, and those who do not, you may be better off without.

If you have to be a bit of a hermit for six months to do what you must do to take care of yourself, be a hermit. You won't need to be on the PWFD forever. One participant on the 3LS found a creative solution for social situations:

> "I had a hard time saying no to my friends who wanted to go out to eat at restaurants not offering whole foods, and I suffered withdrawal symptoms after each outing. Still wanting to be with my friends AND continue my journey to wellness, I decided to start packing my own food whenever I got together with my friends. Even though they teased me a bit, my friends were pretty supportive—especially when I shared my food with them."

Q: If I go on the PWFD, then I'll be eating differently from my family, and cooking two different menus for each meal sounds like too much work. What can I do?

A: Your own health is as important for yourself as it is for the sake of your family, and remember, this will most likely only be for six months. Here are some suggestions for managing this type of situation:

PATIENT A: "I've been on the PWFD for almost four weeks. I live with my boyfriend, who eats terribly. Regarding cooking for my boyfriend: half the time my attitude is this—if he doesn't like it, he can always make himself something else to eat. Not that I am mean about it, but when I do the shopping, I will always ask my boyfriend if there is anything specific he would like to make for himself in the coming week. So I buy him what he wants, and one night a week, he makes his own dinner and I make my own dinner.

"Then, for one or two nights he usually heats up a frozen dinner for himself. He's really happiest when I let him eat 'like a bachelor.' Then, the rest of the time he eats what I make for myself. I usually just wind up making one thing different for him, and one thing different for me. This does take a little more time, but it's not too bad. This usually works pretty well (sharing an entrée, one side-dish, and making another side-dish separately for each of us, or just making one entrée we both will eat).

"Often, my boyfriend is more than happy to help out with some of the prep work (especially if I'm making him a salad he likes instead of trying to get him to eat broccoli). And he's been really good about cleaning up the kitchen on many nights. I think most partners would be generally supportive of anyone who undertakes this. Especially when they see what kind of positive results a whole foods diet can yield."

PATIENT B: "I do the grocery shopping, I do the cooking, therefore it wasn't just my diet that changed, everyone else went along for the ride. Healthful eating is not just for the already unhealthy, and two of the other three members of my family understand and accept that, one being my husband who is actually glad and happy with all the changes. I was not about to buy two sets of groceries or cook two sets of meals, nor do I think anyone else should have to either. The dietary changes upset the twelve-year old. He was most upset at losing sweets, especially pop. My husband had a talk with him about how living in our home means he accepts our rules and our healthy diet. When the kids are not around us, I am sure they get that junk food, when they visit their mom, go to other relatives' homes, and friends' homes, and I know my husband will occasionally, while on the job, buy chips or a pop. So seeing how many breaks from a healthy diet the rest of my family gets, I have no problems laying down the law and serving a liberal whole foods diet for everyone at every at-home eating event."

Also, if your little ones balk, you can put healthy food on the table and when the mealtime is done, take it away. Don't give them any snacks. There has never been a child damaged by a parent only offering healthy foods and letting the child get hungry enough to eat them. This is more of an issue about control rather than a food issue. After all, we are the adults whose responsibility it is to make good choices for our children.

Meal Preparation

Here are some suggestions from a patient about saving time in the kitchen while on the PWFD:

"When I first started the PWFD, I found preparation was time consuming. So I started buying a lot of those single cup or 2-cup pyrex single-serving glass containers (with the plastic lids) and freezing stuff. For example, I will freeze lots of bowls of soup, or rice and beans, etc. I also sometimes make extra (two or three servings extra) meat or whatever entrée I cook and then refrigerate them and take them to work over the next few days. Even things like separating all of my nuts or carrots out into ziplock baggies at the beginning of the week can save on time. For any food that saves well (basically anything except for steamed veggies) I try to always make extra and freeze or refrigerate the rest. These simple things really cut down on the amount of time I spend in the kitchen."

■■■ JAN: Appliances help tremendously when following the PWFD. I use an electric steamer (great for cooking grains, veggies, and reheating food), small electric grill (for fast grilled meat and veggies), blender (makes great nut milks), juicer, toaster oven (for quick and easy baking), a small and large crockpot (for beans, soups, and stews), a food dehydrator (makes great snacks), a bread machine, and an "airpot" (an Oriental appliance for heating hot water for herbal teas). My freezer keeps nuts fresh and holds a wide variety of foods, saving trips to the store. Stocking up when meat is on sale saves money, too.

Cooking several meals at once with the help of many appliances is a very efficient use of time. I make a large quantity of food and put what I don't eat in containers to freeze for lunch on days when mornings are too rushed for preparing food. With the help of my appliances, amazingly I spend less time cooking than before I started the Perfect Diet, and I always have nutritious food to eat. *The Healing Power of Whole Foods* provides additional tips for using appliances to save time in the kitchen. ■■■

Eating Out, Restaurants, and Travel

When eating away from home, one option is to take your own food with you. Here are some other suggestions from patients:

PATIENT A: "I bring my food back and forth to work in Tupperware, used deli containers, 'zip'-lock bags (for carrot/celery sticks) and used grocery bags. It works great. Our grocery stores here have an aisle with all sorts of plastic, sealable containers—all shapes and sizes. Now they even have disposable ones. We have a microwave at work (you could use a toaster oven, I suppose) if I want to heat things up. I don't like to use it too much, and frankly most of the time, I don't mind eating food room temperature or cold."

PATIENT B: "One day, at a conference, I spied one who could only have been a Virgo. He put an ordinary-looking polished square boxy type briefcase flat down on a chair and opened up the top. Well, he took out napkin, knife, fork; all needed utensils from the lid. I swear there was a full three-course meal packed in there, exquisitely. No cooking, of course, as we were in a conference room. But he was totally in control of his food and his body."

It is possible to eat in most restaurants while following the PWFD, although you must be very selective about what you order as many ingredients are not whole. Here are some suggestions from the bulletin board participants for eating out in restaurants:

- "Just order Perrier water and a vegetable plate."

- "Just tell the server that you have multiple food allergies and can't eat anything on the menu. Ask if the cook would prepare a special plate for you and then tell the server exactly what you would like to eat. Be sure to give a nice tip."

- "Many Asian restaurants will serve steamed brown rice and steamed vegetables as separate dishes."

- "My daughter suggests Indian restaurants."

- "Most restaurants offer an acceptable or allowed 'catch of the day.'"

- "Health food restaurants or health food grocery stores often have deli counters with food ready to go (ingredients labeled on each dish)."

- "I took to just saying I had a lot of food allergies when I was dining out—rather than trying to explain my 'eccentric' dieting ideas. I found people sort of felt bad that I couldn't eat wheat or something and would give me more spinach or more rice or whatever."

- "Often the trendy burger and giant salad places are off limits because everything they serve is infused with refined carbohydrates. Salad bars are usually OK, but skip all the prepared salads—just go with the identifiable greens and veggies, and pass on all the dressings. Use plain vinegar and oil as a dressing, if they have it. Ask for no croutons, since they are made with white flour and often seasoned with salt/herb mixes that contain starches, and of course, skip the bacon."

- "Skip anything with a sauce, gravy, seasoning, or breading. Plain meat is usually safe, although prime rib can be injected with broth and seasonings (with starches or sugars). If you order beef/steak, chicken, or fish, ask for it grilled with no seasonings—no seasoned salt, steak sauce, etc. Make sure it isn't marinated which usually means sugar or honey. If you are in a fancy restaurant, ask for it to be seasoned with fresh herbs and lemon on the side (if you eat fruit). Ask for a plain baked potato with real butter on the side, and steamed or sauteed veggies with no seasoning. Always pass on soup—it could be thickened with starch or white flour. If there are no entrees on the menu that look safe, ask for a plain salad to start and for your entree, just a baked potato and steamed or sauteed vegetables. Sometimes some appetizers look OK—ask for those to be served as your entree."

Staying on the PWFD while traveling may take some planning. Here are some suggestions from patients for making trips:

- "For out-of-state type traveling ... just scope out the hotel you're staying in and ask them about special diets. I just learned to speak up and ask for what I wanted. I usually travel with my own food or find a local grocery store, but have found restaurants usually prepare food the way you ask them to—except maybe McDonald's. I always take my own food on the airplane."

- "I've been a traveler for years. It's not easy eating well on the road, but it can be done. An electric wok is indispensable. You can cook everything in it! It's easy to clean (in the bathtub). Getting the food is tough! Keeping it fresh is a challenge! I eat nuts, nut butters, and rice cakes for emergencies. Many health food stores have delis and salad bars. I've found if I just get greens (organic), it's about a buck and a half. That's cheap! You can get a backpacker's stove and head for the town park (weather permitting). Also you can grill food or use charcoal at city parks, state parks, picnic areas, and the like."

- "When I went to Mexico, I was able to get salads, fruit, and rice with chicken."

- "Here are some relatively easy ways to prepare food in a hotel room: a rice/vegetable steamer will cook both. Bring herbs and spices! You will go nuts without variation in flavor."

- "I purchased a plastic pot with a handle, spout and a lid called the Rival Hotpot Express. It is an electric pot with a heat control dial marked from warm to boil. It boils water really fast. To reheat veggies and rice, etc., I put a little water in the bottom, add the food and let it heat. For meat, I boil some water and add the plastic package of frozen meat and cook a couple of minutes. I have even boiled pasta in it for my family. The little Hotpot Express really heats quickly, so don't leave the room for long. The plastic baggie doesn't fall apart in the boiling water, and I even use the cheapie ones. I originally bought the thing for traveling to boil water for herb tea, but now I use it all the time to reheat stuff since I decided not to use the microwave anymore. One thing I discovered: always unplug it after use because it still stays warm even with the dial turned down."

THE LIBERAL WHOLE FOODS DIET

When you have reached the point of feeling much better from the PWFD, and you have gone six months or longer without triggering, you can think about liberalizing the diet and eating small amounts of refined foods on a regular basis. When your system is working better, it can tolerate a portion of your diet being refined, but how much can be tolerated is different for each person.

To change to a liberal diet: After you have gone six months without reaction to traces of refined carbohydrates, test yourself by eating some refined carbohydrates. Make sure the amounts are still small at the beginning when you are doing this testing. Be careful about not overloading your system with too many stressful foods. If you do not have a reaction from a small amount of refined carbohydrates, then you may eat a more liberal WFD. If you do react, then stay with the PWFD for another six months.

Do not make the mistake of going back to your former poor eating habits when you are ready to liberalize. If you do, the benefits you have gained will gradually vanish, your health will suffer, and your original symptoms may return. *The liberal diet is meant to be a whole foods diet without strictly eliminating all traces of refined foods.*

TROUBLESHOOTING FOR THE PWFD

Q: I've been following the PWFD for two weeks, and I'm not feeling any better. I had a reaction to something I ate yesterday. What happened?

A: Here are some possibilities for why or what might be occurring.

1. If you are being perfect with the diet, your reaction is a healing response and this, too, shall pass. See Chapter 5 (about Daily Life with the 3LS) for a description of the healing crisis.

2. If you have been consistently perfect with your diet and have accidentally (or purposely) eaten some refined carbohydrates, your system is telling you that you have eaten incorrectly. Re-examine what you have eaten, and be careful to avoid those refined carbohydrates in the future.

3. If you are sure it is not due to eating some refined carbohydrates, it may be a food hypersensitivity. After several weeks of successfully following the PWFD, your healthier body will help you become more aware of reactions to foods you were hypersensitive to already. For more information about food hypersensitivities, reread page 85, see the Glossary, and refer to the box on page 117.

4. If you have been 100% faithful to the diet and followed it perfectly, you could be one of those few who would benefit from modifying the PWFD by using trial and error testing with some of the dietary approaches that are briefly mentioned in the box below. Entire books have been written about those other dietary approaches, and it would be a good idea to learn more about any approach you think might help you before trying it. There is much to learn about selecting and cooking foods to create the healthiest nutrition plan for yourself.

5. If you are experiencing changes in elimination, read the information on pages 117–118 about dysbiosis. With a change in diet, the colon may take six-plus weeks to adjust.

Troubleshooting Checklist for the PWFD

✓ Have you been perfect in eliminating refined carbohydrates?

✓ Have you been reading every label?

✓ Did you eliminate all caffeine?

✓ Did you eliminate nicotine?

✓ Have you eliminated fruit?

✓ Are you using Appendix B in this book or *The Healing Power of Whole Foods* by Beth Loiselle as a guide to the PWFD?

✓ Have you looked at adding other dietary approaches?

✓ Have you looked at other dietary issues that might be happening?

✓ If after some time the PWFD does not seem to be improving your health, perhaps it's time to add a second leg of the Wellness Program. Not getting enough exercise or relaxation decreases healthy digestive function.

When to Seek Professional Help for Nutrition and Digestion

The Whole Foods Diet is very safe. The situations we know of that may require professional help are:

• Other pre-existing digestive issues become more apparent. Those with long-standing digestive problems may need to start a program of improving overall digestive health. If pre-existing digestive issues are the case, study and learn more about your issue to find the resolution, or seek assistance from a professional health care provider.

- Insulin or medications need to be decreased because you are doing so much better. If you are diabetic, see an appropriate health care practitioner.

- Large quantities of nutritional supplements may be needed to overcome eating a poor diet for many years. See Chapter 8 for information about Orthomolecular Nutrition. Information for consulting with a nutritionist or orthomolecular practitioner is in the Resources.

If your diet seems to be stimulating symptoms, also read the section in Chapter 5 about the healing crisis to understand the body's response to healing.

Other Dietary Approaches

This is a general introduction to a few of the many dietary approaches commonly used to supplement the PWFD. These short summaries are provided to point you in a direction of further learning and study. For specific information, consult appropriate books, wellness practitioners, and other resources.

Hereditary/metabolic diets: (Examples include *Eat Right for Your Type,* Metabolic Diet) Humans, because they have different genetic propensities, metabolize foods in radically different ways. Hence, while some people will thrive on a vegetarian diet and one and only one subset of supplemental vitamins and minerals, this very same diet and set of supplements will worsen the health of the individuals who will need to eat (much maligned) red meat and must take another subset of vitamin and minerals. Thus, this type of diet guides you to eat foods to which your metabolism and/or ancestry is best adapted. Please note that a person's metabolic type may change after a long period of doing Skilled Relaxation due to becoming healthier.

10% fat diet: (Examples include Pritikin Diet, Dean Ornish's Diet) This therapeutic diet (not a maintenance diet) is designed for losing weight and reversing a potentially fatal condition: heart disease. It is perfectly safe to follow this diet for about two years. Then, individuals may increase the fat to 15% for the rest of their lives.

Elimination/provocation diet: This diet tests for hypersensitivities (allergies) to specific foods. A person can have a hypersensitivity to *any* food. The more common a food in a person's diet, the more likely it

continued on next page

continued from previous page

is to be a problem, since we tend to crave and eat the foods to which we are allergic. (In the US, the most common hypersensitivies are wheat and dairy.) Test one food at a time by eliminating it from your diet for four days. Then try eating that food and see what happens. Most (but not all) reactions to food occur within 45 minutes to four hours after ingestion. The elimination diet does not usually cure hypersensitivities since the root cause of allergies is Leaky Gut Syndrome (LGS, see page 37–38 and 116), but it gives your body a rest and relieves symptoms. Some individuals with food allergies will also need to do a rotation diet.

Rotation diet: This is a strategy to space certain foods and certain food groups apart by anywhere from four to seven days to avoid allergic or hypersensitivity reactions. This doesn't mean that on one day you are allowed to have several ingestions of the food allergen. Rather, you eat it only once and then wait four days to a week before you ingest it again. Rotation diets can give temporary relief of symptoms while you resolve LGS (the cause of the food reactions).

Candida diet: Candida-Related Syndrome is due to an overgrowth of yeast in the body. For candida, use the PWFD with no fruit for about three months. Many doctors recommend a very restricted diet to cure candida overgrowth (no vinegar, yeasts, cheese, mushrooms, tamari, shoyu soy sauce, and sometimes no grains). However, not everybody needs to avoid these foods if they have candida, only those people who are actually allergic to those foods. Some people will need to use additional treatment to clear up candida.

Food combining: For some individuals with sensitive digestive tracts, following the protocol of food combining can be helpful. For others, it does not seem to matter much. To follow the procotol, eat simply and do not combine too many different foods in one meal. The basic food combining principle is this: Eat fruit alone, eat vegetables and fat with anything but fruit, and avoid eating protein with starchy food.

Other dietary approaches: Low carb/high protein diets such as Atkins, Zone, or South Beach diet; vegetarianism; Chinese nutrition; Paleolithic diet; macrobiotic diet; high fiber diet; juicing; glycemic indexing; organic foods; raw foods diet; slow foods cooking; eating all fresh foods; drinking sufficient water; paying attention to water quality; and avoiding nightshade vegetables (a family of plants, the Solanaceae, which include the eggplant, tomato, potato, and capsicum peppers). These are

continued on next page

continued from previous page

just a few—there are other dietary and cooking variables or approaches that may help different individuals.

Other variables that might affect health: using microwave ovens, plastic food containers, or aluminum cookware; eating too fast or under stress; not chewing your food enough; improper cooking or storage of food, etc.

Common Digestive Issues

The following is a general introduction to a few digestive issues that can be helped by the PWFD. These short summaries are provided to point you in a direction of further learning and study. For specific information, consult appropriate books, wellness practitioners, and other resources.

Leaky gut syndrome (LGS): Approximately 75% of the US population has LGS.[8] With LGS, you do not process and absorb what you eat in a normal manner because the intestinal lining has become weakened. Therefore poorly digested peptides (proteins) are leaked into the blood supply where the immune system makes antibodies to them. LGS affects almost every system of the body, thus, it's pretty difficult to know if you have LGS. The real problems of LGS are systemic, so other types of symptoms will appear before any gastrointestinal symptoms. If you have food hypersensitivities or GERD, you can know for sure you have LGS, but often people without these conditions have LGS.

To reverse the causes of LGS, practice an effective Skilled Relaxation method and follow the PWFD. When the LGS is treated early, Skilled Relaxation is all that is needed. Complications of long-standing LGS that will not likely clear up by eliminating this syndrome alone are conditions like Crohn's disease, ulcerative colitis, diverticulitis (and its complications), colon cancer, atonic bowel, and polyposis. Skilled Relaxation is still the most important adjunctive therapy for these advanced conditions. However, additional approaches may be necessary, such as taking supplements and avoiding allergenic foods. You will know the LGS is resolved when you don't have any more GI tract symptoms and your other symptoms, including bracing (see Chapter 2), also disappear at the same time.

GERD: Gastro Esophageal Reflux Disorder, also called hiatal hernia, or acid reflux, is an increasingly common condition in which gastric

continued on next page

continued from previous page

contents escape up into the esophagus, causing heartburn symptoms. This tends to be worse when the person is lying down.

GERD (all hernias except traumatic hiatal hernias) is just one aspect of LGS and thus may be cured by the practice of Skilled Relaxation. A ginger root juice protocol is a remarkably safe, inexpensive and effective solution for the symptoms of GERD and has already been described in the book *Saving Yourself From the Disease Care Crisis.*

Food hypersensitivities: These are sometimes called food allergies or food intolerance[9] and are present on different levels. These abnormal responses to food range from acute (which is never resolved and can even kill a person) to chronic (can be resolved by avoidance for a period of time then limiting ongoing exposure, or simply by limiting exposure). The most common hypersensitivities in the US are the foods we eat most commonly: wheat and dairy.

The long-term solution to food allergies is to first eliminate their cause: Leaky Gut Syndrome (LGS), which is resolved through the practice of Skilled Relaxation. The elimination diet and/or the rotation diet (see box on pages 114–115) can temporarily resolve symptoms of food hypersensitivity. However, if you only identify the substances you are allergic to and then restrict those foods, you will not stop the problems, because any new food may eventually start to aggravate the immune system because of the continued leakage of peptides. However, by following the elimination diet and the rotation diet, symptoms will abate, giving your body a chance to heal itself by adherence to the PWFD, Skilled Relaxation, and Exercise. After the healing, sometimes a previously irritating food can once again be tolerated.

Dysbiosis: About 500+ varieties of normal bacteria in the gut work together to create an environment that discourages all kinds of pathogenic bacteria and parasites (including candida). An imbalance of that ecology is called dysbiosis. Dysbiosis is due to putrefaction, fermentation, deficiency, sensitization, or a number of inflammatory diseases within the bowel. Skin and connective tissues may be involved. People who have LGS will likely get dysbiosis and then parasites, which is then usually followed by environmental sensitivities (such as food hypersensitivities). Changes in diet can also trigger dysbiosis.

One can improve the function of the gut somewhat by taking digestive enzymes, replacing the normal colonic bacteria with probiotics

continued on next page

continued from previous page

(available at health food stores), and normalizing the transit time (generally 24 to 48 hours but that is individual) by increasing fiber intake and treating any parasites. The correct practice of Skilled Relaxation is also essential for resolving dysbiosis.

Candida: Candida albicans is a dimorphic fungus. This species is part of the normal gastrointestinal flora. We are all continuously passing the yeast (seed) form of candida through our guts because it is everywhere in our environment. It is only a problem when it sprouts into the fungal form. Candida cannot sprout in our guts unless we already have LGS and the resultant dysbiosis.

One way to determine if you have candida is to take the candida questionnaire that is available in many books and is on the Internet. There is nothing that will reliably eliminate candida faster than first dealing with the causes of the LGS (through Skilled Relaxation and exercise), eating a PWFD (eliminating every trace of refined carbohydrates), taking an antifungal or grapefruit seed extract properly, and supplementing with a good brand of probiotics. Since candida makes LGS much worse, together they produce a vicious cycle that can be reversed by treating either one.

Parasites: LGS comes first, then dysbiosis, then candida or other parasites, which further aggravates the LGS. Getting rid of the LGS (by using Skilled Relaxation) and then dealing with any parasites that might still be present is the best way to become parasite-free. Just eliminating the LGS will not usually get rid of parasites without specific treatment of the different parasites. You can seek specific treatment for parasites from a parasitologist, or, in this country, a holistic physician. Recent research indicates that grapefruit seed extract is at least as effective against parasites as any prescription drug and has no side-effects.

THE AUTHORS' EXPERIENCES

■■■ WALT: I did the PWFD as an experiment since I "knew" it was all hogwash and needed to prove it to myself. Was I surprised! I never planned to do it longer than a week or so, but when it helped me so much, and so quickly, I decided to keep it up longer. I went through this transition myself while I was working a 100-hour week (and doing all my own grocery shopping and cooking), so I know that following it is a matter of discipline and commitment. It actually was a blessing within a couple of weeks because I was getting back so much more than I was putting in, and at the same time it was getting a lot easier to follow. By dealing with it as an experiment—and doing it perfectly—my results were so dramatic they changed my personal and professional life forever. Unexpectedly, many of my own symptoms that I did not even know I had (thinking I was just getting old!) disappeared so fast that I was intrigued.

When I started the diet, I lived on cooked brown rice smothered with chopped, mixed, frozen veggies seasoned with herbs such as sage, parsley, tiny amounts of cayenne pepper (which just sets up the taste buds), basil, garlic powder and mineral salt to taste. The herbs are best put on top of the veggies while they are being steamed for the 10 minutes recommended so that flavors permeate them. That is all I ate for a month. By then I was feeling so good I stayed on this simple diet for another seven to eight months by choice. I never was so healthy in my life.

The withdrawal symptoms I experienced (for three to four days) were, for me, just an exacerbation of some of the symptoms I had been having all along for many years: hunger 24 hours a day; depression; insomnia; frequent colds; acid stomach; severe, and many times debilitating, back pain; chronic constipation; arthritic signs; and other symptoms.

I have always been interested in cooking and was the parent who made the meals most of the time. At the beginning when I started the PWFD, I did not know what I was doing, but I persisted in learning. It took some getting used to.

I continued for several years doing the PWFD. These were the happiest and healthiest years of my life. I believe I no longer need to be perfect, but still rarely eat anything refined. However, the benefits of my doing that for those years have stuck with me (keeping me far from the edge of my cliff) so that I have never felt the need to be so compulsive with my diet today as I was to get healthy in the first place. ■■■

■■■ JAN: I started the PWFD after decades of chronic illness. I experienced only one day of mild withdrawal consisting of a little fatigue and a detox headache, and I was very happy to receive immediate health benefits from starting the diet. I experienced more energy, stabilization of blood sugar levels (which had been a huge problem), and I lost weight, which everybody noticed.

By doing both Skilled Relaxation and the Perfect Whole Foods Diet together, I became more in tune with and aware of my body. Soon I noticed I was having hypersensitivity reactions to many different foods. I then added other dietary approaches: first the elimination diet and then for a few months, the rotation diet. (See pages 114–115 for more information on those diets.) I discovered that I was allergic to wheat, soy, dairy, corn, and eggs. After I stopped eating those foods, my food reactions stopped almost completely and I started making a habit of feeling good!

Now, after four years of the perfect diet, I still avoid refined foods. I stick to the perfect diet about 99.5% and have small amounts of refined foods in social situations. Therefore, I continue to see steady improvement in my overall health, and I feel that the PWFD is making a great contribution to my wellness. The effects seem to be cumulatively increasing over time, and I feel better the longer I follow the diet. I'm delighted by and really enjoy eating the delicious whole foods. My plan is to follow this diet for the rest of my life.

Interestingly, I am aware that the PWFD nurtures and nourishes me on more than just the physical level of the food itself. It feels as though I have been released from some kind of trap, and now I can enjoy my life. This means more than just having extra health and energy. For example, I have learned how to become a better cook since I started this diet—it's so much fun to prepare delicious and interesting meals. Plus now almost every meal seems like a feast to me in contrast to how I was eating before. This diet makes me feel happy, abundant, and whole. I am so glad to be following this nutrition plan. ■■■

Chapter 3, WHOLE FOODS DIET—SUMMING IT UP

Finding the correct foods to eat is a very individual process, since each person has different nutritional needs and each diet has a different purpose. A true diet reflects a lifestyle change to healthier eating habits rather than a temporary way of eating.

The one nutritional improvement that helps most people improve their chronic illnesses and their health with minimal effort is eating whole foods.

A food that is whole has all the parts intact. Food that is refined has had parts removed, depleting it of nutrients necessary for the body to use the food. When nutrients are missing, chemical reactions inside the body known as the Krebs cycle become less efficient, resulting in decreased energy, disease, or functional impairment of parts of the body.

Refined carbohydrates are those that cause the most trouble. The effects of eating refined carbohydrates are made apparent when a person stops eating them. This is known by experiencing withdrawal responses (indicating that eating refined carbohydrates causes some kind of addiction) and/or immune system responses (indicating that eating refined carbohydrates causes some form of allergy).

You can follow a Whole Foods Diet (WFD) in two ways. A Perfect Whole Foods Diet (PWFD) is total avoidance of refined foods. A Liberal WFD includes occasional small quantities of refined foods. The former is the most curative way of eating whole foods and the latter is best used for health maintenance. It is recommended that you start with a PWFD and change to a Liberal Diet after six months. Benefits of a Whole Foods Diet include reversal of unusual symptoms or conditions, increased energy, weight loss, increased enjoyment of food, decreased symptoms, feeling better, self-empowerment, and more positive emotions that come from increased enjoyment of life.

Typical foods to eat on the PWFD include vegetables, whole grains, beans, nuts, seeds, fruit, eggs, some fats/oils, meats, poultry, dairy, some condiments and seasonings. Foods not eaten on the PWFD include all sugars (including fruit for some people), refined foods, caffeine, alcohol, and use of nicotine. *The Healing Power of Whole Foods* by Beth Loiselle is a recommended resource for following this diet as it contains lists of allowed foods and other details helpful for success with the Perfect Diet.

continued on next page

continued from previous page

Planning strategies for following the PWFD may be helpful for social situations, meal preparation, eating out in restaurants, and traveling.

When digestion and nutrition improve after starting the PWFD, other pre-existing digestive issues may become apparent, which may require you to further adjust what you eat. Continued learning and study about food and nutrition, and professional help, may be helpful.

See the summary on the next page for instruction for following the PWFD.

Perfect Whole Foods Diet—STEPS TO TAKE

1. Think about the timing of starting the diet. For example, waiting until after holidays or after a vacation is a good idea.

2. If you are diabetic, seek medical supervision as your need for insulin or hypoglycemic agents may drop dramatically.

3. Find out if this diet is worth your while and will help you by doing a two-week trial (some people find out in just a few days). That means being 100% perfect on the diet for two weeks. One way to do a two-week trial is to eat a very simple menu consisting of whole grains, vegetables with their peels, protein foods, spices or herbs, nuts for snacks, and mint tea or chamomile tea and water. Another way to do a two-week trial is to read *The Healing Power of Whole Foods* and create a meal plan that works for you for the two weeks.

4. Carefully document how you feel each day. (Remember, for the first several days, you may experience symptoms of withdrawal such as fatigue or headaches. After the withdrawal clears, you can expect to feel much better.) If you follow the diet perfectly, you will know it is worth your while by your experience of some benefits in four days, lots of benefits in a week, and even more in two weeks. If you are not feeling better after two weeks, examine everything you are eating more carefully and be sure you are eliminating all refined carbohydrates.

5. Once you know it is worth your while to follow the PWFD, you can decide how to continue. As you learn how and where to shop as well as how to use spices, eating all whole foods will get easier. You may find it helpful to remove all refined foods from your kitchen. Read *every* label to avoid eating all traces of refined foods.

6. Further learning and study about diet, nutrition, and cooking may help as you become more sensitive to your body. If necessary, at any time after the two-week trial, adjust your diet. Consider adding different dietary approaches.

7. You will continue to see more benefits for about three months so long as you follow the diet perfectly, although the improvements come slower

continued on next page

continued from previous page

as time goes on. It then typically takes six to twelve months to get your health to the place where your symptoms will not return easily.

8. The Whole Foods Diet is only one part of the 3LS. Do all three aspects of the Wellness Program for fastest results, greatest health, and numerous wellness benefits.

APPRECIATION FOR THE WHOLE FOODS DIET

I started the PWFD back in January 2002 (it is now March 2004). Within two weeks, my persistent and painful plantar fascitis, from which I had been suffering for two-plus years, disappeared. My asthma symptoms diminished, and a wonderful bonus of excess weight dropped off with no effort.

—L.C., Graphic Designer, Rockville, MD

A little over four years ago, I had receding, bleeding gums, with no improvement in sight. From what I understand, I was in the early stages of this nasty problem. Of course, my rheumatoid arthritis was a much bigger issue for me at the time. For me, changing to a Whole Foods Diet gradually cleared up all of my gum/tooth problems. I also did other things, primarily for the arthritis, but the end result is that both the RA and the dental problems went away (along with some other things). I do still take three grams of Ester C per day, and I'm sure this has helped me, but I feel that the diet is probably more of a contributor to my improvements. I've had no dental issues since I made these changes. I rarely floss and my dentist knows it (I do get regular cleanings and brush regularly, but I have always done this), but it's obvious to me the reason for my continued dental health. I'm in much better shape than many of his diligent flossers.   *—Joseph Hackett, IT Manager, Louisville, KY*

Walt, look what you've done to me. I'm spending all this time reading books and labels, and going to the health food store, and rearranging the kitchen. I find myself meal-planning at odd times during the day and thinking about what I'm eating. Worst of all, I talk about it a lot. Just ask my wife. She may not have suffered enough from her chronic sinus problem to take the cure, but she's sick enough of hearing about it from me that she has begun a Whole Food Diet. Of course she's watched my health being restored, so she knows it works. Seriously I know this sounds weird, but I stopped in the middle of what I was doing and realized I was feeling great. Not good, great! And it really has been so long since I felt that way.   *—Jim Hare, Teacher, Laughlin, NV*

We went on a whole foods diet and that has really helped me and my husband with cholesterol and many other things. I never really had high cholesterol, but his was at 220 at 25 years old. With the change in the diets, it is down to a healthy level. We both have a lot more energy, and it helps us for our exercises. The main thing that happened for me was my PCOS [polycystic ovary syndrome] with resulting acne (heavy), mood swings (bad), weight gain, no periods, and hair loss. Most all of it is regulated now. I think with healthy eating and exercise, my body will continue to improve.

—*L. H. Welch, Arlington, TX*

I was afflicted with rheumatoid arthritis in May 2003. The progression of RA started as a single joint pain in the knee and within a month, had spread to the rest of the body. Every single joint was affected (including knees, wrists, shoulders, jaws, hips, spine, and the small joints of hands and feet). Extreme pain & tenderness accompanied me for about six months. I found Dr. Walt Stoll, who advised me about the 3LS Wellness Program. I followed the 3LS, especially the skilled relaxation. The e-diet changed the whole story (done in Nov 2003). I discovered my food allergies and have been quite strict about the diet. Four months after the elimination diet and a few herbal medications, I've almost recovered and am pain free. I see improvements everyday and have gained a more expansive outlook towards life. My joint pains are almost gone now. This was my goal and I'm almost near my goal and had picked up a few additional benefits like more energy, ability to deal with stressful situations, and currently helping other people to discover true health. There is tremendous power in the 3LS!!!

—*Chandu Siram, Senior Software Systems Engineer, Los Angeles, CA*

I have written before about how good the diet has made me feel and wanted to share a few more comments. I often find if I get cravings of ANY kind I can satisfy them by eating something else. For example, if I feel like having rice or chips or something that I am not allowed, I will instead have a rye cracker with goats milk cheese on it, just something to fill that craving space inside of me. I think it's when we get cravings, and do NOTHING to satisfy them, that they get stronger. Just eating something healthy can help it pass so much quicker. I want to do whatever I can to get healthy again: physically and mentally. Sometimes it's a struggle, and sometimes it feels so very natural, but we can overcome and regain our health with perseverance and determination.

—*Maria Keswell, Service Assurance Consultant, Beldon, WA, Australia*

Four months ago I started the whole foods diet and Skilled Relaxation, and my life changed dramatically! My acne and hypoglycemia disappeared and I lost eight pounds in no time. —*Anonymous*

I tried Moducare for Rheumatoid Arthritis. I got minimal relief. I have since done the elimination diet and the follow-up food testing (metabolic diets) and I am doing incredibly well. I spent almost $3,000 on supplements last year alone (including Moducare), and I haven't spent more than $25 since doing this diet…It's hard, but worth it.   —*Rebecca W., Actress, New York, NY*

I have been on the PWFD since January 1998 (this is May 2003). The last two years I have liberalized it, in a sense that I don't worry if I have to eat out. Most times, I am able to get a satisfying meal (not afraid of making fussy orders!). At home, I eat two cooked meals a day, always made of perfect whole foods. My husband has been doing the same as me, and although he was not ill to begin with, he has experienced big improvements in his general condition. We don't find it difficult at all. We have never eaten better food, really. Both of us have become quite accomplished at making good food, and eating in restaurants became even somewhat disappointing. The most important—and difficult— thing was to see the world through new eyes. Some of the things I used to buy, I now regard as poison. Occasionally I do get upset, like when I see children who scream at the register because they can't get their soda fast enough, or when I think about the junk people are made to believe is food.

—*Sonja Sunde, Social Anthropologist, Bergen, Norway*

You know what's great about the PWFD? You have to be perfect. There's no room for cheating and therefore you can't say, "I'll cheat a little bit now, it can't hurt me." Since you have to be perfect, you can't get carried away with the cheating! I really think that's what makes it easier than any diet where you cut back on things, because cutting back is relative so you can get away with justifying having stuff that you shouldn't have. I like the structure and definite boundaries of the PWFD. There's no gray area.   —*J.S, Student, Boulder, CO*

I suffer from CFS [chronic fatigue syndrome]/candida/depression and have been on a Whole Foods Diet now for some time. Every time I touch refined sugar, carbohydrates, drink alcohol, etc., my body reacts to it in a negative way: bloating, increased pulse rate, fatigue, etc. It's my body's way of telling me, "You no longer need this." Our bodies are not meant to take refined foods and alcohol. Once you become attached to feeling good in your body, you become willing to keep doing what it takes to keep it healthy for the demands in your daily life.   —*Anonymous*

Before starting the PWFD, I hadn't considered myself unhealthy. I had no need for prescription medications; I was exercising on a somewhat regular basis; and my weight, cholesterol, and blood pressure were acceptable. I was your average "healthy American." I first started the PWFD over a year ago by being fortunate enough to have a roommate who was already following it. I had a lot of support and an endless supply of delicious recipes and whole foods preparation tips. After the first several weeks on the diet, I couldn't believe how much more energy I had! I was studying a lot at the time and became able to maintain full steam on just six hours of sleep per night whereas before the diet I needed eight hours and at least one nap.

Another significant change I experienced with the diet was increased clarity and focus. I hadn't realized how much brain-fog I had until it started to clear. My classmates observed the change too, noting how clear my eyes were and how focused I was in school. Everyone was wondering how I was able to remain healthy during numerous spells of cold and nasty flu bugs plaguing the school. My joint aches began to dwindle and I noticed that even with no change in my physical workouts, I became more limber. As I began to feel better and better, I realized how "unwell" I had felt before the PWFD days.

As I started to feel better on the PWFD, and as I learned more about health and my body in massage therapy school and from Jan and Dr. Stoll, I looked back at my old days with a new perspective and began to see how many indicators of "dis-ease" my body had been showing all along. They ranged from feeling sluggish after eating, to catching colds several times a year, to suffering headaches multiple times a month. I wasn't a heavy drinker, but I ended up having to eliminate alcohol altogether because a single beer caused a severe hangover.

I was also facing over a year of slightly abnormal lab tests. Since none of these signs were serious, I shrugged them off as signs of growing old or just bad luck. In hindsight, however, all these indicators of "dis-ease" were adding up, and I now realize how close I was to the edge of the cliff. I'm just happy I ran into Jan and Dr. Stoll who, by their examples and teachings, began to steer me in the right direction before I began having more serious health issues. With the PWFD and continuing my exercise, the red flags began to disappear. I'm also happy to report that after six months on the PWFD, my lab test came back normal.

—Julia M. Schloesser, Licensed Massage Therapist, Colorado Springs, CO

■
■
■

The Right Exercise
For You

This chapter covers:

1. How exercise, especially aerobics, helps reverse chronic conditions and enhances and maintains health
2. How to set exercise goals and select appropriate forms of exercise to meet them
3. General instructions for starting an exercise program

EXERCISE—LOVE IT OR HATE IT?

■■■ WALT: One of my precepts in offering the 3LS Wellness Program has always been to let the patient know it does not much matter where they start (which part to do first), since any of the three practices eventually produces energy to do more. Ironically, if exercise ranks as the last of the three legs you would consider, this probably means that it is the single most important thing that you could do for your health. This is because people tend to avoid doing the very thing that would help them the most. However, even if you begin with the aspect of the Program you find easiest, my bet is that within a year, you will find yourself doing what you thought in the beginning you would never consider doing: exercise.

As we have developed into a nation of "couch potatoes," it has become increasingly important to exercise. The important thing is just to *begin* exercising regularly, even if you choose something simple and easy. Today, with all the different kinds of exercise available (even some you can do while sitting on the couch watching TV), people have many choices for starting an exercise program. Most people who begin one kind of exercise eventually become interested in adding other types. After becoming aware of how good it makes them feel, and the other encouraging messages they receive from their muscles and body, they want more.

Once people understand that they can multiply by three the benefits of their Whole Foods Diet (WFD) and Skilled Relaxation (SR) just by adding Exercise, especially aerobics, more of them will be able to pry themselves off the couch. Don't use your age or condition as an excuse not to do some movement. There's no time like the present to start exercising. ■■■

Choosing an Exercise

Exercise has been known since the days of Hippocrates to be an essential part of a healthy lifestyle. Every bodily system that has been studied has been shown to improve in function with simple exercise. It doesn't matter what health problem you have, you'll be farther along the road to recovery if you start doing *any* kind of exercise on a regular basis. In the past 4,000 years, many types of exercise have been developed for different results and benefits.

The dictionary defines exercise for health as activity, such as in a regular series of movements, designed to train, strengthen, or develop some part of the body or faculty. Exercise does two main things: it increases metabolism (which, among other things, promotes burning calories), and it burns fat and builds muscle (which does not always show on the scales but is visible in measurements).

Aerobic exercise (AE) receives prominence in this chapter, because it was the first really effective and medically documented approach to exercise. Of all the types of exercise that exist, AE provides the greatest enhancement to health and offers the most comprehensive wellness benefits for those who are able to do it. Aerobics is superior for cardiovascular and anti-aging effects.

But just because aerobics is best for preventing heart disease, it is not necessarily best for meeting all health goals. Several other exercise concepts are available that can be added to a health or wellness program. Some exercises complement and can be done alongside AE. Any exercise may be chosen by people who are unable to do aerobics. Examples of non-aerobic exercise (anaerobic) include activities that don't get your heart going fast, like *gentle* rebounding (mini-trampoline), progressive strength exercise, non-aerobic walking, t'ai chi, qi gong, yoga, stretching, and Alexander technique.

They all have varying effects and benefits, and are suitable for different individual capacities. Much variety exists, so you may select one or several types of exercise that are right for you.

The concept of "choose the right exercise for you" is not widely promoted in the commercial marketplace. We believe this is mostly because people who promote any type of exercise have benefited from a particular one, and consequently they tend to believe that their exercise is the best and only. However, each type of exercise has different benefits that meet different goals, and a large percentage of people need exercise variations. Just like the other two parts of the 3LS Wellness Program, exercise cannot be "one size fits all."

What's the Right Exercise?

∎∎∎ JAN: In my massage practice, I have found that many people hold a deep and ingrained belief that vigorous exercise is the only really healthy kind of exercise. However, during different stages of life and healing, vigorous exercise may be what a person does *not* need. For example, people who are strongly bracing may initially benefit more from stretching or doing gentle movements to alleviate muscle tension rather than exercises that tighten muscles or create stress. That was my experience. Similarly, a person who has been ill or has had restricted movement may need to start slowly to re-strengthen muscles, release connective tissue and restrictions, and restore healthy movement. Thus, less vigorous exercise offers more benefits than aerobics at certain stages of healing.

Some people receive advantage from following very specialized or individualized exercise programs to resolve specific health conditions or to maximize good health. For example, now some health clinics and sports medicine centers offer "prescriptions" for exercise programs that are individualized and scientifically-based. Physical therapists, personal trainers, and Pilates teachers may also provide such instruction. Survivors of life-altering catastrophic illnesses such as multiple sclerosis, heart disease, stroke, and cancer have formed a network for camaraderie in athletic competition (see Resources). Other similar group programs may be helpful for individuals with specific conditions.∎∎∎

Setting a Goal for Yourself

Goal-setting often stimulates motivation and results in greater achievement. It can be helpful to write down these aspirations to make sure you know what they are and don't get sidetracked from meeting them. Set easy-to-moderate goals for yourself so that you will be successful. After you meet them, set new ones.

Goals may be chosen in terms of achieving certain results in strength, time, or distance. Some examples are walking one mile in 20 minutes instead of 30 minutes, getting strong enough to change from lifting two-pound weights to three-pound weights, or lengthening your AE sessions from 20 to 30 minutes. Goals may also be set in terms of health benefits. Some health goals include:

Achieving cardiovascular fitness

Alleviating emotional states such as depression or anger and enhancing positive emotions such as self-confidence or contentment

Attaining a higher level of physical health or fitness

Bettering one's quality of life

Boosting energy flow in the body

Building stamina

Conditioning for a particular sport or activity

Detoxifying and circulating lymph

Developing physical strength

Enhancing body-mind integration

Decreasing musculo-skeletal pain

Developing better posture

Enhancing coordination

Heartening optimism

Improving balance

Increasing awareness of body

Losing weight

Overcoming specific illnesses

Pregnancy fitness

Preventing specific health conditions

Recovering physical function

Re-educating the body in non-restricted movement

Rehabilitation from injury or illness

Restoring range of motion (flexibility)

Reversing or delaying the effects of aging

Reversing specific symptoms

Strengthening the immune system

Toning muscles

Here's an overview of applying exercise for optimum health:

Goals for Enhancement of Health Through Exercise

1. Maintain or improve range of motion of various body parts
2. Maintain or improve sufficient strength in the major muscle groups
3. Maintain or improve sufficient reserves of function of the cardio-vascular and other metabolic support systems
4. Maintain or improve the balance between food intake and energy output
5. Maintain or improve the balance between muscle groups

How about just feeling better and having more energy? In this chapter, we will focus on using exercise as part of the 3LS Wellness approach to health. We encourage you to learn more about exercise, thus we have chosen the book *Fitness for Dummies,* by Suzanne Schlosberg and Liz Neporent, as a key resource for learning more about starting an exercise program. It is a practical reference that covers a wide variety of exercises and describes them in detail.

Key Resource: *Fitness for Dummies*

by Suzanne Schlosberg and Liz Neporent
This reference is the best exercise book we have seen. It covers a wide variety of exercises and describes them in detail. The book covers cardio, strength, and flexibility exercises (including different types of yoga, for example), setting exercise goals, buying equipment, choosing an exercise class, health club, or exercise videos, hiring a trainer, exercising at home, fitness rip-offs, common injuries, and more. (Wiley, John & Sons, 1999.)

A Note to Athletes: The 3LS is for You, Too

If, as an athlete, you wish to enhance your physical performance, adding both the regular practice of Skilled Relaxation and a Perfect Whole Foods Diet to your training would be highly beneficial. Two largely important factors affecting the progress of a training routine are diet and rest. Insufficiency in either can sap your energy, and doing both can improve bodily function and thus your athletic ability.

World-class athletes know that doing Skilled Relaxation, with or without imagery immediately prior to competing in their event, can improve or maximize their performance. The greatest athletic professionals use Skilled Relaxation and imagery on a regular basis to enhance the quality of their game. The book *Mental Tennis,* by Vic Braden, helps with understanding the use of visualization and Skilled Relaxation in athletic competition (see Resources). Any kind of mind training, i.e., meditation, imagery, self-hypnosis, and/or visualization techniques, can bring about a great change or enhancement in performance.

■■■ WALT: The Perfect Whole Foods Diet (PWFD) would be the best diet for optimal athletic performance during the six months of eliminating a refined carbohydrate addiction. After that, the liberal Whole Foods Diet would work fine. Either way, we would recommend supplementation with whole food concentrates (see page 95). It is not a refined carbohydrate addiction by itself that reduces athletic performance, but the reason behind the addiction (less efficient Krebs cycle, for example) that makes the Perfect Whole Foods Diet so beneficial for athletes. Nutritional improvements result in enhanced metabolic efficiency and higher performance levels. By the way, if you read the labels on performance snack bars and sports drinks, you will find that they do not meet the requirements of the Perfect Whole Foods Diet.

If athletes understood that putting their energy into diet and Skilled Relaxation would improve their performance more than increasing the amount of aerobics they do, they might change their allotment of energy expenditure. They might first put more time into Skilled Relaxation and a Whole Foods Diet, and expect to experience improvement in function and more productive energy to then put back into their sport. Fitness professionals would better help the athletes they train by promoting the 3LS Program to them.

In addition to adding the other two aspects of the Wellness Program to your training program, consider adding variety to the exercise portion to enhance the body's overall function. Such a holistic approach may also enhance performance of your main activity or sport. Integrated exercises (like qi gong or t'ai chi) enhance energy, focus, and concentration, and conditioning exercises (like stretching and weight-lifting) prevent injury, promote endurance, and also improve performance. Athletes who participate in non-aerobic sports, such as weight-lifting, would benefit from adding aerobics. As team physician at the local high school of the town where I first practiced medicine, and later from teaching at the women's athletic department at the University of Kentucky, I know clearly how much conditioning exercises that are different from your main sport can prevent injury and improve performance. Professional athletes practice them consistently. ■■■

AEROBICS! THE FOUNDATION OF ANY WELLNESS PROGRAM

The form of exercise we believe is optimum for overall health and fitness, and the exercise we recommend for most people is Aerobics. AE is a special type of exercise that is many times more effective for the promotion of health, well-being, and management of stress than any other form of exercise. Yet AE is so simple to do that many people find it hard to believe that it could produce all of the benefits claimed for it.

What is aerobic exercise? Aerobics is any extended physical activity that increases heart rate and breathing while using the large muscle groups at a regular, even pace. Some common examples of aerobic activities are jogging, bicycling, and swimming.

Benefits of Aerobic Exercise

Aerobic activity is a powerful force for health. Even this partial list of the proven benefits of AE sounds almost too good to be true. Regardless of the direction of your deviation from wellness, aerobics will draw you toward health. If you are fat, you will lose weight; if you are skinny, you will gain weight. If you are depressed, it will cheer you up; if you are nervous, it will calm you down. If you are fatigued, it will give you energy; if you have insomnia, it will help you sleep at night. If you start AE by the age of 40, it slows your aging 20 years; start by the age of 50, it slows aging 15 years; by the age of 60, 10 years.

Some of the physiological effects of aerobics are listed below.

Aerobics decreases:	Aerobics increases:
Blood lipids (cholesterol, triglycerides, etc.)	Amount of blood ejected with each heartbeat
Blood pressure	Blood volume and total hemoglobin (overall oxygen-carrying capacity)
Emotional disturbances (anxiety, depression)	Bone density and joint strength
Exercise heart rate	Coordination and endurance
Insulin requirements in diabetes	Digestive efficiency and bowel function
Percent of body fat	Heart and skeletal muscle vascularization
Posture problems and low back pain	High density lipoprotein ("the good guys")
Resting heart rate	Lung capacity
	Oxygen extraction at the tissue level during maximum work
	Percent lean body mass
	Return of heart rate and blood

Among other things, people who do aerobics have more energy, sleep more soundly, and wake up more refreshed with fewer hours of sleep. Aerobic activities use more calories than other activities and reduce the chances of catching viral infections to nearly zero (this means you will catch fewer or no colds at all). Aerobics increases sex drive, strength, and produces a positive mental outlook. It speeds up

continued on next page

continued from previous page

the healing of injuries by 15% to 25%. And Aerobics is also powerfully effective in stopping smoking (within six months of beginning an AE program).[1]

If this partial list isn't enough to interest you in learning more about this remarkable process, we suggest you file this information away until you are ready to get healthy, or... just keep reading and learn how to start aerobics anyway.

How to Do Aerobic Exercise

The basic steps for starting AE are outlined below. There are a few simple things to learn and do before beginning your aerobics program.

First step: It is best to do a little reading or research about aerobic exercise before trying aerobics on your own. That way you will become more knowledgeable about what you are doing. Some suitable books and websites are listed in the Resources section at the end of this book.

Second step: Before you start doing AE, check with your doctor to see if you need a stress test. Aerobic exercise is used to help people prevent heart attacks. However, if you are already at risk of a heart attack, your pulse rate requirements will be different, and you will need to know about that to prevent injury. Also, if you are taking prescription medications, smoke, have problems with your back, have diabetes, or have experienced chest discomfort, consult a physician or other qualified practitioner before beginning any exercise program as you may need to either adjust your medications or adapt your training program.

■■■ WALT: Since heart disease is now happening earlier and earlier in life, it is probably wise for anyone over 20, or those who are overweight, to get a stress test. This is especially true since it is always good to have a baseline stress test on record to compare with one later in life should a diagnostic record be needed. To keep a baseline stress test on record means that you should insist upon having a copy of the tracing to keep at home. Definitely, anyone over the age of 30 wishing to do aerobics needs a stress test if they have led a sedentary life. If an individual is over 40, has not exercised much and has never had a stress test, he or she should get one whether or not contemplating starting an exercise program. ■■■

Third step: Check your pulse rate for ten seconds immediately upon awakening in the morning. This is your awakening pulse. Use one of these methods:

1. Neck. To feel and count the carotid pulse, place the index and middle fingers gently on the side of the neck, next to the throat. This is usually a fairly easy place to find the pulse.

2. Wrist. The radial pulse can be taken by placing the first two fingers lightly over the radial artery of the wrist, directly in line with the thumb.

3. Temple. The temporal pulse can be felt by lightly placing the first two fingers on either temple located just in front of the upper part of the ear. This one is harder to find.

4. Chest. The apical pulse can be felt, after heavy exercise, by placing the palm of the hand over the left side of the chest.

Write your pulse rate on your calendar every day. This will give you a baseline to compare your improvements after you've been doing aerobics for a while.

Fourth step: Choose an activity that you can do continuously for at least 20 minutes. *Any* activity that keeps you moving non-stop for 20 minutes and elevates your heart rate is perfectly adequate. Here are some examples:

Some Aerobic Activities

Bicycling, stationary biking, or spinning (exercise class stationary biking)

Dancing (aerobic)

Jogging/running

Jumping rope

Rebounding (mini-trampoline—vigorous)

Rowing

Running in place

Skating (ice or roller)

Stair climbing

Step classes

Swimming

Treadmill

Walking (brisk)

While aerobics is a specific metabolic *process,* there are many different activities that can be used to *produce* that process. You can do your favorite activity, even if it is not listed, as long as it keeps the heart rate at the correct level for the 20 minutes (described in the Fifth Step below). Activities like baseball, however, where you have bursts of activity and then stand around most of the time, would not be suitable for an aerobic exercise program.

Fifth step: Learn and follow the basic concept of keeping your heart rate at the correct level when doing your aerobic exercise. To do so, monitor your heart rate so you can keep it at the required level. Do this by checking your pulse at various times during your exercise, and immediately afterwards.

Some people find taking the pulse manually while exercising to be confusing, easily miscalculated, or difficult. An option is to purchase a simple heart rate monitor that you wear on your wrist to constantly tell you your pulse rate. These are available at sporting goods stores.

The correct heart rate for aerobic exercise is summarized in the chart below, from the International Fitness Association.[2]

Target Heart Rate Chart

Age	Beginner 60% to 70%		Intermediate 70% to 80%		Advanced 80% to 90%	
	Beats/ Min	Beats/ 10 sec*	Beats/ Min	Beats/ 10 sec*	Beats/ Min	Beats/ 10 sec*
to 19	121–141	20–24	141–161	24–27	161–181	27–30
20–24	119–139	20–23	139–158	23–26	158–178	26–30
25–29	116–135	19–23	135–154	23–26	154–174	26–29
30–34	113–132	19–22	132–150	22–25	150–169	25–28
35–39	110–128	18–21	128–146	21–24	146–165	24–28
40–44	107–125	18–21	125–142	21–24	142–160	24–27
45–49	104–121	17–20	121–138	20–23	138–156	23–26
50–54	101–118	17–20	118–134	20–22	134–151	22–25
55–59	98–114	16–19	114–130	19–22	130–147	22–25
60–64	95–111	16–19	111–126	19–21	126–142	21–24
65–69	92–107	15–18	107–122	18–20	122–138	20–23
70–74	89–104	15–17	104–118	17–20	118–133	20–22
75–79	86–100	14–17	100–114	17–19	114–129	19–22
80–84	83–97	14–16	97–110	16–18	110–124	18–21
85+	81–95	14–16	95–108	16–18	108–122	18–20
*To use six-second counts, multiply by 10 to get beats/min Chart courtesy of International Fitness Association						

Your fitness level determines which of the three intensity levels, Beginner, Intermediate, or Advanced, should be maintained. Try to maintain that level during exercise. Start with Beginner if you have not exercised for a while. At least four to six weeks should be spent in each category before moving to the next level if doing three aerobics sessions a week.

Instead of using the chart, you may also calculate your target heart rate. Take the number 220 and subtract your age from it. The number that you get is your maximal heart rate or the highest recommended rate for your heart at all times. This is the level that must never be exceeded. Never exercise even near the maximum heart rate. Up to 90% of your maximum heart rate is safe.

During aerobic exercise, you want to work out at a percentage of your maximum heart rate. Beginners would best start exercising with a lower number (in different references we've seen this number range from 50% to 75% of your maximal heart rate) and increase the rate after you've exercised over a length of time (weeks to months). Average aerobic conditioning is in the intermediate level (we've seen this figure range from 70% to 85% of your maximal heart rate). High-intensity continuous exercise or interval training, which is not for everybody, is done on the higher end of the scale (from 80% to 90% of the maximal heart rate).

Your pulse during the entire 20 minutes must be in the heart rate range calculated for your age and ability level, so check it several times, especially when you are new to aerobics. After stopping your exercise, check your pulse only during the first ten seconds so that your pulse has no chance to slow down. You want to know what your pulse was while you were exercising, not after you have finished.

By frequently checking your pulse when you exercise, you may begin to develop sensitivity for what your pulse is all the time and will be able to adjust the intensity of your exercise program accordingly.

Sixth step: Choose a suitable length of time to exercise. For most people, it would be wise to begin an aerobics program at 20 minutes, three times a week (not including warmup and cool down; see the Seventh Step below). Some people will need to start with less time and increase gradually. Be sure to listen to your body and exercise in a manner that is suitable and comfortable for you.

Seventh step: Be sure to add a recommended warmup and cool-down period right before and after the exercise.

- Warmup makes your workout feel smoother, prevents injuries and helps your body move efficiently from a low to high metabolic state. Perform the same activity you'll be doing for aerobic conditioning at a much lower level of intensity for five to ten minutes. Gradually increase the intensity of exercise until you are at the range of your target heart rate.

- Cool down is a gradual reduction in the intensity of your activity. This slowing of activity helps return blood which has been sent to the working muscles back to normal circulation. To cool down, reduce the intensity of your exercise gradually for five to ten minutes at the end of your exercise.

Eighth step: Monitor the actual improvements in your health. Do this by checking your pulse rate for ten seconds on awakening in the morning and continue to write the number on your calendar every day (which you started in the Third Step above). Four to six weeks after starting your aerobics, you will most likely notice that your awaking pulse rate has dropped 15% to 25%. The changes reflect improvements in your stress level and metabolism from doing AE.

Ninth step: When you do aerobics (or exercise of any kind), if something doesn't feel right or hurts, have it checked. Pain is not good, especially in joints, bone, and chest. Muscle soreness is normal, but not to the point of causing difficulty. Never continue a workout with soreness; instead, give the muscles a chance to repair and rebuild. ■■■ WALT: For example, a problem I experienced when starting AE by jogging was shin splints—painful muscle spasms due to inflammation in the attachments of the shin muscles at the bone. Because of the shin splints, I had to stop my aerobics until I got better, then I restarted. ■■■ Most other pitfalls or common mistakes would be mentioned in basic books about aerobics and in *Fitness for Dummies.*

Aerobics: What You Should Know

Aerobics can be done by all ages. However, older people may need to start quite slowly (shorter time and lower heart rate). Here's a health tip for older adults: Until about the age of 50 to 60, doing aerobic exercise for 20 minutes three times a week is sufficient for general health. At that older age, adding Synergetics (described in a section below) or other stretching activity would be helpful to maintain flexibility.

Look for results in six to eight weeks. You will be able to tell if you have reached the "full benefit" after six to eight weeks of regular aerobic exercise by how much better you feel. Additional benefits will be seen even after three to six months. However, the accrual is much slower.

Start slowly and gradually increase. Either a shorter time or a lower heart rate can be used for starting until your body becomes accustomed to exercise. Listen to your body to know what intensity and duration of exercise is right for you. A reasonable mechanism of self-awareness should alert you if you need to adjust your exercise.

Avoid exercising with a full stomach. Generally, it is better to exercise before eating. We have all been told for years not to go swimming after eating, or we might drown or experience problems like nausea, vomiting, gas, or stomach cramping. Some people, if they have eaten, wait to exercise until they don't feel any sensation of food in their stomach to know that they won't have any problems. We would recommend waiting about two hours after eating before you exercise, mainly depending upon how tough the food you chose to eat is to digest and what kind of exercise you will do. For example, fruit takes but a few minutes, while greasy meat takes more than two hours. It is usually all right to do exercise like gentle walking after eating.

Change your program if you experience excessive fatigue. Fatigue after aerobics is normal for about a week or so into the program. Some people, however, will be fatigued due to Krebs cycle difficulties (See Chapter 3 about diet for information on the Krebs cycle). These individuals experience more than normal fatigue after each exercise period, and weeks later, still experience fatigue from each exercise session. For them, it would be advantageous to discontinue Aerobic Exercise and begin the 3LS by choosing the Perfect Whole Foods Diet and Skilled Relaxation to help correct the Krebs cycle function and reduce the fatigue. You also might use a more gentle form of exercise for a while before starting aerobics. Walking and rebounding are good exercise choices to start with initially. Other kinds of mild exercise are listed later in this chapter.

It's okay to exercise longer than 20 minutes. After you have been exercising for some months, it is all right to increase the time you spend. If you wish to exercise more, we recommend gradually (over a year) working up to an hour, five days a week.

If you don't have extra time in your schedule, know that the most benefit per minutes spent is received from sessions lasting 20 minutes three times a week. People who have little time for exercise can do just that much and know that they are still getting great health benefits. If more is done, there will be some increase in benefits, but there is less benefit per minute spent.

Vary your exercise program. Mix high-impact activities (like jogging, step aerobics, and activities with jumping or hopping) with low-impact, weight-supported activities (like swimming, rowing, and cycling) to avoid continual stress on joints and muscles. Some fitness specialists recommend low-impact activities over high-impact activities for all aerobics.

Remember the other aspects of the 3LS Wellness Program for total health. The "smart shopper" who is really interested in improving health, after doing aerobics for 20 minutes three times a week for six to eight weeks, will then consider spending some time focusing on diet or Skilled Relaxation to provide balanced health benefits. The three aspects of the Program are multipliers of each other, and it may be a better decision to spend the extra time on the other aspects instead of just increasing exercise. This is just as true for people wishing to improve health as it is for those wishing to improve performance, as we mentioned in the section for athletes.

INCREASE YOUR METABOLIC EFFICIENCY FOR HEALTH

The idea behind aerobics is to exercise long enough and hard enough to use up all the oxygen stored in your tissues to get into your "second wind" (to kick in the little-used aerobic metabolic pathway) and then to keep that going for a few minutes. The second wind occurs approximately $12^{1}/_{2}$ minutes after reaching your target heart rate,[3] and that's actually when the major benefits of aerobic exercise accrue.

You see, there are two metabolic pathways in the body:

> **Anaerobic metabolic pathway:** Normally, oxygen goes from our lungs to be a stored type of oxygen in our cells and then from that stored form into action. It is stored so that we will instantly have oxygen available to us, so when the sabretooth tiger lunges (remember "fight or flight"?), we will not have to wait until we can breathe fast enough to spring into action and start running.

> **Aerobic metabolic pathway:** When we do sustained exercise at the specific heart rate for our age, after that average $12^{1}/_{2}$ minutes, we have exhausted all the stored oxygen in the cells. Then, we switch into directly using oxygen from our lungs. This is called reaching the second wind or aerobic metabolic pathway.

By regularly using this mechanism of taking oxygen directly from the lungs (aerobic pathway) many wonderful things happen to help our health. The aerobic method of using oxygen is an oxygen transfer system that is actually 15% to 25% more efficient than the method of using stored oxygen.[4] This is one reason why you feel so energized when the second wind hits and why the second wind feels so wonderful, like you could run or exercise forever.

It only takes four minutes of using the aerobic metabolic pathway to create the health benefits of aerobic exercise. However, it is still very important to do aerobics at your target heart rate for at least 20 minutes. This is because the average time for getting rid of the stored oxygen in the body occurs after $12\frac{1}{2}$ minutes of sustained exercise at the correct heart rate. However, some people deplete the oxygen and achieve the aerobic metabolic pathway in only eight minutes, and others take 16 minutes. Thus, to be certain that you are getting at least 4 minutes of the aerobic metabolic pathway, in case you are one of the 16-minute people, do at least 20 minutes of exercise. By exercising aerobically for 20 minutes, the 16-minute people will get at least 4 minutes of the aerobic metabolic pathway. Those who reach the pathway in eight minutes could actually quit after 12 minutes and do as well, but it is fine to do the full 20 minutes.

What Is Metabolism?

Metabolism is a key concept for understanding how aerobics (and the 3LS) functions to help you achieve wellness and good health. Your metabolism is the interactive combination of all the thousands of chemical reactions that have to work in a certain way in your body, as well as all of the electromagnetic and structural reactions. These reactions produce energy and basic materials needed for important life processes.

All life forms are dependent on many hundreds of simultaneous and precisely regulated metabolic reactions. Each reaction is triggered, controlled, and terminated by specific cell enzymes or catalysts, and coordinated with the numerous other reactions throughout the organism. Each living cell has a metabolism (cell metabolism) and humans have a "total" metabolism that can differ from that of the individual cells. A person's metabolic efficiency can be assessed through many laboratory tests.

Metabolism is often described as a two-part process.

- Anabolism, or constructive metabolism, is the process of using these substances to build or mend cells.

- Catabolism, or destructive metabolism, is a continuous process of using these substances to produce the energy required for all external and internal physical activity.

Both types of reaction have a certain order or pathway to produce specific, life-essential end products. Each process involves the uptake and digestion of some kind of food (this is why nutrition is so important) or oxygen (this is why aerobics is so helpful), and also the disposal of waste products.

It might interest you to know that when anabolism exceeds catabolism, growth or weight gain occurs. When catabolism exceeds anabolism, such as during periods of starvation or disease, weight loss occurs. When the two metabolic processes are balanced, the organism is said to be in a state of dynamic equilibrium.

The anaerobic and the aerobic pathways are both metabolic processes, as is the Krebs cycle.

Your metabolism is determined both by your genetics and lifestyle to this point. Anything that is really healthy for individuals will tend to bring their metabolism back towards normal (wellness). Doing any part of the 3LS, or all of it, creates healthy effects by altering these thousands of chemical reactions towards optimal function.

Aerobics is a metabolic approach to exercise. One of the main purposes of doing aerobics is to improve metabolic efficiency. Kenneth Cooper, M.D., the original expert on aerobics, was not clear how this metabolic improvement happens, and there is still a lot of uncertainty among the experts exactly how aerobics works. However, there is no question that it does work. Perhaps aerobics provides better circulation and distribution of vitamins, minerals, enzymes, etc., for all the metabolic processes in the body. Another possibility for why aerobics benefits the body may be because AE simply provides more oxygen. Energy production (the Krebs cycle) requires oxygen, and the more oxygen available to the cells, the more energy can be produced.

When one has regularly been exercising aerobically, a person feels better all the time and not just during the exercise session. Thus it does seem that aerobics also improves the anaerobic function. The body exercised aerobically seems to "act" as though it was using oxygen aerobically at all times.

AEROBICS Q & A

Q: Should I cross-train in my aerobics practice, i.e., do different types of AE regularly to use different muscle groups, such as bicycling to use leg muscles and rowing to use arm muscles?
A: In terms of getting the metabolic benefits, it does not matter. What's most important for the metabolic benefits is for the pulse rate to be achieved for the 20 minutes.

Varying your exercise can be a good idea, however. Cross-training is good for conditioning different parts of the body and can keep your interest level high so you don't get bored. Mixing high-impact activities like jogging or step aerobics with low-impact, weight-supported activities like rowing and cycling will also decrease the impact to joints and muscles.

Q: I have been doing aerobics every day, seven days a week. Do I need to take days off? Does the body need to have a complete rest sometimes?

A: This seems to be individual and has something to do with the way your body can handle exercise. Some people do well exercising daily, but others need a break. If the time comes when you feel tired and need a rest, take one.

Q: Can a person do too much aerobic exercise?

A: Too much of anything is not a good idea. Gentle to moderate exercise is beneficial for everyone, but a narrow-minded focus on exercise can be unhealthy. Excessive exercise can stress the body's reserves and lead to depletion and health problems. Currently, some professionals are recommending an hour a day, seven days a week of cardiovascular activity as a healthy level of exercise, but we think exercising more than that may be over the line.

Q: But isn't the amount of exercise each person needs an individual matter? What about athletes or people who do triathalons, run marathons, and do long distance bicycle races? They have to train intensively to participate in these events and might be doing aerobics more than one hour a day.

A: How much you exercise depends upon your goal, of course, but doing too much of anything is not advisable. For example, over-training can lead to hormonal abnormalities. The absence of menses in many female aerobic practitioners exercising at high levels tells us they may be substituting ego for health. Professional athletes are also known to have a shorter life span than other people and many must retire early because they "burn out." Some people also use excessive amounts of exercise as a crutch or drug to avoid facing their life problems, and this is a misuse of exercise.

Problems can also occur from exercise not balanced with other healthy activities such as Skilled Relaxation and nutritious diet. Moderation and balance are two good principles to follow for reaching the goals of achieving and maintaining good health.

Q: Should I stretch before or after aerobic exercise?

A: Stretching before and after exercise accomplishes different things. Stretching before exercise tends to prevent exercise-related injuries, and stretching after exercise gives the muscles the most effective stretch.

A Massage Therapist's Experience with Stretching

■■■ JAN: *Before* your workout, warm up your muscles with gentle exercise, then stretch. Focus your stretches on the muscles you use most in your particular workout. Move slowly into each stretching position, pay attention to your body, do not overstretch or bounce, and breathe deeply. Avoid stretching when muscles are cold and tight, or they have contracted because of pain or fatigue, or when a joint aches or has been twisted.

Stretching before exercise increases blood flow to muscles, increasing the temperature of muscles and joints and allowing muscles to extend further. Stretching before exercise also makes joints more flexible and prevents strains, for example, when running on uneven ground.

After exercising, wait until after your cool-down (to allow the body's blood flow to normalize so you do not become light headed or nauseous), then stretch.

Stretching after exercise keeps stressed muscles from contracting hard and cramping, and facilitates the removal of metabolic waste products. Stretch both after cardiovascular (aerobic exercise) and strength training.

Stretch daily if possible, even on the days you don't work out, to keep muscles flexible, prevent injury, improve performance, and to help muscles respond more quickly and powerfully in all circumstances. It's nice to learn a variety of stretches and vary your flexibility routine to stretch your muscles at different angles. Remember that the development of flexibility takes time, so be content with slow and steady results from stretching.[5]

Other stretching protocols are available, but I have found this one to be very effective. Stretching can also be a form of exercise in itself. See the second half of this chapter. ■■■

Q: If I only stretch once, is it better to do it before or after exercise?
A: Possibly before, since if you are injured, you will not be able to exercise at all. Of course, if you stretch both before and after, you get the maximum benefit.

Q: I work all day and I don't have enough energy or time to start doing aerobics! I'm too tired after a day at work. What can I do?
A: If you use the excuse that you are too tired for aerobics, you are just kidding yourself. If done correctly, after a few weeks, you will have more energy following aerobics than before you started. If you are tired or fatigued, AE is most likely exactly what you need to get your energy back (unless your fatigue is due to Krebs cycle problems, see pages 83–84 and 141).

Also, people who do aerobics tend to end up sleeping more soundly and wake up more refreshed with fewer hours of sleep needed. Thus, the 60 minutes or so spent each week doing aerobic exercise is typically returned several times over in additional hours available for activity. The fewer hours spent sleeping and the increased efficiency in accomplishing tasks because of more energy and alertness can help your daily time management. Therefore, the excuse that "I don't have time to do this" is exactly that—an excuse.

Q: Can I do aerobics once a week for 60 minutes instead of three times a week for 20 minutes?

A: Aerobics once a week does not bring the desired health benefits and also increases the potential of recurrent injuries.

Q: I work four days a week, ten hours a day. If I do AE on my three days off, which is three days in a row, will I still get the great benefits of doing aerobics?

A: It is better if your exercise is spaced out, as much for prevention of injuries as for effectiveness. However, doing AE this way is certainly better than not at all. Even doing it this way, you may find within a few months that each night you will need about an hour less sleep than before, giving you the extra time to do aerobics on your workdays.

Q: I have problems with my knees. Can I do aerobic exercise?

A: Yes, however be selective about the kind of exercise you do. When a person has arthritis, baker's cysts, old traumatic damage to the knee, chondromalacia, or other condition in a knee joint, weight-bearing exercise like dancing, climbing stairs, or even walking increases the pressure within the joint. In the worst case, such exercise grinds away the cartilaginous surfaces of the joint. Every joint movement under load may be just one fewer movement that joint is capable of making during your lifetime. In a way, with those conditions, the number of steps you have left to take in this lifetime may be limited. You need to consider how you will spend them.

We recommend water exercise for people with such conditions. The water supports much of the weight of the body, allowing the exercise to strengthen the muscles without further grinding away the joints. Many communities with indoor pool facilities have water aerobics programs. Rowing and certain exercise machines (like elliptical machines or recumbent bicycles) might be other options. Do anything that takes the weight off the knees.

If you have a particular health condition or need, consult with a personal trainer or fitness expert about finding other kinds of exercise that will not cause further progression of your condition. The key concept with exercise, and all of the parts of the 3LS, is "Do what works for you."

Q: I have not been able to tolerate exercise for a long time because of illness. Lately I've been doing gentle rebounding, and I would now like to start doing actual aerobics, slowly. Would it be better to start with ten minutes at a time, three times a week (which I know won't allow me to reach the aerobic metabolic pathway), or 20 minutes at a time, once a week?

A: When you are recovering from a chronic illness, and are just starting to exercise, it does not matter how long or how often. Start with as much as you can do, one or more times a week. At the beginning, you can even do five minutes at a time. What you are doing is getting your muscles and your body accustomed to this.

Work up slowly to longer and more frequent exercise sessions until you can sustain 20 minutes three times a week. By slowly, we mean you may need to stay at a certain level of exercise for several weeks or even several months. Do not be in a hurry to increase the intensity or length of exercise sessions, but take your time to avoid placing unnecessary stress on the body. People who try to add too much too fast often have to stop exercising to recover, and so they lose their safe and steady momentum and health benefits.

Q: Aerobics is famous for helping reduce stress. Does AE alleviate the stored-stress effect in the hypothalamus?

A: ■■■ WALT: Good question! It is well known that the resting pulse is a good indicator of stored stress-effect.[6] The higher your resting pulse, the more stored stress-effect is present. The drop in resting pulse rate that occurs around six weeks after starting aerobics is a direct measure of discharge of accumulated stress and increasing metabolic efficiency.

The simplistic explanation for the drop in pulse rate has been that exercise is similar to fleeing and fighting, and so it discharges the stored-stress effect. While this may be the case, I do not think this is the majority of the good effect brought by the weeks of aerobics. The drop in the resting pulse after doing AE over a period of weeks happens too fast for it to be all due to the reduction of stored stress-effect. I think aerobics mainly increases the horsepower (increased physical strength and energy) the individual has to handle the stress load. ■■■

Aerobic Exercise—Points to Remember

- See your doctor for a stress test before starting aerobics.
- Read a book about aerobics to learn more about it.
- Be sure to start slowly, and listen to your body.
- When doing aerobics, if something hurts or doesn't feel right, have it checked by a sports medicine specialist, massage therapist, or physician.
- Make sure you are achieving the correct heart rate for 20 minutes so that you get the benefits.
- Do not exercise within two hours after a meal.
- Exercise before your Skilled Relaxation practice to enhance the benefits of both. Exercising after Skilled Relaxation nullifies the effects of the Skilled Relaxation session.
- Aerobics is many times more effective in promoting health than non-aerobic exercise.

OTHER EXERCISES AND THEIR EFFECTS

This section introduces you to other forms of exercise that you can do according to your goals, ability, and interest. Each type of exercise uses the body in different ways and so gives different results and benefits. So far as we know, the health parameters for non-aerobic exercise are just now beginning to be investigated and determined scientifically. For example, some recent reports have come to light of the benefits of just walking three to five times a week for 30 minutes. There will be a lot more information available in the future as more studies are completed.

Exercise physiologists can talk for hours about the individual benefits of the specific exercises we have listed, and entire books have been written on each of the exercises. Therefore there is no need to duplicate that information here. This section of our book is mostly meant to help you choose something to do, and interest you in learning more about it. We will describe the most important effects of each and refer you to the Resources section at the end of this book for learning more.

The following paragraphs describe basic categories of exercise (besides aerobics) and mention some health conditions that are likely to improve with their use. For total health, doing something from each of the three categories of exercise is best, plus aerobics, if you have enough time to do them all. You might also alternate them.

Non-aerobic (Anaerobic) Exercise

Exercise that is milder than aerobics is mainly for prevention of cancer, diabetes, aging, breathing problems, and rehabilitation. Non-aerobic exercise does not increase the heart rate to a significant degree, and so it does not have cardiovascular benefits like aerobics. However, it builds stamina that can help anyone battle stress and help prevent disease. Examples of anaerobics include Alexander Technique, balancing and coordination exercises, Feldenkrais, gentle rebounding, qi gong, Pilates, stretching exercises, strengthening exercises, Synergetics, t'ai chi, walking, and yoga.

Strengthening Exercise

Strengthening exercises are for building muscular strength in parts or the entire body. Strength training is generally non-aerobic. Strength can mean many different things, and another variable to strength is the area or part of the body being strengthened. Examples of strength training include isometrics, Pilates, progressive resistance exercise, and weight training.

Flexibility Exercise

People who do not maintain a normal range of motion of all muscles slowly lose their flexibility. Any health book will tell you how important full range of motion is for maintaining health and youthfulness as you age. Remember the principle of "use it or lose it."

Flexibility exercises are effective for conditions like bracing, chronic fatigue syndrome, fibromyositis, invalidism, musculoskeletal disorders, prevention of arthritis, recurrent back or neck pain, reducing the effects of aging, and stiff-man syndrome. Examples of stretching exercises include: Pilates, stretching or flexibility exercises, Synergetics, and yoga.

■ ■ ■

Some exercises fall into more than one category. To help you get started, here is a list of some activities and exercises that can be fun to do:

Adventure racing	Canoeing	Exercise (fitness or
Aikido	Circuit class	physio-) ball
Alexander Technique	Coordination exercises	Exercise boot camps
Backpacking	Cricket	Exercise videos
Badminton	Dancing (how about	Feldenkrais
Balancing exercises	hip-hop, belly	Football
Basketball	dancing, or square	Frisbee
Body sculpting	dancing for some fun?)	Fun runs or walks
Bowling	Downhill skiing	Golf

Handball
Health clubs
Hiking
Hockey
Isometric exercise
Jazzercise
Karate
Kayaking
Kick-boxing
Martial arts
NIA
Pilates
Ping pong
Prenatal exercise

Progressive resistance
    exercise
Qi gong
Racquetball
Rebounding (mini-
    trampoline)
Rock climbing
Roller skating
Rollerblading
Soccer
Softball
Snowboarding
Snowshoeing
Stretching

Swimming
Synergetics
T'ai chi
Tennis
Trampoline
Triathlons
Ultimate frisbee
Volleyball
Walk-a-thons
Walking
Walking hills
Water exercises
Weight machines
Weight training
Yoga

Below is a short description of several of the exercises mentioned above and their benefits. We're detailing a few here because of their usefulness. If any of these exercises interest you, we recommend that you learn more about them before you actually start by reading an appropriate book (see the Resources section at the end of this book), take a class, or seek the guidance of an exercise professional such as a personal trainer.

Alexander technique and Feldenkrais are for bodymind integration. Alexander Technique is a simple method of movement designed to teach awareness of how we move as we go about our everyday activities. Its goal is regaining the natural grace and balance of a child, and discovering easier and more efficient ways of movement. Feldenkrais is an approach that expands a person's repertoire of movements, enhances awareness, and improves function. This is done by expanding the self-image through movement sequences that bring attention to the parts of self that are out of awareness and by improving the relationship to gravity.

Balancing and coordination exercises are for enhancing core stability, balance, coordination, and reflexes. Whether you are a high performance athlete, dancer, or an older individual, balance is a critical function for completion of activities. Medications, poor vision, gait, balance disorders, and chronic medical conditions may indicate the need for balance and perception training. The simplest device used is a balance or wobble board. Certain yoga postures and balance beams may also be used for balance training. Bodymind coordination may be improved through activities like dance and specific drills.

Isometric exercise is a form of active exercise that raises muscle tension by putting pressure against stable resistance. This may be achieved by opposing different muscles in the same person, as by pressing the hands together, or by making a limb push or pull against an immoveable object. There is no joint movement and the muscle length remains the same. Isometrics can be helpful for a goal of building muscle mass quickly.

Pilates is a series of exercises that involve slow, precise movements, either using your body weight or specially designed equipment to work your muscles. You might work your abdominal and leg muscles, for example, by pushing against a bar on springs or by raising your legs when they're attached by straps to a pulley. Some exercises are conducted on a mat which may be taught in a class. Many people benefit from using Pilates for rehabilitation from accidents or injury, and for strengthening the core muscles of the body (abdominals and back muscles) for improved posture and stamina.

Progressive resistance exercise consists of using low weights with a high number of repetitions. It is a new technique that has been found to be effective at reversing the effects of aging and sarcopenia (muscle wasting).

Resistance is essential for making a muscle stronger. When a muscle has to work against a load placed on it, it adapts to the stress by creating new muscle fibers and making neurological changes that ultimately make it stronger. Progressive resistance exercise is believed to be the most effective strengthener for people for whom aerobic exercise is not practical or older people who have allowed their muscles to atrophy.

Start with the amount of weight that is easy and do 10 reps. Then, each week (or after several weeks), add a little weight. Stop adding weight when it becomes even a little hard to do the 10 reps. Then a week or a few weeks later, add a little more weight.

Rebounding is a low-impact exercise done on a rebounder (mini-trampoline). It has many health benefits. Rebounding is excellent for stimulating lymph circulation, which greatly assists with detoxification processes. It can be done at any level of fitness and may be aerobic if done vigorously. Even though muscular exercise may be derived from rebounding, the greatest health results come from the movement itself. Even very gentle rebounding (just gently bouncing up and down without lifting the feet from the mini-trampoline) produces benefits due to the circulation of fluids including lymph and blood.

Rebounding for ten minutes, several times a day, can be very beneficial for health for those who have been ill or are weak. One of the nice things about rebounding is that people who are very weak can even have someone else do it for them at first. The weakened person can just sit on the mini-trampoline and the other can create the bouncing motion. Similarly, if someone has leg or knee problems, the good benefits may be derived by standing on the rebounder and moving the forearms up and down just enough to create a rhythmic movement with the body going up and down.

Stretching relaxes muscles, therefore it decreases tension and muscle spasms, restores flexibility, and increases range of motion. Regular stretching can be useful for any specific area of the body. For those who are bracing, great benefits come from daily stretching of all the major muscle groups (full-body stretching). Full-body stretching relieves tension in the entire nervous system and is marvelous for enhancing bodily self-awareness.

Stretching also increases the ability of a muscle to contract, so it is helpful for athletes who wish to improve their performance.

Synergetics is a gentle series of movements that are no-impact and no-stress. Synergetics can be easily done in the midst of everyday activities and is very effective with very little expenditure of time. Synergetics is designed to gently stretch and strengthen all 600 muscles and not spend much time outside daily activities to do it (12 minutes twice a day). We especially recommend it for people over 50. A video and book are available (see Resources).

T'ai chi, qi gong, yoga, and many of the thousands-year-old Eastern disciplines that are gentle to do, are marvelous for relaxation, development of energy flow in the body, and general health. These exercises are widely available for learning in classes, books, and videos.

T'ai chi and qi gong are traditional Chinese exercises that combine controlled breathing, gentle movements, and mild stretching together to harmonize the bodymind.

Yoga is a gentle exercise that uses posture and breathing to build strength, endurance, and flexibility, as well as increase your breath capacity. Yoga can be done every day and at any age.

Walking. Today overwhelming medical research exists that shows significant benefits from simple walking. Even something as casual as a walk around the block can help you burn off some of the tension that you carry around. Gentle walking has different benefits than aerobic walking. Aerobics can be achieved with brisk walking and provides all the benefits of aerobics mentioned earlier in this chapter. Gentle walking is effective for general metabolic health for those unable to do aerobics. If you can, walk at least 30 minutes, three times a week, but it is appropriate for you to start with however much you can.

Water exercises (swimming, water aerobics). Communities with an indoor pool now have water exercise programs taught and supervised by physical therapists or fitness instructors. Chest-high aerobics and swimming are the important ones. Water aerobics can provide a vigorous workout and are especially wonderful for exercise if a person is overweight, experiences generalized arthritis, or has conditions where weight bearing would make your condition worse. Localized issues such as knee, hip, ankle, or foot conditions are also best treated or exercised under water. The water exercises have been almost unbelievable for arthritic patients.

Weight-training (weight-lifting) is for building muscle strength and mass. It is using high weights with low reps (the opposite of progressive resistance, which is low weights with high reps).

■ ■ ■

You can find many opportunities for exercise. Seek out YMCAs, community recreation centers, health and fitness clubs, mall-walking programs, clubs for all kind of activities, videotapes, TV programs, sporting goods stores and other venues.

Alternate types of exercise for balanced training. One possible regimen for combining different types of exercise would be doing AE three times a week and walking on the off-days. Another combination is doing Synergetics or stretching every day, and progressive resistance exercises at least three times a week. Design an exercise program to suit your goals!

TROUBLESHOOTING FOR EXERCISE

Troubleshooting Q & A

Q: I'm having trouble getting started exercising. Do you have any suggestions?

A: The truism in holistic healing that "people tend to put off the very thing they need the most until the very last" applies to exercise as well as the other parts of the Wellness Program. We have found that those who will just do *something,* even if very easy, frequently will adjust their standards and goals upward as their level of fitness progresses. Start with something very simple and non-vigorous like rebounding, synergetics, or gentle walking. Just get

Not a Fitness Pro? Here Are Some Tips

- **Get a medical exam** if you are beginning an exercise program for the first time or after a long pause from exercising, to clear you for exercise.
- **Consider previous injuries** that might be affected when selecting an activity.
- **Begin slowly,** and do not overdo. Plan to get in shape during several weeks and months, not in days. Follow common sense and don't push past exhaustion. The older you are, and the heavier (% fat) you are, the slower you should start your exercise program. Take it easy at the beginning with reduced speeds and short exercise sessions.
- **Listen to yourself** before you do something that seems too challenging even if recommended by coaches, teachers, experts, or friends. Exercise is like good medicine for you, but you have to find the correct dose for your individual needs. Go at your own pace and do the amount that feels right for you and according to your capability.
- **Monitor your progress.** Taking your time will help you be careful not to flare up existing conditions. Troubleshoot in three to four weeks and modify your exercise plan as needed.
- **Wear good quality, supportive shoes.** Your joints and back will appreciate it.
- **Avoid eating** two to three hours before engaging in vigorous exercise. Also, try to avoid eating for about one hour after exercising.
- **Do not drink cold (55° F) beverages** while perspiring or right after exercising.
- **It's good to exercise outdoors** in the fresh air whenever possible, and be inspired by nature, too. However...
- **People with certain illnesses** or conditions, who are very sensitive to the external environment, may feel better exercising indoors where they can control the temperature, workout, humidity, etc.
- **If the weather is bad,** have a backup plan such as a fitness club, home equipment, exercise videos, or TV shows.
- **Exercise safely.** Avoid jogging or walking alone in the dark or in desolate areas. While taking care of your health, don't forget your safety.
- **Use the chart** in Chapter 5 to keep track of your pulse rate and aerobics program.

into the habit of doing these activities daily or several times a week to start with, then build your exercise program by adding more and different kinds of exercise later.

If you're having trouble getting started or staying motivated...

- Start with something very easy.
- Figure out your obstacles to starting an exercise program and make a plan to overcome them.
- Know the benefits that you are looking for and work toward achieving them.
- Find an exercise buddy to help you both keep your schedule and have more fun. But try to avoid exercising with a partner who differs greatly in age or physical condition than you.
- Consider a session or two with a personal trainer. Or join a fitness club and make some friends there to help keep you going.
- Buy yourself some fun or flattering exercise clothing.
- Take it one day at a time.
- Reward yourself for continued discipline with some kind of healthy treat.

Q: Do things like dancing, gardening, backpacking, and going up the stairs count as exercise? Does exercise done on the job, i.e., lifting boxes, doing massage, painting, and construction work count as exercise?

A: You'll benefit from getting any kind of exercise in the regular activity of daily life. However, most articles we have seen compare those exercises with being a total couch potato. Certainly it is an improvement.

If there is no exercise in your life at all, even making small changes like parking at the end of the parking lot so that you walk farther to the store and back to your car, or taking the stairs instead of an elevator, is an improvement. Some individuals use a pedometer to count the number of steps they take each day to document these small improvements for the sake of encouragement.

Remember that none of these are aerobic activities unless they meet the standard for pulse and time.

Q: Is it more important to have physical strength or cardiovascular strength? One needs both kinds of strength, right? Which is more important for basic health?

A: Cardiovascular health will keep you alive long enough to do the other exercises for the duration necessary enough to get their results. So far as is presently known, the other exercises do not prolong life but only improve the quality of life and health while the person is living.

Q: Can exercise help heal chronic illness? I am 21 and recently I have had two spinal fractures. From the look of the x-rays, the radiologist and doctor think my bones are not dense enough and that I may have osteoporosis in spite of my age. If I do lots of weight bearing exercise and take calcium supplements, will my bones get dense again?

A: Exercise can be used to help reverse many chronic conditions. Osteoporosis is just one of many examples. In your case, osteoporosis is reversible, but you are going to have to embark on a very different lifestyle. You have a genetic susceptibility, or this would not be happening to you at your young age. Besides Practicing Serious Wellness, I also think it well worth your while to find a good holistic practitioner and a sports medicine specialist. Take a copy of your medical records and the bone density report. If you do these things, you will totally change your life for the better.

Q: Patient A: I am recovering from an illness, are there any considerations about exercise to keep in mind? Patient B: I'm too weak to exercise or my body feels worse after exercise than before. What should I do?

A: As mentioned previously, people who feel very fatigued from exercise may have Krebs cycle difficulties and would benefit by beginning the Relaxation and Diet legs of the 3LS first before beginning an exercise program.

If you have been seriously or chronically ill, or if you cannot exercise at all, start with non-aerobic exercise and build up slowly. Start with five to ten minutes of walking or gentle rebounding, once or twice a day. If you cannot even do rebounding, sit on the mini-trampoline and have someone make the bouncing happen for you. Just do what feels comfortable.

If your illness has not been severe, or if you are starting to feel better and want to start aerobics, begin with a reduced intensity of exercise for a short length of time. Start with five minutes of easy aerobics. When you start feeling like you want to do something more strenuous, your body will tell you it is time: "My goodness, this energy is fantastic, I need to get out and jog up a hill." Then slowly build up to 20 minutes, three times a week.

Otherwise, the kind of exercise that would be most beneficial for you depends upon your condition. We have mentioned the general benefits of each type of exercise, and you can choose which one to experiment with first.

Consult a sports medicine specialist or personal trainer for additional help with selecting an exercise.

Q: Yesterday I went cross-country skiing, and today I'm so sore and tired I can hardly get out of bed. Why?
A: Most people tend to overdo any exercise in the beginning. It can feel so good to be exercising, sometimes it's easy to overdo it. You will get in aerobic shape soon enough, so there is no need to try to do it instantly.

You have overdone it if:

- 10 to 15 minutes after having stopped the exercise, you still feel out of breath.
- Two hours after the exercise you feel unusually fatigued.
- You cannot sleep well that night.
- The next morning you feel physically fatigued and sore.

If you experience pain during or after exercising, you have likely injured yourself. See an appropriate practitioner if needed.

Q: I've been exercising for months and then took a week off. I was incredibly sore when I started up again, which surprised me. What happened?
A: What I have experienced and what patients have shared with me is what you have probably noticed yourself: if you miss a few days of a regular exercise program, your muscles begin to tell you about it. This is normal.

Q: My problem is maintaining momentum because depression causes me to get sidetracked from exercise.
A: Some individuals who lose momentum due to depression have found that practicing Skilled Relaxation can help pick them up and give them energy to get moving. We have also given you many suggestions in this chapter for finding ways to get moving and stay interested. Also see the question below.

Q: Patient A: I still can't get off the couch. Patient B: I still can't find the time or opportunity. Patient C: I don't have any money for a health club or exercise equipment.
A: No motivation, time, or money? But you'll feel so good after you start…

Getting motivated: If you are having trouble beginning your exercise program due to lack of motivation…

- Remember that doing something, no matter how little, is always better than doing nothing.

- Find *anything* that will be easy or fun for you to do. If you enjoy something, you're more likely to do it consistently. Find some activity that feels comfortable.

- Don't look at exercise as a routine you have to do. Consider it your fun time and find ways to make the exercise enjoyable and make you smile.

- Start with even five minutes each time.

- Start by doing just enough so you feel better instead of tired, and you will soon come to enjoy the exercise and your motivation will increase.

- Find an exercise buddy and make a commitment so you will be obligated to be there and not let someone else down.

- Start your exercise program when you're on vacation.

- Get a little extra energy by eating a small healthy snack before you exercise.

- It's true that dramatic changes from exercise take time, but subtle changes happen immediately and can give you the encouragement to do more. After just one workout (whatever workout means to you), you will reap the psychological benefits of enhanced mood, an increased sense of relaxation, a decrease in anxiety, and a surge in self-esteem. Do at least enough so that you get this good feeling!

- Remember to find a healthy way to reward yourself for exercising regularly.

Time or logistics issues: Plan a strategy to make time and space for exercise. Some possible strategies:

- Exercise first thing in the morning, before you start your day, on your lunch break five days a week, or the first thing you do when you get home from work.

- Combine activities, such as exercising while watching TV, or walking to the bank to make your deposit instead of driving.

- Use social events as opportunities for exercise. Instead of playing bridge or going to movies, take walks, go golfing, or watch an exercise video or DVD with your friends.

- Schedule a regular appointment in your day-timer for your exercise session.

- If child care is a concern, think about a babysitting exchange. If you work, exercise at lunch or during the workday when child care is already in place. Or, exercise together with your kids.
- Make exercise a priority and schedule other activities around it.

Keeping costs down: Many forms of exercise are free, including walking, jogging, hiking, jumping rope, stretching, isometrics, dancing, and stair climbing.

- Hold a book or can of food for arm exercises. To make a heavier weight, fill a bucket with cans, rocks, or bags of beans.
- Squeeze a tennis ball.
- Do stretching. Use a belt, sash, rope, or towel if you need to gently pull into a stretch.
- Use a sturdy step stool to do step-ups or climb your stairs.
- Turn on the radio and dance.
- Follow along with TV exercise shows.
- Go for a brisk walk or jog around the neighborhood.
- See if your community has a walking, hiking, biking, or jogging club, or a softball league.
- Some YMCAs offer a financial assistance program for those who cannot afford to pay the full membership fee.
- Borrow some exercise videos or DVDs from the library.
- Go mall-walking.

Exercise and injury

■■■ JAN: The incidence of sports injuries is higher now because more people are exercising these days without having the benefit of the kind of health care support given to professional athletes.

Since weekend warriors (people who exercise only on weekends) don't always know much about how the body works or how to care for it, injuries and problems can be more common for them. For example, when beginning exercise of any type, many people have connective tissue restrictions, which limit their movement and make them feel stiff, sore, and tired. Visits to a massage therapist can help loosen up these restrictions, help you learn how to take good care of your body, prevent injury, and give you feedback about problem areas. There is even a whole area of massage called sports massage, which caters specifically to the needs of athletes and weekend warriors.

One example of injury from even mild exercise is the "yoga casualty" I regularly see in my massage office. New yoga students sometimes stretch beyond their limits, possibly due to desire to compete or from trying to emulate the teacher, who has probably been doing the practices for many years and is very flexible. If you take up yoga, or any exercise activity, listen to your body and only do what is comfortable for you rather than using a predetermined idea or following an instructor's direction too closely. Therapeutic massage can be used by anyone who exercises for increasing awareness and prevention of injuries, and be an opening to a lifetime of wellness. ■■■

Troubleshooting checklist

✓   Are you starting out slowly enough?

✓   Have you read more information about the type of exercise you are doing to make sure you are doing it correctly?

✓   Are you doing your exercise before, not after, regular meals and Skilled Relaxation practice?

✓   Are you getting proper nutrition and drinking extra water?

✓   If your activity does not seem to be helping your condition, consider trying a different exercise activity. Try one that is, for example, less vigorous or uses your body in a different way. Also try beginning your wellness program with a different leg of the 3LS Wellness Program or adding a second part of the 3LS.

When to seek professional help with exercise

With care, exercise can be very safe. Below are the few situations we know of that may require professional help.

•   Not starting slowly enough or not listening to your body may aggravate old injuries or cause new injuries. Injuries are usually characterized by sharp or localized pain experienced continually or when you do certain movements (as contrasted to aching feelings from sore muscles). Stop doing the activity, because continuing exercise can turn a minor injury into a major one needing months of rehabilitation. *Fitness for Dummies* has a good description of common injuries, descriptions of home remedies, and information for knowing when you need to consult a physician or sports medicine specialist.

- Avoid serious conditions like a heart attack by consulting your physician before starting an exercise program.

- Many conditions or diseases have contraindications for exercise. For example, people with detached retina possibilities (or a family history of them) should never do yoga that puts their head in a low position, people with low blood pressure should avoid activity that makes them lightheaded, and so on. We cannot list all health concerns in this book, so check with a physician, personal trainer, or sports medicine specialist if you have specific health conditions, and always inform your exercise instructors of your health problems.

If your activity seems to be stimulating health problems, read the section on pages 188–192 in Chapter 5 about the healing crisis to understand the body's response to healing.

THE AUTHORS' EXPERIENCES

■■■ WALT: As a team physician, I began to apply the approach of conditioning training to the high school team in the little Ohio town where I launched my medical career. Fortunately for the team and for me, the coach was amenable to my innovations. The football team, the only sport deemed to need a team physician at the time by the city fathers, had a tradition of coming in last every year. The result of my approach of recommending year-round conditioning exercises was that within three years, the incidence of injury went almost to zero, and we won the championship. Within two more years, all the other football teams in our conference had adopted my conditioning program! This was in the early '60s, and this conditioning program rapidly spread until Ohio was one of the first states in the country to adopt it as a high school policy.

The results I saw clinically with the football team began to take the concept out of purely professional interest and into the personal. If it did this much good for kids, how much good might it do for me? I had never been athletic, except for ping pong and tennis, but this was about the time that Dr. Cooper published his landmark book, *Aerobics,* so I started jogging. However, within a week of starting my running program, I suffered shin splints and had to quit. I studied the causes of shin splints to keep them from happening when I began jogging again.

After I dealt with the shin splints, and started my aerobics program more slowly, I was routinely reaching an aerobic level within a few weeks.

Once I felt the "second wind" phenomena, I could not wait to exercise on my aerobics day.

Within six weeks after starting my aerobics program, the benefits were so dramatic that even my very conservative medical colleagues began asking me what I was doing. Of course, they had heard about the crazy new doctor running out on the highway at all hours of the day and night, but they seemed to want to hear it from me. So far as I knew (and still know), I was the only person in this town of 10,000 people who was jogging at the time. Remember, this was in the early '60s, long before the exercise for health attitude caught on. The upshot was that I was asked to run an aerobics program for the county. Most of the docs joined the program, and their example made it very popular with patients. It was the most successful preventive medicine program in the county for years. We jogged on the high school track in good weather and ran in the high school gym during inclement weather. Too bad there was no indoor pool in this little community or we would have had the first water aerobics program in the state as well.

Aerobics became a lifetime practice for me. Within six months of beginning my program, I experienced every benefit on the list at the beginning of this chapter. Meanwhile, I became aware of other kinds of specialized exercise techniques over the years from my trainers and coaches, since I maintained my interest in practicing sports medicine. I enjoyed qi gong and t'ai chi by going to conferences in holistic medicine. I learned about rebounding from Al Carter and was urged to actually try it by Terri-Lynn Johnson, one of the clinicians at my center. All these forms of exercise were beneficial. However, my favorite choice remained aerobic exercise. I have yet to see anyone who did aerobics who did not think it was the best thing since sliced bread. ■■■

■■■ JAN: I really enjoy physical activity, and at different times in my life I have derived pleasure from hiking, backpacking, swimming, jogging, dancing (many kinds), snowshoeing, and bicycling. However, until recently, I never exercised regularly three times a week as Walt recommends. I wish I had known what I was missing!

Several decades ago, when life circumstances became very difficult and I was unable to exercise at all for many years, my health declined significantly. When I finally started my recovery, I couldn't do aerobics. My body was functioning so poorly that a four-mile easy walk or easy bike ride left me so fatigued it would take me four days to recover. At that time, I was bracing tremendously.

Fortunately, I figured out that stretching really helped alleviate my bracing. Stretching was the only form of exercise my body could tolerate at this time. Thus I began my exercise program with stretching 30 minutes every day without fail. At first I could only do a few stretches. As my flexibility increased through daily practice (the stretches I did regularly became easy as I became more mobile), I kept adding more and more new stretches to my routine. After about a year of daily stretching, I was able to stretch all the major muscles of my entire body in less than half an hour, and I consequently felt so much better!

By this time, I had found Walt's website, and he suggested that I add daily rebounding and gentle walking to my exercise program. Just adding those two activities made me feel great! Rebounding and Skilled Relaxation really complement stretching for the purpose of relieving bracing.

Starting rebounding was the simplest and most effective lifestyle change I've ever made. There is a world of difference between a day with no rebounding and a day with 15 minutes of gentle rebounding. It takes *no* energy to do some gentle bouncing. On a day with rebounding, I'm more relaxed and energized, my body feels better aligned, and I feel happier. What a difference even this tiny bit of exercise makes! I have even taken my mini-trampoline with me in the car when I go on vacation. The effects of doing simple exercises *on a regular basis* like rebounding, stretching, and walking were cumulative, and helped tremendously with my recovery. This stage of exercising made me feel like I was reclaiming and in control of my body rather than being at its mercy. What a *wonderful* feeling that was.

I then had a lot of false starts with the next step of my exercise program. I kept overdoing it whenever I tried to start aerobics or weights, and would not feel well afterwards and had to stop. It took some time before I found the right kind and amount of exercise for this stage of my recovery. I learned that only a very small amount of gentle exercise *once a week* was what I needed. I started taking a yoga class one day a week at the YMCA. The stretching, strengthening, and breathing of yoga were magical in helping my nervous system work better. At the beginning, I had to stop and rest frequently in class, but after six months of just once-a-week yoga practice, I had much more stamina and rarely had to stop and rest, if at all. I hadn't thought exercising only once a week would provide any benefit, but it was just the ticket!

From the yoga class, I became well enough and strong enough to start adding more exercise. It really surprised me that such a small amount of regular exercise—the yoga class—could open the door to better physical function. Now besides yoga, I'm lifting 10 to 15 pounds on the weight machines once a week without experiencing fatigue, and sometimes also taking a 3-mile hike. I feel great!

From my own experience, I am convinced of the miraculous power of regular exercise. I hadn't realized that my muscles had become weak from my being ill for so long, and how much that physical weakness was in itself a continual stressor keeping me ill. I am now learning how to become a personal trainer so I can help guide other people to find and enjoy the right exercise for them, too. ■■■

Chapter 4, The Right Exercise—SUMMING IT UP

Exercise is an essential part of a healthy lifestyle. Regardless of the type of health problem you have, you'll be further along the road to recovery if you start doing any kind of exercise on a regular basis. Every bodily system that has been studied has been shown to improve in function with simple exercise.

Aerobic exercise was the first really effective and medically documented approach to exercise, and provides the greatest enhancement to health. However, aerobics is not best for meeting all health goals, and other exercises may be done alongside or instead of aerobics. Each type of exercise has varying effects and benefits, so it's important to choose the right kind of exercise to address your health goals.

Athletes, who of course already exercise sufficiently, would benefit from adding the other two parts of the Wellness Program, Skilled Relaxation and Perfect Whole Foods Diet, to their training.

Aerobics is any extended physical activity that increases heart rate and breathing while using the large muscle groups at a regular, even pace. Aerobics makes you healthy by increasing your metabolic efficiency. Metabolism is the interactive combination of chemical, electromagnetic, and structural reactions in the body. Aerobics improves both the aerobic and anaerobic metabolic pathways in the body.

Other types of exercise include the broad categories of non-aerobic (anaerobic) exercise, strengthening exercise, and flexibility exercise. There are many varieties of exercise in each category. New exercise methods and combinations are being invented all the time. There are many possibilities and ways to find exercise opportunities.

To help you learn more about different types of exercise and select the one that is right for you, we recommend that you read *Fitness for Dummies,* by Suzanna Schlosberg and Liz Neporent.

Aerobic Exercise Summary—STEPS TO TAKE

1. Check with your doctor to see if you need a stress test before you start doing aerobics. Also, read *Aerobics,* by Kenneth Cooper or any other book about aerobic exercise.

2. Every day, before you get out of bed in the morning, check your awakening pulse rate for ten seconds, and write the number of heartbeats on your calendar.

3. Select an activity that can be done continuously for 20 minutes (to keep your heart rate up). Examples include bicycling, jogging, rope-skipping, rowing, stair-climbing, swimming, and brisk walking. The best one for you will usually be the one you enjoy the most (or hate the least) so you will be more likely to continue it.

4. Your fitness level determines which of the three intensity levels, Beginner, Intermediate, or Advanced, should be maintained. Try to maintain that level during exercise. Several times during, and immediately following your exercise, check your pulse. Your pulse must be in the appropriate range for the entire 20 minutes. To calculate your target heart rate:

Take the number 220 and subtract your age from it. The number that you get is your maximal heart rate or the highest recommended rate for your heart at all times. This is the level that must never be exceeded. Never exercise even near the maximum heart rate. Up to 90% of your maximum heart rate is safe.

During aerobic exercise, work out at a percentage of your maximum heart rate. Beginners start exercising at 50% to 75% of their maximal heart rate) and increase the rate after exercising over a length of time (weeks to months). The intermediate level ranges from 70% to 85%, and high-intensity continuous exercise (or interval training), which is not for everybody, is done on the higher end of the scale (from 80% to 90% of the maximal heart rate).

Your pulse during the entire 20 minutes must be in the heart rate range calculated for your age and ability level, so check it several times, especially when you are new to aerobics. After stopping your exercise, check your pulse only during the first ten seconds so that your pulse has no chance to slow down. You want to know what your pulse was while you were exercising, not after you have finished.

5. Do the exercise for 20 minutes, three times a week. Listen to your body; start on a slower schedule if necessary, and if something hurts or doesn't feel right, have it checked.

6. Continue checking your pulse rate in the mornings. It takes six weeks after starting your aerobics program to see the true benefits. Around that time, you will notice a 15% to 25% drop in your awakening pulse rate. This reflects a discharge in accumulated stress and an increase in metabolic efficiency. At least four to six weeks should pass in each category (beginning, intermediate, or advanced) before moving to the next level if doing three aerobics sessions a week.

General Exercise Summary

1. Choose one or more activities that you enjoy.
2. Get a good book and become knowledgeable about it, take a class, etc.
3. Start slowly, especially if you are older, have been ill, or are over-weight.
4. Frequency? Regular exercise is best, every day or three times a week, in 20-minute intervals. But do whatever you can. Listen to your body and slow down or change exercises if necessary.
5. Enjoy!
6. Exercise is only one aspect of the 3LS Wellness Program. Do all three practices for fastest results, greatest health, and numerous wellness benefits.

PEOPLE SPEAK ABOUT THEIR EXERCISE EXPERIENCES

With exercise I lost approx. 30 pounds and have wonderful energy that I thought I never would have. My skin feels and looks better, and I only need six hours of sleep a night to feel refreshed. Need I go on? I basically just do stretching, some aerobics, and a 12-minute walk/run mile. I do the stretching every morning, the walking three to four times a week and the aerobics probably once a month. I don't really have time to do the aerobics more right now.

—L. H. Welch, Arlington, TX

I have had problems with low body temperature and periods of lethargy. My thyroid tests are always within the normal range but a bit on the low side. I have been studying for the past three years, which means a lot of sitting. I dislike medicines, so I started to run every day. At first it was very hard. I was out of breath after five minutes, and then I walked home. But I continued, and now I can run for 15 minutes without stopping, and five more after a small break. My body temperature went up from day one. Sometimes it can be a bit on the low side, but jogging helps right away.

—Sonja Sunde, Social Anthropologist, Bergen, Norway

My mum, at 86, started her first regular exercise program last year on her therapeutic rebounder. Much progress since: remission of heart disease (say no to nitro), remission of arthritis (say no to painkillers), and now, wonder of wonders, she reported to me tonight that she has had enough improvement in her feet that she was able to entertain company today. To do that, she wore her SANDALS, which she has not been able to wear for at least five years due to the numbness in her feet. It should be emphasized this process has taken over one and a half years. Nonetheless, she feels it is somewhat of a miracle for, as she puts it, "an antique like me." As far as we are aware, there is little or nothing else that will help out those who are on a downward spiral of neuropathy, a condition that generally leads to incapacitation. *—Anonymous*

I started jogging when I was 20, and then continued jogging and working out at a gym with aerobics and weights. I found that while I did aerobic exercise I exercised all parts of my body. I definitely burn calories with aerobic exercise, and it is a great stress release. I also build up energy. Twenty-seven years down the line and I am still working out and still loving it. It has become a part of my life.

—Eleni Savva, Larnaca, Cyprus

Exercise got out my extra energy. To help release stress, I do yoga, tae bo, and walk. I also play ball with my daughter in the yard. I laugh and exercise this way which helps a lot. I feel happier and healthier.

—*Jennifer Boals, Veterinary Technician, Boise, ID*

I walk daily, averaging two miles a day. I've been walking regularly for over six years and have not missed a day in over four years. It is the only thing my pain and energy levels allow me to do on a regular basis. But I did lose 55 pounds doing that, and I have gained muscle strength, balance, endurance, and self-satisfaction for sticking with something for so long. I walk as much for the emotional benefits as for the physical ones. I love my sacred time every day and always come home feeling better than when I left, on one level or another. If I have a decision to make, feel stressed, or need to think something over, I head for the park to pound it out.

—*Mary Lilga, Environmental Scientist, Richland, WA*

I use a NordicTrac, Total gym, light free weights and Pilates. The most important thing is to find some form of exercise you like and will do. I try to do something every day, even if it's only a walk with my wife and dog in the park. —*Stephen Hockenberry, Westfield, MA*

I have found exercise to be a great addition to wellness. I have found it very helpful for relieving stress, and also putting me into a good frame of mind, i.e., gets those "feel good" endorphins flowing. I tend to rely on rebounding for my exercise. I want something simple and convenient, and I can do at any time. Just being able to put on my sweats and exercise at home is very convenient and plays a huge role in staying focused and disciplined on a goal. Rebounding is so simple. I just get on there for 20 minutes, whilst watching television or listening to music.

—*Maria Keswell, Service Assurance Consultant, Beldon, WA, Australia*

I had been a long-distance runner (six or more miles per day, at least five days per week) from the ages of 17 to 39. At that point, I was unable to run anymore due to chondromalacia of both knees. I was not able at the time to find a form of aerobic exercise that did not further injure my knees. So I sat around for three years and gained weight and got sicker. (Weight gain to the tune of 60 lbs.) I felt absolutely awful. No energy, more aches and pains, terrible depression, and I seemed to have less resistance to every virus going around. I was sleeping 14 to 16 hours a day and still feeling exhausted. Part of that might have been due to untreated developing hypothyroidism, which is now being treated, but I believe a portion was due to not exercising.

I finally found an exercise I can do. I've only been at it now a little over a month, but in that time on the elliptical trainer (an hour a day) I have lost 16 lbs., regained my energy, sleep eight to nine hours a day, have much less depression, and fewer aches and pains. I am thrilled that I found an exercise I could do that does not aggravate my knee condition, because I am certain that regular exercise, at least 20 minutes three times a week (ideally even more than that) is absolutely necessary to good health. My mother, by my age, had cancer that had spread to her lymph nodes (the doctors did not expect her to live) and three heart attacks. My sister and many other relatives are morbidly obese, or were so before they died. I believe that exercise has saved me from these ailments.

—*L.L., Freelance Watercolor Artist, Former Army Officer, Washington, D.C.*

At 53 years, I have chronic rheumatoid arthritis. I've come a long way with how I exercise or do physical activity. Before I got RA I enjoyed walking, fishing, swimming, and snow skiing. Then I got RA and my whole world changed. It was hard to do anything because I was in pain and agony. But I knew I needed something to help me keep moving as I didn't want to become a house prisoner.

My first PT told me that they had the best results by getting people like me on a horse. I thought he was plum loco—I was in intense pain, severe panic, walked like a stiff board, and I was to get on a horse? Yes! Now I ride horses for therapy. I've ridden with people who have MS, brain injuries, and other chronic injuries and diseases. Horse motion is the closest thing to human motion. It allows my body to relax, stretches muscles, strengthens me, and challenges my brain. I have become one with my horse. Horseback riding is not my only activity. I swim, do water aerobics, and snorkel. I just started Pilates, on the equipment since I can't get down on to the floor, but that may come. And what has all this physical activity done for me? One thing I can say is this disease is not stopping me from enjoying life. I am not totally handicapped since I've not shut myself off from the world. It has allowed me to meet others who are in the same predicament, and we enjoy ourselves without concentrating on the fact that we are sick or disabled or have a handicap.

Don't let people tell you that you can't do something because of your physical condition. Find someone to help you modify it so you can try it. Find some activities that get you moving. If you are interested in therapy riding as a rider or as a volunteer contact: North American Riding Handicap Association (NARHA) for more info. Enjoy yourself.   —*Joanne Catlin, Boulder, CO*

A slow-growing navel orange-size benign brain tumor was successfully removed when I was 32 years old. Thus by age 33, I developed altitude intolerance, heat intolerance, labile hypertension, rapid heart rate, and acute panic attacks. I, an athlete who had at one time lived, hiked, and jogged in the 100-degree plus summertime heat of California's northern Central Valley, was now terrified of having a heart attack or panic attack if I so much as walked to the mailbox on a balmy morning. My temperature dysregulation was so acute that I can only surmise my hypothalamus must have suffered literal structural damage due to compression from years of slow tumor growth. Seven years later, my thyroid decided to reveal a large nodule, and I had a hemithyroidectomy. I gained 40 pounds in two months. I must also say I was living and continue to live a typical overworked, overstressed American life. I'm a self-employed mother of two young kids, a wife, and the only child of elderly parents.

So when I embarked on the 3LS, I was a stressed out, physical wreck. A year later, perfect whole-foods eating, lots of massage, a full course of Rolfing, and twice-daily twenty-minute sessions of long-neglected meditation were beginning to put a slight dent in my symptoms. I was no longer housebound and had lost some heat intolerance. Encouraged by being outdoors again, after a year on the 3LS without much exercise, I began first to walk and then to swim. Every day I walked or swam, and pretty soon my body achieved its optimal homeostasis. Now, nearly eight years after embarking on the 3LS, I'm still tied to allopathic medicine. There's no question, however, that the 3LS has contributed to my well-being, in the sense that eating right and meditating allowed me to exercise again. In my case, regular aerobic exercise above all is the key to health maintenance. It's the one thing I can't stint on.

—*Kyra Kitts, Psychic/Energy Healer, Los Osos, CA*

After almost two full years of bothersome hives, what has worked best for me so far is a combination of controlled breathing, meditation, and basic self-hypnosis. I've even gone back to the gym—and as long as I keep my workouts light, I've had no real problems with hives. Thanks a million.

—*Sam Wong, Graduate Student, Portland, OR*

Chapter 5

The 3LS and Your Daily Life

Key points in this chapter:

1. Living with the 3LS
2. How to relate to family and friends
3. How healing progresses while using the 3LS

ARE YOU PROCRASTINATING?

By now we're hoping that you have already started one aspect of Practicing Serious Wellness. If you haven't felt sufficiently motivated to begin the 3LS yet, think of it this way: how much do you love your chronic condition? Imagine or remember what it was like before you had health problems, or what it might be like if you didn't have them at all!

Making a choice to begin any of the practices that comprise the Wellness Program really comes down to having the desire to feel good, and a willingness to put some effort into achieving that goal. When you are firm and clear about your decision to do something, then accomplishing it is generally just a matter of finding the way that works easiest. Typically, only indecision makes accomplishment difficult, much more so than actually doing a practice. Once you have firmly made up your mind that you are going to do this, you may well discover that making the lifestyle changes necessary to accomplish any of the practices is much easier than you previously thought.

Staying with the Program

Starting is the most important step in the process of helping your health. Making changes often feels awkward at first, but soon after you start, the new routine will start to feel comfortable. As you become healthier and more sensitive to your bodymind, you'll likely find yourself eager to add the other legs of the 3-Legged Stool Wellness Program to your new lifestyle.

Engaging in any of the practices is really just a matter of creating a new habit. After you do it for a little while, the new habit becomes self-sustaining. In six months, your new habit will feel natural as a part of your daily life, and then if you skip your practices, you'll feel unusual!

Ponder this wise person's words: "If you always do what you have always done, you will always get what you have always gotten." The source of this quote is unknown. However, the message is profound.

Start the Program any way you can. Since people differ greatly, what works for one person may not be the best approach for another, so the aspect of the Wellness Program you select to begin and how you integrate it into your life will be as individual as you are.

For example, some people need a structured approach with the 3LS. For these individuals, we have included some charts at the end of this chapter for keeping track of activities related to the 3LS. For those who like structure, you can follow the program exactly, but nevertheless, be flexible enough to listen to your bodymind and make adjustments where necessary.

Other people need less structure and find using charts and exact instructions too rigid. These individuals can find a way to make the 3LS spontaneous. Listen to your body's feedback and be natural with accomplishing your practices, but still follow the instructions for the Wellness Program accurately enough to ascertain you will get the benefits you desire.

Some people may feel the instructions for practicing the 3LS seem vague, or they haven't quite caught the concept and feel uncertain about how to start or what to do. Others might be wondering whether or not they are doing it right and wish for a class or summer boot camp for learning this three-part Program. If this describes how you feel, you would probably do well to find a health care practitioner knowledgeable about the 3LS Wellness Program or the individual practices, and work under his or her guidance. See the Resources at the end of the book.

However you approach it, feel free to experiment to discover how this 3LS can work best for you. Do what works!

Maintaining Steady Progress

The following tips may help you make the 3LS a part of your daily life. You may learn from the mistakes people commonly make and avoid them. Let us just mention that the biggest mistake is not starting one of the practices, but by now you've already begun, right?

Mistake #1: Failing to follow the instructions exactly

People often thwart their healing efforts by failing to follow the instructions accurately. There is a *world* of difference between the results of twice-a-day and only once-a-day Skilled Relaxation, just as there is a *world* of difference between thrice-a-week and twice-a-week Aerobics, and a *world* of difference between a Perfect and Liberal Whole Foods Diet. You will never believe the difference until you try these practices exactly, according to the instructions that we have so carefully described for you. The greatest lack of success we have seen occurs with people who think they can shortcut on the instructions by doing a lot less than what is recommended and still achieve good results. This healing program is set up exactly the way it is because, done correctly, you can start seeing results in the shortest period of time possible. We want you to see significant results in six months to a year, not five years.

Mistake #2: Giving up too soon

Another way people slow down their healing is by giving up before any benefits accrue. There is always a risk that a person will quit before realizing he is finally on the right track. Thus, we encourage you to keep practicing the Wellness Program even if results are not greatly apparent for a while. Sometimes the benefits are subtle. At other times, it takes an accumulation of doing the practices for a while and then suddenly, dramatic results are experienced. So continue, and do not stop, even if benefits are not immediately visible.

For some people, healing occurs slowly, and patience and persistence are required. The natural history of any chronic condition is that it gradually gets worse over the years, so for a very few individuals, just staying the same might actually be an improvement. Just doing the practices one day at a time will likely mean continuing to do them a month from now and a year from now, and that can only help your health condition.

However, progress will not be slow for everyone. Some of you will be surprised by experiencing changes and health improvements soon after starting any of the aspects of the Wellness Program. For some people, the changes will be almost immediate and dramatic.

Mistake #3: Expecting fast changes to a decades-old health problem

Again, if anyone practicing the 3LS finds that progress is slow and gradual, it does not mean that your practices are not working. After you've double-checked to make sure you are using the practices correctly, keep doing what you're doing. Just the fact that you are making any progress at all is a sign that you are working in the right direction. Some people have very deep-seated problems after many years of illness, and a condition as entrenched as that can easily take years to totally resolve. Some people still see improvements after ten years of practicing all three parts of the Wellness Program faithfully.

Furthermore, some tissues and functions take longer than others to respond. Everyone's chronic symptoms disappear at different rates and not everyone can expect to reverse *all* of the patterning of a lifetime of unhealthy habits in a year or so. The hope is that the slow improvements you see will be the carrot on the stick that keeps leading you forward.

Just as it takes years for the damage of a chronic condition to reveal itself, it can also take years for such damage to *totally* stop showing after the stressor is gone. However, for most people, it does not take very long to see initial results from use of the Wellness Program. In our years of experience, we have found that for most people, a Perfect Whole Foods Diet demonstrates significant results within two weeks, aerobics within six weeks, and Skilled Relaxation within a couple of months. We doubt that anyone would be interested in doing any of the practices of the 3LS if they had to wait for years to see any benefits.

If progress seems unusually slow, continue looking for other ways to help yourself. There may be other factors involved since there is generally more than one cause to any chronic condition. See Chapter 6 (about causes of illness) for ideas about other contributing factors. More information about other resources and methods of treatment is in Chapter 7 (about getting additional treatment) and in Chapter 8 (about healing mind, emotions, and spirit).

Mistake #4: Avoiding the most important practice for your condition

Many people who want health improvements sometimes try everything except the most important and beneficial practice for their condition. You have already heard us say that frequently people will do anything and everything except for the very practice that will help them the most. This happens so often, it has become a truism in holistic healing. What needs to be done may be obvious to others, but the person will not believe it and will certainly avoid it. So one clue that might help you make faster progress is to know that if one aspect of this Wellness Program seems exceptionally uninteresting to you, that exact practice may be the one that proves the most helpful to your recovery.

However, even if you do not begin with what you need to do most, any wellness approach will move you in the right direction. *Any* movement toward health will make it easier to later add the aspect you avoided to your regimen. Remember that many people get better by practicing only two aspects of this Wellness Program, and some even by doing only one.

Do you remember that we named this program after the sturdy image of a 3-Legged Stool? We consider that balancing on three legs is more stable than on just one or two. However, even practicing just part of this Wellness Program can still benefit you. A one-legged stool (such as those used by golfers, cobblers, or harvesters) can still provide some rest for a weary person. Although trying to balance on a two-legged stool sounds awkward, practicing two parts of the Wellness Program will definitely move you towards health. While we think doing all three legs of the program is the most beneficial, we applaud any movement you make towards health.

It is human nature that sometimes nothing is going to get us to do the thing we dislike and really need to do until we are convinced in our heart, by trying everything else first, that we really *have* to do it. However, we encourage you to take your reluctance to do a certain practice as a clue that it may benefit you greatly.

Mistake #5: Stopping the practices after feeling better

Another way of short-circuiting the healing process happens when people start feeling better after using the 3LS for a while. When symptoms improve, sometimes people stop the practices. Unfortunately, stopping the practices usually brings about a relapse, and symptoms return. What is usually necessary to resolve chronic conditions is for the individual to continue doing the program that helped, faithfully and without fail, for at least a year after all symptoms are gone. However, recurrences do happen, especially if the person stops all their efforts. Remember, this program is a lifestyle change.

How Long Should I Practice?

A question that people often ask us after they use the 3LS precisely for six months to a year is, must they continue to be so meticulous with it forever? Well, that depends. Humans are very different in their genetic horsepower. A small percentage of people will get over their health problems with a less-than-perfect Diet, no Exercise, and haphazard Skilled Relaxation. However, some people have to be perfect in *everything* to move away from the edge of the symptomatic cliff and get back in the middle of the field and stay there. Some people simply have to work harder than others to maintain their health.

In general, the longer a person is perfect in practicing the 3LS, the more a slight mess-up can be tolerated before having a setback. This is true of all three aspects of the 3LS—Diet, Exercise, *and* Skilled Relaxation. A good working guideline is that any imprudence during the first six months is likely to quickly set you back to the very start. After six months, the rule gets pretty fuzzy *depending* on how long you have had problems and how bad those problems were. After a few years of meticulous practice of the 3LS, or any of the aspects of the 3LS, most people rarely need to be perfect, as long as they are reasonable. Practicing Serious Wellness is a lot like regularly putting money in the bank—the longer you do the 3LS well, the longer you can make a withdrawal (not be so meticulous) without going broke.

We have yet to see a person who has done the 3LS accurately for more than *six months* who had to go back to the start from any small indiscretion, unless he persisted in testing fate by overdoing it. Usually, after this long, it takes only a week of accuracy to get back to where you were before.

After a year, some people might get away with dropping the Skilled Relaxation to once a day and following a more liberal Whole Foods Diet. Even after a year, stopping any part of the Wellness Lifestyle is a calculated risk. It is true, that to be 100% sure of permanent resolution, one cannot relax a strict wellness lifestyle a bit. It is a lifetime commitment. If the individual does not do at least some of the healthy things that brought about a cure in the beginning and do them for the rest of his or her life, he or she is more likely than others to have it recur. This is because the genetic susceptibility for exactly what happened has already been proven.

Some people have a recurrence of their symptoms or illness if they stop doing strict wellness even *several years* after their problem has cleared up. These people seem to have a genetic need to work harder at being healthy than the rest of us. At least by this time, they know that they *can* be healthy and what it takes to get there. Or, this may happen in these few individuals because a different, significant cause of the health problem exists that has been missed or overlooked. An example would be a strong hypersensitivity to or heavy burden of pesticide exposure that has continued in a person's life even as he was doing the Wellness Program. The wellness helped in spite of it, but eventually the missed cause finally overwhelmed even that. However, the continued Wellness practice usually makes it much easier to find that

3LS Wellness Program—Points to Remember

- The synergistic effect of practicing all three parts of the Program is the fastest way to improve your health. However, you don't have to *start* all three legs at the same time.

- The 3LS gives your body what it needs to heal itself. The body's capacity for healing is nearly unlimited – given a chance.

- Most chronic conditions will clear up just by the careful practice of the three aspects of the Wellness Program. However, some people will need additional treatment.

- Some people ask about the correct order for coordinating the 3LS with taking a shower in the morning. We recommend: 1) exercise, 2) Skilled Relaxation, 3) eat, 4) then shower.

- Eating right before Skilled Relaxation is not recommended, but the relationship with eating is not a very important consideration.

- Exercise done right before Skilled Relaxation is a wonderful combination. It is multiplicative in its effect. Doing them in the opposite order is not helpful. While Skilled Relaxation before exercise feels good, it seems to short-circuit the long-term results of the SR. Thus, if you have been doing SR before exercise, consider rescheduling both. If you must do your SR first, wait for two hours before exercising.

external cause, and the bodymind has more strength and resilience to help with any required remedy.

After doing the 3LS for six months to a year, if you let yourself go back to the lifestyle you had and the way you felt before you started the 3LS (heaven forbid!), your experience on the 3LS will have shown you that your health condition is a choice. Hopefully, you will then choose to return to Practicing Serious Wellness consistently.

For those who have a recurrence of any kind, cutting the frequency of practicing the 3LS is generally not considered worth it. **Caution: a very few individuals find they cannot get the same results the second time as they did the first time because they are older and their unaddressed causes have had longer to work on them.** If there is a recurrence, and restarting the program does not clear the problem as it did before, the likelihood exists that something was "broken" beyond your bodymind's capacity for healing it. Restarting the program will still greatly improve how you do, though.

To summarize, there are two main reasons why the 3LS may not bring the desired results.

1. You didn't understand and carry out the instructions accurately.
2. You didn't practice the techniques consistently over a period of time.

TROUBLESHOOTING Q & A FOR THE 3LS, NOW THAT YOU'VE BEGUN

Q: I've been doing everything you recommend for a year, and I'm still not feeling any better.

A: This is very unusual. The most important thing about this Wellness Program is applying it perfectly and accurately. So, go back and re-read the instructions for each aspect of the Wellness Program, especially the trouble-shooting sections, and make sure you are doing everything correctly. Unless you practice each of the three aspects of the Wellness Program as described, you will not be able to count on certain results.

The other thing that comes to mind is that you may be exposed to some kind of daily stressor that is exceeding your efforts to reverse the effects. For example, if you are taking a prescription medication whose side effects are headaches, and you are doing SR to try to resolve your headaches, it is unlikely that your headaches will go away by just practicing SR.

Q: I practiced the 3LS for a year and it helped a lot. However, six months later, my problem came back.

A: ■■■ WALT: I hope what I share next doesn't describe you, but I have seen this too many times not to mention it. The majority of people tend to forget how bad they really felt, and once they have done a lot better for a while, stop doing what they did to get those benefits. Afterward, they are surprised when the problems come back. This happened to me, and it was the rare patient to whom it did not happen (until they learned to keep up their curative ways long enough to avoid relapse). For many people, Practicing Serious Wellness will need to be done for their entire lifetime.

Many people go through this kind of start-and-stop experience. We all tend to forget how bad we felt and many have to backslide to learn our lessons the hard way. Imbedding new habits takes time and effort. If you've relapsed due to carelessness, forgive yourself and get back on track. If you keep a brief diary of how you are feeling daily, you will more easily remember how you felt before putting in the wellness effort. ■■■

Q: I was practicing all three legs of the Three-Legged Program faithfully and even went to see a biofeedback specialist so I knew I was producing the right kind of brain wave. But my condition worsened. Maybe the situation I was in was so stressful (domestic violence) that no amount of SR helped.

A: You are right that there is a limit as to what can be done if the psycho-social stress level is high enough. However, if extreme stress is the reason your condition worsened, working with the stressor is the first essential thing to do. Read Chapter 8 (about healing mind, emotions, and spirit) to learn about and find resources for improving your social situation. That is the first step for you to take.

After the stressor has been resolved, then you still need to do the SR to reverse your health problems.

Later in this chapter is a discussion of the healing crisis, which may be another reason you are not feeling better—yet.

Q: I've had some successes thanks to the 3LS, but still seem to have such a long way to go since my problems seem to be so deep.

A: At least you are on the right track. Persevere in doing the practices and be patient if your progress is slow. Our suggestion is to carry on with your wellness and continue looking for your path to the top of the mountain. Most chronic illnesses have more than one cause. See Chapter 7 (about seeking additional care) and Chapter 8 (about healing mind, emotions, and spirit). What you have achieved can only help any other treatment you might need.

People who Practice Serious Wellness can and do emerge from physical and psychological disorders with increased rather than impaired function. You *can* get in control of your life and your health. Many people who think they will never return to normal, actually become supernormal. Persist.

RELATING TO FAMILY AND FRIENDS WHILE PRACTICING

So many people have questions about how to relate to others while they are working to improve their health condition that their concerns merit a discussion. Many individuals wish to help friends and family embark on a path of healing with the 3LS, and so we discuss that, too.

A Healthier Family

■■■ JAN: Some people believe that they are taking time away from their families, especially their children, if they practice the 3LS Wellness Program.

However, by practicing the 3LS yourself, you can enrich your family life. You set a good example for your children and spouse by engaging in healthy activities. Not only will you be a happier, healthier person (nicer to be around), but children and other family members will also benefit from having a positive role model. They can look up to and learn from your actions, your taking care of yourself, and your integrating healthy activities and habits into daily life.

You will not lose time with your family members if you include them in your healthy activities and involve them in Wellness. For example, some families enjoy SR practice together, spend time in the kitchen collectively creating interesting Whole Foods dishes, and Exercise as a group or team. Such family activities can encourage closeness and good relationships.

Some people think that the way to give and receive love with family members is to bake sugary cookies, give a box of chocolates, etc. Think how much *more* you will be loving them by giving them the true treat of good health and healthy lifetime habits. ■■■

■■■ WALT: I agree with Jan about involving the whole family in learning and practicing wellness whenever you can. Here is another good reason for introducing family members to the 3LS.

One of the things they got right in medical school was: if your grandfather got his disease (diabetes, arthritis, hypertension, or other illness) in his seventies, your father will get his in his sixties, and you will get yours in your fifties. I was taught that 40 years ago. Now, in the new millennium, they are teaching: if your grandfather got his in his seventies, your father will get his in his fifties and you will get yours in your thirties! This is apparently due to the incredible increase in eating only refined foods (thus accelerating aging and reducing immune reserves) in the past 50 years. Daily articles in the media are already bemoaning the epidemics of chronic illnesses in our young people, illnesses that used to be only present in people past middle age. The refined diet has greatly accelerated the decline in health witnessed in the first half of the last century. The health-diminishing diet and lifestyle is, of course, greatly aggravated by the dramatic increase in environmental pollution and the resulting burden of toxins our reduced capacity has to cope with day to day. This means we carry a greater toxic load and have fewer reserves. However, living the healthy lifestyle of the 3LS can delay and even sidestep the onset of many illnesses. Without wellness, what will your quality of life be in the future for you and your children?

It is interesting how the three aspects of the 3LS Wellness Program mimic the healthy everyday lifestyle of several hundred years ago, when people had more time to relax, refined foods were not available, and there were no cars, so exercise in the form of walking was part of daily life. ■■■

3LS and other people Q & A

Q: My job and family life are just too stressful. I think first I need to make some major changes in my life right now before I can get well using the 3LS.

A: ■■■ WALT: When I started patients towards Wellness at my holistic center in Kentucky, I used to routinely caution them not to make impulsive or sudden changes simultaneously. They would come to me saying that they were going to quit their job, get a divorce, move to Mexico, etc., because they just couldn't take it any more. Knowing that any of those choices would greatly increase their stress, at least at first, I would tell them to wait until they started feeling better before taking that step. Even though they might have eventually found that any one of those drastic steps was necessary, they would be much more capable of handling the stress of such a taxing change if they allowed themselves the opportunity to become healthier first.

However, after Practicing Wellness for a while, many of them found that the boss (wife/husband, etc.) who was supposedly intolerable yesterday was suddenly, somehow, not so bad that next month. The change occurred because the patient was no longer living so close to the edge of his or her cliff and was not overreacting to everything. The boss had not changed, but the patient had. I experienced this with many patients. So I advise you to practice the 3LS and get healthier before you make any major life changes. ■■■

Q: I'm getting healthier all the time, but my friends can't deal with it. They invite me over for a (sugary) meal and get on my case when I hardly eat anything. So when I opt out on said dinner dates, my wife gets on my case. I can't talk about SR without being viewed as a weirdo, despite the times. When I'm at the gym, my coworkers laugh at my (wussy) 20-minute walk every 2 days. It wouldn't be so bad if half of them weren't falling apart healthwise. Still they try to punch themselves up with coffee and then down with prescription drugs. I get to watch my own family decay long before their time. My wife isn't even 30, and she's already headed for

serious health problems. It comes up daily anymore, so I can't put it out of mind for too long. What shall I do?

A: ■■■ JAN: Congratulations on your own healing progress and your increased awareness. Someone as astute as you would benefit greatly from finding support for yourself for living a healthy lifestyle. Later in this chapter and in the Resources at the back of the book, we mention some ways to get support from Dr. Stoll's website (www.askwaltstollmd.com) and by cultivating relationships with practitioners familiar with the 3LS Wellness Program. Also helpful in your situation would be doing some personal growth work to learn some advanced relationship skills and how to gracefully and tactfully maneuver through some of these challenging situations. Chapter 8 has some suggestions as to how to learn these skills.

Also, as you get healthier, you will change as a person and as a result, you will make new friends. Healthy people want to become friends with other healthy people, and then you will not be so alone in what you are doing.

We cannot make other people change, but we can serve as a good example to others through our own diligent practice. Continuing on your own path to health is one of the best ways you can inspire your family and friends to do the same. ■■■

Q: I am amazed at the negative reaction I have been getting from friends and acquaintances about the physical changes they see in me. I have found that getting healthy is not always supported by those around you, in fact, often not.

A: ■■■ WALT: You are correct about people (family, friends and associates) frequently having a hard time adjusting to those who experience radical improvements in their health. Getting healthy can be one way to find out who your real friends are.

I have seen relationships change dramatically because one partner suddenly got healthy. I have even seen marriages break up because one partner practiced wellness and far outgrew the other partner. In those cases, the connection was to a sick person and the spouse did not have any idea how to relate to a healthy person.

However, take heart. Getting healthier can also improve and enhance relationships. There is nothing more attractive (and sexier) than a vigorously healthy person. Plus, I have also seen many spouses grow and change along with the healthy one. Read on…■■■

Q: Do you find that family members are supportive or understanding of someone starting the 3LS?

A: Definitely. To answer this question, here are some examples from several patients.

> PATIENT A: "My husband has been a great support. He cut out sugar and coffee immediately, and went on the whole foods diet gradually. He took all the parasite cures and the vitamins along with me. My (female) colleagues at work were fantastic. They knew I did this on my own and were skeptical of the outcome, but they supported me nonetheless. I was able to cook in our little kitchen at work, and soon they grew envious at the lavish lunches I was having. I would have done the same thing even without support, but it was so much easier with it! I appreciate it so much."

> PATIENT B: "I started the 3LS two years ago this coming March. I have had a lot of support from my family during this time. Gradually, they have also started to include more healthy foods in their diets. They eat more fruit, veggies, and salads. My husband is my biggest supporter. Along with new changes in his diet, he is also doing yoga with me for Skilled Relaxation. I have also been able to help many friends by sharing what I have learned."

■■■ WALT: Here is my personal story: I had been practicing medicine for years when I became convinced that sugar was a basic cause of much that ailed me. I started the Perfect Whole Foods Diet. At the time my four children were living with me, as I had just been through a divorce from their mother. At first, they thought their dad had lost his mind. However, when they noticed how much better my health was, after just a few weeks, they changed their minds. I arrived home from my office one night to find brown bags full of groceries sitting all around the kitchen. They had rummaged through all the cupboards and removed everything that had a trace of refined carbohydrates. After that, they chose to eat only what I ate. ■■■

Q: I would like my loved ones to follow this Program, but I'm having trouble getting them to be interested.

A: We suggest that, as much as you love your family and friends, that you put all your effort into helping yourself. You will serve as a shining example for them, and that will help them be interested. After they see your changes, they are more likely to come to you for what you know and will be ready to hear it. Until then, you are probably wasting your time.

An interest in health is one thing that you cannot give to or do for anyone else. Each person has to be the one actively seeking and be ready to do what is required. Many conditions are easy to resolve, but *only* if the individual is willing to become a student. When our loved ones are willing to learn more, then we can help. Until then, nothing any of us has to say will make the least bit of difference. After they become convinced by your example, they will be able to use their own motivation, not yours, for personal wellness changes.

Q: Somehow I feel responsible to tell my husband of the dangers of his current unhealthy behavior. But I know exactly how he will react. He will tell me that I worry too much and I am so negative in my thinking. But I am going to give it a try, because what if he does have a stroke? I will have to live with the guilt of knowing that I never warned him about it. I just don't want to get into an argument with him about it, as he can be very critical and sometimes just doesn't think rationally or want to hear the truth.

A: All you can do, which should save you from any guilt, is speak what you know, telling him only once or twice. This is not a stress *as long as* you are not attached to his doing anything you have suggested.

The best thing you can do to help your husband is to take excellent care of yourself by practicing this 3LS Wellness Program. Just serve as a genuine example for him. Although we would like it to be different, each person must find his own way.

Q: My wife is having serious health problems. I know she has to be the one seeking her own answers, but how can I convince her? I am just now trying to get going in the right direction myself, but I have a feeling it is going to take some time. Also, when compared to most people around me, I am already in really good shape and really healthy. So she might end up saying that she doesn't see any significant improvement in my health.

A: People must often experience pain before they will do something to help themselves. In the case of health conditions, it is nature itself (i.e., illness) that gets people's attention. Therefore, in some cases, people's ability to use the 3LS may depend entirely upon how much they are suffering (i.e., does their health condition get their attention?) and how many practitioners they've gone to who have been unable to help. At that point, they may be ready for a new approach.

Unfortunately, some people are so sick by the time they have suffered enough to consider other options that they cannot make healthy decisions for themselves. If they are not willing or are no longer able to do the learning and practices for themselves, you must accept that this is "as good as it gets." You are just going to have to love them exactly the way they are. Some people may even decide that they would sooner die than learn something new. That is their prerogative. If they are not ready to learn, just love them as they are until they die. No one can force anyone to grow and change.

HOW HEALING PROGRESSES WITH THE 3LS

The actual reversal of a chronic condition using the 3LS is a creative process that happens over time. The earlier you start working on becoming healthy by practicing the 3LS, the easier it will be, and the sooner you will have more energy to apply to Wellness.

All who are actually reversing the causes of their chronic condition by Practicing Serious Wellness see faster improvements in the beginning and slower, though progressively increasing, results for years thereafter. These improvements can continue until they are healthier than their so-called healthy friends.

As mentioned in earlier chapters, if you are doing all three aspects of the Program, you will probably notice immediate improvement. None-the-less, it will likely take six to twelve months before significant changes occur, although many will notice significant results in three months or even less. This time period will be longer for some and shorter for others. Remember, though, results can come quickly from doing any aspect of the Wellness Program, and most people will feel some results almost immediately.

The human bodymind tends to heal any injury or condition if given enough time and the correct resources to do so. Sometimes the healing

Moving Towards Wellness

Wellness is a wonderful process that happens gradually. First you start to feel better and have fewer chronic symptoms. Then you feel happier and more coordinated. Exacerbations may continue but may be followed by even greater well-being. As you become healthier, you become more aware of what is actually going on with your body (you can feel it more clearly) so you can take steps to resolve other health problems. You become springier and more responsive. You like yourself better. Your mind becomes clearer and you make better decisions. Gradually you feel well more of the time. Your tastes and interests change, and you become a new person. It feels good to be alive!

progression occurs in a certain pattern according to Herring's Law of Cure: "Healing starts from the head down, from the inside out, and in reverse order as the symptoms have appeared." Some healing experiences are uncomfortable, but these are usually short, sporatic, and are a necessary part of the healing process. Some people are caught off guard by the healing changes, and do not understand that these bodily experiences come with a transformation to a healthier lifestyle. Read on to learn more about the body's natural process of healing.

Exacerbations and Remissions

While practicing the 3LS, you will most likely experience a trend of gradual improvement consisting of remissions (times when your symptoms are better or gone), and exacerbations (times when symptoms recur). This is the natural progression of the healing process. Thus you can expect slow, steady improvement, but do not be surprised if there are days when symptoms return, especially at the beginning. All chronic conditions that are actually being resolved progress this way, with remissions and exacerbations. Don't stop, but *it is a good idea to keep a dated record of remissions and exacerbations of all your symptoms.* (You may use the charts at the end of this chapter.) With this written record, you will see that as your health is regained, exacerbations become farther apart, less severe, and of shorter duration. Your remissions are longer, more frequent, and you feel better as time passes.

Exacerbations (including any setbacks that happen because you have strayed from the program) are only minor encumbrances if the program stays on course. As long as you are moving in a healthy direction, you are still on the right track. Mainly, the exacerbations are reminders of the importance of practicing your wellness program.

If you obtain very quick results after starting the 3LS, you will probably experience a few exacerbations until your condition is finally resolved. Do not let the exacerbations discourage you. Just the fact that you saw results very quickly is proof that you are on the right track.

The "Healing Crisis"

During the course of reversing a chronic condition, occasionally people experience what is generally called a healing crisis. Healing crisis symptoms are good in that they herald a positive outcome. Healing crises are temporary and are a normal part of the healing process.

The healing crisis may be a return to experiencing symptoms of the past, but symptoms have less intensity than the original experience. It is interesting to note that some people experience this on a 12:1 timetable. For example, if you experienced a period of headaches six years previously that lasted for 60 days, then six months from the time of starting to get well, you might experience five days of mild headaches.

Healing crises may also simply be times of reorganization and integration in the bodymind, which may manifest as fatigue, disorientation, emotions, or a change in the expression of symptoms. Even though you are moving on a healthy path, any shift in direction requires adjustment, and as you adapt, sometimes you will experience some discomfort. For example, most people will feel worse for a while when going through withdrawal of sugar or nicotine, or feel fatigued when starting an exercise program after a long time of inactivity. Encountering such healing reactions, even if uncomfortable, does not mean you should stop your healthy pursuits, though. They are a normal part of the healing process. It is important at this time to rest and sleep more.

Occasionally, doing one of the aspects of the 3LS or other healing practice can be a catalyst that opens up historical emotional or spiritual issues needing to be addressed in a person's bodymind. With sufficient patience and reasonable health practices, most people who have these issues appear find that the issues generally take care of themselves and they return to some sort of balance. However, a few individuals will need to directly address these issues as part of their path of healing. An example might be someone who quiets down when practicing Skilled Relaxation suddenly noticing the intensity of his or her underlying chronic anxiety. Such a person may need to seek professional help to work through the old underlying feelings. Having such historical issues arise (and then resolving them) is a sign of increasing wellness and is part of the journey to the top of the mountain.

■ ■ ■

Starting a wellness program is a considerable change for anyone, especially if you are using all three aspects of the 3LS Wellness Program. Be assured that all the healing crisis reactions we have mentioned are temporary, because it just takes the bodymind a while to adjust to changes. Despite any exacerbations or healing crises you may experience while practicing the 3LS, you will most likely still have the sense that you are improving and are on a right path.

What's the difference between having healing crisis symptoms while doing the 3LS and actually getting worse from a health condition? The truth is that doing healthy things does not make anyone worse. If you are truly feeling worse, you may have an acute or emergency condition, which is something different from the symptoms of your chronic illness. If so, go see a doctor or other health care practitioner.

Here is another reason why you may feel temporarily uncomfortable during the healing process despite the fact you are truly getting better. A brief relapse or exacerbation (which is to be expected as part of healing) feels a lot worse after you've been feeling good for a little while. People tend to forget how bad their symptoms were when they had them constantly. The dramatic contrast between feeling great and then relapsing is actually a positive sign, since it documents your progress and is a pretty good indication of the final benefits you will get from doing the 3LS. Increased sensitivity is the hallmark of getting well. After you are well, the increased awareness is a joy.

There's another thing that often happens during healing. Once you are free from nagging pain or pressing symptoms, you may simply start noticing the lesser health issues and symptoms that have been with you that have not been in your conscious awareness.

If you are in doubt about whether what you are experiencing is a normal part of the healing process, contact a health professional well versed in natural healing (See Chapter 7 and/or Resources).

The natural inclination of all humans is to revel in the recently improved condition and expect to get better faster than the average. However, the healing process usually takes more than weeks or months. Give it adequate time.

Healing crisis Q & A

Q: I got sick in Asia four years ago and have been diagnosed with all kinds of digestive problems. The source of my frustration is that everything I do to try to heal my body seems to make the symptoms I'm trying to alleviate worse. Doing nothing isn't an option because I feel so poorly that way. But each time I start some kind of healing program, I have to stop because my symptoms worsen significantly.

A: It sounds like whenever you start a new wellness program you experience a healing crisis: a temporary exacerbation of symptoms. It will probably take a combination of factors to resolve your basic problems, and Serious Wellness is definitely the place to start. This is probably going to take you a couple of years.

Persist. Also, consult practitioners with experience and training in working with digestive problems (see Chapter 7 Resources at the end of this book).

Q: I've been doing the Perfect Whole Foods Diet for one month after having eaten junk food and experiencing digestive distress for a long time. However, now there's a pimply rash around my mouth! Is that a healing crisis?

A: Here is a very instructive response to this question offered by one of the participants on the bulletin board at www.askwaltstollmd.com. Her answer brings up some significant concerns for people who begin learning to heal themselves holistically.

> "I wouldn't call a pimply rash around the mouth a healing crisis, and it certainly seems less critical than the poor digestion you are trying to heal. You haven't been doing this very long and have apparently made significant changes to your diet. A change in diet can cause its own set of problems for a while, and you may be slightly allergic to something new you introduced. You may want to contact your doctor to rule out any other causes for the rash.

> "If you feel you are moving in the right direction with your health overall, don't panic now and start making wild adjustments to fix this small problem. Make very small adjustments, one at a time, to see what is causing the problem. Give yourself time and don't be impatient, or you will end up with the endless circling and confusion common to impatient people who are actually healing but don't realize it. They throw things at their symptoms weekly, don't stick to a plan, make large instead of small changes and then after doing all that, are constantly frustrated because their body responds erratically. Hang in there and use your intellect wisely, and you will get to your goal much quicker."

Healing is a process that can take time, energy, and attention, and can give you surprises along the way. The next question provides an example of how healing may bring unexpected improvements.

Q: Please advise me. I used to have scoliosis [curvature of the spine], my left leg was about ¼" shorter than my right leg, and my right shoulder was about 1" lower than the left. I was in excellent health except for adhesions in the right upper quadrant following gall bladder surgery. I sought out a Rolfer to reduce the pain of adhesions and had the first session four months

ago. After the first session, I started to experience something that felt like jet lag only 10 times worse. I visited my internist and the ER to find out what it was, but never connected it to the Rolfing until the fourth session, when my Rolfer did my left leg, which resulted in a multitude of problems, too numerous to list here. So I went to my chiropractor, only to learn that the scoliosis of 62 years standing was gone. The problem is that my spine continues to be unstable. Your advice and feedback would be welcome.

A: This type of healing response or healing crisis is a common and normal reaction to long-term bodymind imbalance. Granted, your symptoms are more dramatic than most, but that is just an indication of how much you needed this and how much good you will finally obtain. Clearing up scoliosis of 62 years standing is already a medical miracle and a blessing.

It would not be a surprise if you needed 30 Rolfing sessions rather than the usual ten. You may need to begin a guided exercise program to strengthen your spinal muscles as well. Since the 3LS Wellness Program helps everything work better, begin the practices. Also, ask your Rolfer for more advice, and consider starting Alexander Technique or Feldenkrais to speed up this healing phase. All of your current symptoms are good signs and will be temporary if you persist in moving forward with diligence in healing.

Changing Techniques as You Heal

As you heal, you may have to change paths, since each of us becomes different as we get nearer to the top of the mountain (Wellness). Thus, healing approaches that worked in the beginning may lose their effectiveness, and so you may have to select new techniques to continue to see progress.

Here are some examples of the kinds of changes we are talking about:

1. The SR technique that was working for you in the beginning may stop working so well.

2. After a long period of doing SR, your metabolic processes will likely change. Therefore, any dietary approach used along with the Whole Foods Diet that helped when you were over-stressed may need also to change. Staying with that previous diet might actually make you sick, and so you must adapt to the new situation.

3. Most people who start on any kind of exercise program eventually get interested in adding other varieties, so your exercise program will likely change as well.

Change is what you want to have happen, so all of these events are good signs that you are moving forward with your healing program.

Some Positive Signs That You Are Healing

1. Your exacerbations are shorter and you recover faster from them.
2. Sometimes your exacerbations feel worse than before. They are not actually worse—this is due to the fact that you are now comparing them to what it is like to feel good, rather than just feeling sick every day!
3. You begin noticing things "wrong" with you that never bothered you much before. You now notice your smaller problems since your main problems are resolving.
4. Your main symptom hasn't yet disappeared, but some of your other symptoms are gone.
5. Changes in your condition don't necessarily feel like improvements, but you are aware that change is happening.
6. Improvements don't seem to last, but at least they start happening.
7. An intense exacerbation is sometimes followed by improvement.
8. You still have exacerbations, but there are periods of time when you are symptom-free.
9. Exercising slowly becomes easier.
10. Your body loses the numbness caused by bracing, and you become more sensitive.
11. Emotions surface. This is the healing crisis.
12. Treatments that didn't work before suddenly start working.
13. You start getting used to feeling good and feel really frustrated when you have an exacerbation.
14. As your health condition improves, you may become a different person. You will likely see changes in both your body and your personality.

TWO ESSENTIAL TOOLS FOR HEALING

While using the 3LS, you can maximize your efforts by making use of two healing tools that are already part of your own repertoire of natural resources. These tools are 1) your awareness and 2) your mind. They are very powerful tools, and using them will make everything else you do for your healing more effective.

Tool #1: The Power of Your Awareness

One of our favorite recommendations for healing is to practice self-awareness by "listening to your bodymind." The wisdom of the bodymind is one of the most reliable tools we know for finding your own personal pathway to health. When healing is happening, rather than symptoms being suppressed, listening to the messages of the bodymind is a powerful way to choose what works best for the stage of healing you are in at the time. Insight for listening to the signals your bodymind constantly gives you can be easily understood in the following experience of one patient.

One patient's story: "It has occurred to me that in health and healing (or wellness—using Walt's term), all it takes is to do ONE thing right as a start. With enough commitment to this one thing, gradually (and eventually) the other right things will happen almost automatically, so the right pieces will fall into the right places, providing a whole, perfect picture of wellness in the end. If this sounds too vague, here is some clarification, using my own experience.

About seven years ago I wasn't feeling healthy, both physically and mentally, so I decided to start running. After running daily for a month or so, I felt the NEED to stretch after the run (I wasn't aware of the need for warm-up and cool-down at the time—very ignorant of me), so I began to stretch before and after the run. It helped a lot in getting rid of the stiffness in the legs afterwards, so I enjoyed my running even more.

Later, in order to run better, I felt an intuitive/instinctive need for healthy foods such as whole foods and more veggies. It just happened on its own, without anyone pushing me or teaching me. Then this interest in healthy eating led me to explore health food stores and health books. After reading tons of materials on this subject and experimenting with bushels of whole grains, I realized that whole foods ARE the best food for me.

Hence, I reached the stage of knowing all I need to know about how to eat and how to exercise. After this, it just felt natural to unclutter my life and simplify everything. And once I simplified everything, including getting rid of the TV, it naturally became necessary for me to commune with nature, paying a lot more attention to the beauty and enjoyment of nature, which gives me far more wholesome pleasure than modern entertainments. Meanwhile, there was also the urge to learn how to avoid, as best as I could, other toxins in modern life (and I found answers to previously unexplained headaches I experienced whenever I went to clothing stores, shoe places, home improvement centers, and ozone alert cities).

What's more, I've recently felt a need to look inside myself— searching for an inner aspect of me. I'm guessing this is possibly the beginning of my spiritual level (a concept I used to laugh at!).

So you see, one simple act of running has led to a whole chain of events and actions, with the possibility of reaching the spiritual level. I don't know what's going to happen eventually, but I feel I'm on the right track."

People with unhealthy bodies are pretty numb and at the beginning, don't always do well with self-awareness. However, by following the 3LS Wellness Protocol, your health will most likely improve enough for you to begin to feel what's happening in your bodymind again. As improvements continue, you become further aware of internal changes. Listening to your bodymind makes it your own personal testing laboratory to determine your own answers for healing, and naturally, you come to find your own next steps for furthering your health.

Using the "bodymind laboratory"

This is the process of trial and error, or using awareness with specific treatments or therapies. You use your bodymind laboratory by listening to what your body and mind are telling you as you pursue a course of cautious trial and error. Your body's response gives you information about whether a particular course of treatment is helpful. For example, if you think you might have a hypersensitivity to wheat, you might avoid eating all wheat for seven days, and then eat it to see if you have a reaction or symptoms. The reaction or lack of reaction gives you information about whether eating wheat is beneficial for you or not.

With trial and error, even if a healing method you try doesn't work to improve your condition, you can still consider it a useful experience because you have ruled out one among many possible treatment options. The trial may also give you further clues about the nature of your condition. Both getting hints about what your problem is and ruling out what your problem is not can be quite useful in guiding you towards resolution of your condition.

Often, using the bodymind as your testing laboratory (using trial and error) is more practical, accurate, and reliable than clinical laboratory testing. Use clinical testing (standard laboratory tests) if you think it might help you obtain useful information about your condition. However, many clinical or laboratory tests are not always accurate, are often expensive, and cannot always give a holistic or whole body answer. The bodymind is infinitely more complex than any commercial laboratory can ever completely test.

With trial-and-error approaches to healing, or self-help of any kind, be cautious. Do not hesitate to consult a qualified practitioner for advice at any time. Some people and conditions need personal attention from one or more health care professionals rather than a self-help approach. Other individuals do very well planning their own healing with or without the assistance of health care practitioners.

As you become healthier and your body becomes more sensitive, the feedback you get from your bodymind laboratory can be one of your greatest healing tools. As you heal and go through changes, it becomes essential to respond to your body's current experience. This is why it is important that you listen to your bodymind, stick with whatever healing approach works the best at the time, and not be afraid to change techniques if the one you are doing stops working. The more you learn along the way, and the more self-awareness you have, the better equipped you will be to choose your next approach if that becomes necessary.

Increase your self-awareness

■■■ JAN: In the holistic healing model, everything is connected to and affects everything else, thus, self-awareness of all aspects of your life can be a very useful aspect of healing. Here are a few insights on how to increase your self-awareness.

Awareness of your body, and what feels good and what hurts, can help you make decisions enhancing your health and well-being. Since many people are somewhat numb due to bracing, they may have lessened awareness of what feels good or hurts them until something finally becomes quite painful. Bracing, disease, cultural habits, and symptom-suppressing approaches to health care can all contribute to this lack of ability to feel. Dedication may be required to learn to relax, become aware, and feel your body again.

How to become more aware of your body: One way to increase awareness is to constantly bring your attention and awareness to your body. As many moments of the day as you can, check in to see how your body is feeling. It can be helpful to start with awareness of just one part, or you can check in with your entire self. If you become aware of discomfort somewhere, keep your awareness upon the physical sensations and see what they tell you. It may be helpful to put words to these sensations by describing what you feel on paper or telling a practitioner or friend. The action of describing may yield clues about what your body is trying to tell you, and provide insight and possible solutions.

Body awareness can also be enhanced through activities like receiving massage, stretching, self-massage, practicing SR, exercising, and generally becoming healthier. Some people even use a watch with an hourly beeper to remind them to check in and feel their body. Your awareness may lead you to know what your body needs for optimum well-being.

Awareness of your emotions, combined with skills for understanding them, can make your feelings a useful message system and ally for achieving your life goals. Having a full range or repertoire of all emotions, and using them well, can enrich your life and benefit your physical as well as mental health. Healthy use of emotions involves experiencing and understanding what you feel, and sometimes taking appropriate action. Your feelings give you clues about your state of balance, integration, and harmony with the world and yourself. Feelings that are ignored cause health and life problems. Sometimes emotions are the result of an imbalance in lifestyle or body chemistry.

Many people are uncomfortable with emotions, especially the so-called negative ones. However, emotions are signals about whether your life is manifesting appropriateness or disharmony. Emotions reflect external conditions (in the psychosocial environment) or internal conditions (in your mind or in your own body/biochemistry).

Becoming aware of the two parts of emotions—physical sensations in your body and the thoughts that accompany those sensations—can help. By considering these two parts of emotion separately, you can learn more about what your feelings are trying to tell you.

How to become more aware of your emotions: When emotions arise, it can be helpful to stay with the feelings for a while (rather than trying to make them go away). Sometimes, emotions come fast and mixed. At those times, knowing exactly what you are feeling may not be easy. It can be helpful to go to a quiet place where you can be alone, slow down, and fully experience your emotions without distraction.

To feel the physical sensations, focus your attention on your body for a while. Directing awareness to the physical sensations keeps you in touch with your present experience and often yields much helpful information about how and what you are actually feeling. This awareness of your body can also help calm down highly charged emotions and help feelings evolve and change.

Next, focus your attention on your mind to find out exactly what you are thinking. It's often helpful to write down your thoughts so you can evaluate their relevance to your present situation.

Emotions may arise in combination or be experienced in various sequences. Each emotion has a different function and message. See what you learn from how each emotion feels in the body and what thoughts are stimulated in the mind.

Sometimes when feelings are strong or confusing, discharging emotional energy can help you attain clarity. Some ways to discharge emotional energy include repeatedly talking to a safe person about the factors contributing to the feelings, or engaging in constructive physical activity (such as running or chopping firewood). After the emotional charge is released, it may be easier to understand the feelings and thoughts. Do not make the mistake of stopping the exploratory process after feeling calmer! Return to practicing awareness to hear the messages of the body and mind.

Emotions also have the aspect of expression. Expression of emotions can be productive and appropriate, or ineffectual and harmful. Effective communication of your feelings and needs to others is a skill that takes practice.

To learn more about healthy emotions and positive communication, seek out helpful books on the topic. There is a special healing power in sharing with another person, thus you may also find it helpful to seek out a counselor, therapist, friend, or wise elder.

Clarity of mind and body is a great power. Becoming aware of and being fluent in emotions is one step towards total health and well-being.

Awareness of your thoughts, and how they affect you both positively and negatively, can guide you to use the mind's creative power to support you. Many people are unaware of what they think and the power that their thoughts hold over their behavior and success. For example, repeating negative thoughts about yourself, the past, and others may create self-defeating behavior and undermine plans and goals. The good news here is that repeating positive thoughts about yourself, the past, and others can support healthy behavior and lead to success in achieving plans and goals. You can learn to create thoughts that are helpful to your life. A change in thinking pattern occurs by becoming aware of what you think, knowing exactly what you want for yourself, and guiding your thoughts to support your goals.

How to become more aware of your thoughts: Pay attention to mood changes and look for clues as to how your thoughts may have created the change. Become aware of which thoughts immediately preceded any shift in emotion.

Another way to enhance awareness of thought is to simply sit down for an hour and write down every thought you think during that hour. You might be very surprised to find out exactly what is in your head. As you go through your day, see if you can catch any thoughts that repeat over and over, have the same theme, or do not seem helpful.

You can make a plan to create and generate positive, uplifting thoughts that enhance, energize, and move you forward in a creative way. This can be done specifically through preparing positive statements, such as affirmations, or by examining your beliefs and changing them to be constructive and supportive. Write them down and tape to a mirror or someplace you will see them, and practice using them. Many books about improving the quality of thought are on the market. Counseling or therapy is another way to obtain support for positive thinking. Retreats, including guided retreats, may be helpful for providing time and quiet space in which to refocus your thoughts and rework your belief structures.

Awareness of your spirit, and what feels right for you in the deepest sense, can multiply the peace and joy in your life. Many people do not allow themselves sufficient time, space, and quiet to listen to their own hearts and spirits. Thus, they miss their own deeply abiding inner source of joy, peace, calm, happiness, wisdom, guidance, harmony, and contentment.

How to become more aware of your spirit: There are many ways, both formal and informal, to learn how to connect with your inner self or spirit. More formal ways include seeking out spiritual or religious activities and education that promote mindfulness or experience of the spirit. Participating in community service activities (service to others) may also bring you closer to your higher nature. Informal learning may also be done alone. Becoming aware of your inner feelings, such as when something feels very right for you or wrong for you, can be one way of listening to your heart and spirit. Having feelings of joy, compassion, and love indicate a connection to the spiritual nature. To create opportunities for such connection, consider spending time quietly alone, visiting nature, and scheduling time for calming practices such as prayer and meditation.

■ ■ ■

Self-knowledge and self-awareness are beneficial for both maintaining health and for healing chronic conditions. If you continuously pay attention to both dramatic and subtle changes in your bodymind as you heal, you can learn more about yourself, plus adjust your treatment efforts correspondingly, in a timely and effective way. ■■■

Tool #2: Constructive Use of Your Mind

The mind is one of the most underused healing tools we have available. Most brain physiologists and psychologists agree that humans use less than ten percent of their brain potential. Just as we mentioned earlier in Chapter 4 (exercise) that imagery and other mental techniques can be used to enhance one's performance at tennis, and in Chapter 2 (relaxation) how the use of the mind in practicing Skilled Relaxation can help you heal, you can also use the power of your mind in other ways on your path to health.

Knowledge is power

Body and mind directly affect each other. Their close relationship is one reason why we use the term bodymind in our book. Since they are so integrated, your mind can be a great resource for your own healing.

Let us give you an example. "Here, take this" is not the most effective method of taking medicine, even if the remedy you are using or taking is what you actually need. After knowing *what* to do to help your condition, you can further use the power of your mind by knowing *why* you are using that particular remedy, and *how* it works. This actually makes for a more complete cure. Your understanding increases awareness, so that the energies of your mind become part of your healing power. This engages more of you in the healing process, facilitating healing and making treatments and therapies work more effectively.

Besides understanding the treatments, understanding the nature and cause of your condition can enhance your healing efforts and recovery. Engaging your whole being in your healing process brings greater power to your recovery. Please note that understanding more about your condition and treatments is different from any kind of futile attempt to search for answers instead of practicing Wellness.

We're suggesting here that you understand while you practice Wellness. Learning and studying on your own can bring this knowledge to you. However, doctors and other health care practitioners you work with should also be teaching you and helping you find information about your condition and your remedies. If they don't, be sure to ask. After all, the word doctor means teacher.

The mind can also be used directly in healing and doesn't cost anything to use. There are many healing techniques that directly make use of the power of the mind, such as affirmations, self-hypnosis, visualization, awareness, and prayer. We have included descriptions of some of these techniques in Chapter 7 (about using additional care). Read on to learn more ways to increase your knowledge for greater healing power.

■■■ WALT: **Research, Learning, and Study:** Many people would benefit from becoming more involved in their own health care and decision making beyond just going to see a practitioner or physician. If you have a chronic health problem that seems to defy resolution, the solution most likely rests in your concentrated personal effort. This means becoming a student and learning as much as you can about your condition and the basic mechanisms causing illness and health. By doing so, it is likely that you will encounter the lifestyle changes and modalities that will benefit you the most, and move to a more direct path of healing.

Truly achieving wellness, for many people, takes personal commitment and work. If this process of learning seems daunting to you, just read and study a little bit every day and you will slowly begin to see the whole picture. There comes a time in the accumulation of knowledge when everything seems to just fall into place and, eventually, everything gets simpler and easier. Actually, we have already made this process considerably easier for you by condensing as much information into this book as we could.

Here are several valuable resources to assist your learning and study. The first resource is www.askwaltstollmd.com. My website contains numerous articles I have researched and written with specific information about diseases, conditions, and remedies. Extensive archives on the website contain other articles about certain conditions and treatments from various sources, plus questions and answers I and others have given on those topics. You may benefit from other people's experiences, both what helped them and what didn't, and read a wide range of viewpoints and opinions. My website has its own search engine for finding information on different topics. After studying the articles and archives, and searching the website, if you still have unanswered questions, you may post your question on the website's bulletin board. Answers are given by me and also volunteers who contribute their time, experience, and expertise. Volunteers include individuals who have resolved their own chronic health conditions and also professional and retired health care practitioners. The website and bulletin board are non-profit, and everything offered is donated. People who recommend different approaches on the bulletin board are unbiased in what they say because they don't receive financial gain if you follow their suggestions.

Another resource is my first book, *Saving Yourself from the Disease-Care Crisis.* Look for the revised, updated second edition, co-authored with Kathleen M. Diehl, which will be entitled *Beyond Disease Care.* It contains information about the root causes of many chronic conditions. The second edition has more depth and a wider scope of information, and may be considered a companion book to *Recapture Your Health.*

On her website, www.lifespringarts.com, Jan has helpful resources for the 3LS Wellness Program, including Internet links, information for self-help healing, and instruction for helping musculo-skeletal conditions. See also the website for Sunrise Health Coach Publications at www.sunrisehealthcoach .com for possible new titles on holistic health. ■■■

Another good place for study and research is your public library. There, you may find articles, magazines, and books relevant to your condition. No books we know of are 100% right, not even this one. We are still learning, too, but most have some truth to them and can often serve you very well. The Internet also often has the most up-to-date information available. Just realize when you are researching the Internet that sometimes it is necessary to sort through a lot of junk to reach the treasures.

To narrow your searches, see the Resource section at the end of the book. Also, do not overlook reading the informative Glossary.

THE AUTHORS' EXPERIENCES

■■■WALT: I started practicing the 3LS Program with Aerobics. After more than 10 years of perfect aerobics, however, I still had a half dozen chronic conditions and was taking four prescriptions from my four physicians. It wasn't until I added the Perfect Whole Foods Diet to my wellness program that I suddenly was remarkably improved (of course the diet was done while I was still doing aerobics—perhaps it was the combination?). Then, I added SR. Within six months of following the Whole Foods Diet, practicing Silva Mind Training (a form of SR) and continuing to do aerobics three times a week (as I had been doing for ten years already), almost all my symptoms disappeared and I was off all medications. I learned the importance of practicing wellness every day.

I would say that I always had an average energy level. However, with a few months of practicing wellness, I only needed about two hours of sleep a night. Just that alone more than made up for the time I was spending with SR, aerobics, and shopping for and cooking whole foods meals. The results were so astounding and quick that I soon had even more hours just for play than I had previously.

I felt better than I ever had in my life, and then my patients began asking me what I had done to get so much healthier. That was when I realized that I did not know what to tell them. I only knew what had helped me and really had no idea how to individualize programs for each patient. Intrigued, I wanted to learn more. I ended up going to so many holistic postgraduate courses that it wasn't long before I was being asked to present at those courses as a nationally recognized expert. I became a founding member of the American Holistic Medical Association and served on its board of trustees for many years.

In essence, my efforts at healing progressed from healing my personal life, to healing my patients, to participating in healing the nation. My interactive website is just an extension of that process. ■■■

■■■ JAN: After I started looking for help with my health problems, it didn't take me long to figure out that the allopathic doctors didn't have all the answers I needed. I also tried a number of other healing approaches and obtained some clues and some help, but still did not make much progress. However, as soon as I began doing the 3LS, I immediately began getting and feeling better. I started with SR and quickly added the Perfect Whole Foods Diet and RE. During my first three years of using the 3LS, I experienced slow yet steady health improvement that ended up as a dramatic result. I believe it took the synchronistic combination of all three aspects of the Program to make such great changes in my long-time health condition.

The results from the 3LS were amazing! After only about a year of practice, people were noticing the changes and said things to me like: "Jan, you have lost weight!" "Your complexion is much improved." "You look ten years younger! You carry yourself differently, and there is a spring in your step that wasn't there before." "You seem like a totally new person!" "You are 100% different than you were last year at this time." "You are much calmer than before." "Your entire persona has changed." "You look slim like a model."

I found that all aspects of my life had improved. One wonderful example was a decrease in hypersensitivity to noise—previously I could not even tolerate eating in restaurants because the noise bothered me so much. Another was having social situations become much more pleasant for me, because I felt so much more relaxed and more energized. It is a joy to be free from fatigue and feeling so poorly, which I experienced for so very long. My emotions also improved greatly, and many areas of living which were formerly out of reach have now become part of my daily life.

Now after three years of the 3LS, I am pleased to find that my life continues to improve in an upward spiral of continually increasing health. I plan to make the 3LS a lifetime practice, and it is interesting to see the changes I make in how I use each aspect of the Program. For example, I learned through trial and error that the best time for me to do SR is after meals, because it helps my digestion (no more Leaky Gut!). Also, as you will read in the next chapters, I added some other treatments to my healing program. I know without a doubt that they would not have worked so well without my having practiced the 3LS first for several years.

Another bonus from learning the 3LS is how it has done more than just help my own health. I have also been teaching it to my clients, friends, and family. The reward for doing so is the privilege of observing people all around me becoming healthier and happier in their lives, too. It is a real joy to be able to share something so useful with others. ■■■

Chapter 5, THE 3LS AND YOUR DAILY LIFE—SUMMING IT UP

Practicing Serious Wellness is a matter of replacing harmful habits with healthy habits. Be accurate in practicing the Wellness Program, but listen to your bodymind and be flexible enough to make adjustments where needed.

Common mistakes in practicing the 3LS Wellness Program include: avoiding the most important practice for your condition, giving up too soon, expecting fast changes to a decades-old health problem, failing to follow the directions exactly, and stopping the practices after feeling better.

How long you need to do the practices is very individual. For a long-term resolution to your condition, make a lifetime commitment to the practices.

Share and involve your family and friends in the 3LS Wellness Program to give them the gift of learning a healthy way of life. Some people will be supportive of you, others will not. Be an example to others.

Wellness happens gradually and includes exacerbations and remissions as normal parts of healing. A healing crisis is a return to experiencing past symptoms with less intensity or is a time of reorganization manifesting as fatigue, disorientation, emotions, or change in symptoms. Give the bodymind time to adapt to the healthy changes you are making. As you heal, it may be necessary to change techniques because of changes in your bodymind. This is true of all three aspects of the Wellness Program.

You possess two tools that can increase your healing power.

1. Awareness of your bodymind will most likely increase as you become healthier, and awareness can also be a great tool for your healing journey. Awareness includes body, thoughts, emotions, and the non-physical aspect of health or spirit. There are many practical things you can do to increase awareness.

2. Using your mind is a second useful tool for healing yourself. Knowledge of how your condition is caused, plus understanding how the healing methods you use work, can increase your healing power. Mind techniques like affirmations, self-hypnosis, and visualization directly use the mind's power for healing. In addition, study and research make more options available for your recovery and can streamline your path of healing.

The charts provided at the end of this chapter can help you be consistent in your practice of the 3LS Wellness Program.

Making Changes Step-by-Step

If you feel challenged to get going and unsure what steps to take, here is a structured, step-by-step plan to follow to begin the 3LS.

1. Know why you are doing this wellness program and the benefits you want to receive. Write down the consequences of staying the same, what will happen if you change, and the goals you'd like to achieve.

2. Choose just one aspect of the 3LS Wellness Program to start with. The one that seems most interesting to you will be fine. Remember that change occurs in steps, so for this Program it's okay to take your time. Just get started.

3. Write down the steps you need to take for your chosen activity. To simplify the process, consider each step as a separate mission. After you do it, think: Mission Accomplished! Below is a sample outline of steps. You can make up your own steps and add them to the list.

STEPS TO TAKE

Skilled Relaxation

a) Choose a practice to try (or read the *Relaxation and Stress Reduction Workbook* to get some ideas).

b) Start doing that practice 20 minutes once a day for a week.

c) Increase to two times a day for the next week.

d) If that practice doesn't seem to be working for you, try another one. Repeat if necessary.

e) Reread Chapter 2 (or the summary) to make sure that you are following all the steps.

f) Continue practicing.

g) After one month or so of twice-a-day practice, go for biofeedback testing.

Whole Foods Diet

a) Plan a simple two-week trial of only eating whole foods. Use the Quick Start Guide (or obtain *The Healing Power of Whole Foods* book) for knowing what foods to eat.

b) After you know from the trial that the diet can help you, organize ways to continue following it.

c) Clean out all refined foods from your kitchen, pantry, and refrigerator.

d) Make a meal plan for a week.

e) Make a shopping list according to your meal plan. Be sure to include foods for snacking if you get hungry between meals.

f) Go to the health food or other grocery store and buy the whole foods according to your list.

g) Schedule extra time for cooking and organizing your kitchen. Follow your meal plan, one day at a time.

h) For the next week, repeat steps d – g.

Right Exercise

a) Choose an exercise that you will enjoy doing (or read *Fitness for Dummies* for ideas).

b) Set a small goal that you can easily reach and be successful with, such as exercising three times a week for five minutes each time. Set a schedule for yourself and write it in your day-timer.

c) Obtain any necessary equipment or sign up for a class.

d) Start your exercise program and see how it goes.

e) Adjust or reduce your exercise goal if necessary to keep you exercising regularly. After you achieve your goal, set a higher goal.

4. Make sure that each change or accomplishment is positive and enjoyable. Reinforce the change by admiring the outcome (Hurray! I exercised for five minutes today! Or Hurray! I ate pistachios instead of a candy bar!) and enjoy your success. Reward yourself with both good words and healthy treats.

5. Protect your new behaviors by controlling your environment or using memory aids like calendars or charts. Remove distractions. Bring in anything that helps you. Enlist the support of family and friends to help you stick to your plan.

6. Be flexible and adapt or change your plan where necessary. Identify what works well and continue doing those things. Find new ways to work with what isn't helping you.

7. After you have done one aspect of the Wellness Program for some time and feel comfortable with it, choose and do a different part.

COMMENTS ON THE 3LS WELLNESS PROGRAM

I came to Dr. Stoll's bulletin board because I was diagnosed with autoimmune disease. My ANA was 1200 and it was recommended that I see a rheumatologist. I was also told that I would probably have to take some medications for the autoimmune. I know that those meds are terrible for your body, and they only take care of the symptoms (not get to the root cause), so that's why I started the wellness. After reading the archives, I decided I had Leaky Gut Syndrome and candida too. Now my ANA has gone down by almost half (currently still working on that). I'm free from indigestion, stomach pain, free from gas most of the time. I used to have arthritis pain; I control that with my diet. I was having hair loss, brittle and dry. Now I have thick hair…Had to get it thinned (that was after adding healthy fats back into my diet). I ride my bike five to ten miles every other day. I walk one hour a day. My daughter paid me a wonderful compliment the other day. I'm turning 50 this year, she told me I look 40.

Now I have to tell you, I don't follow this perfectly. I have my rough times. I get tired of the routine and I deviate… and then I feel horrible. So, back on I go. It's a daily process that I work on. There are some foods I didn't mind giving up at all. But, there are others I miss. Like Walt always says, how much do you want to feel good?

—*Barbara A. Freedle, Secretary/Office Assistant/Homeschooling Mom, Merlin, OR*

I'm amazed at how simple but powerful Dr. Stoll's 3LS Wellness Program is. I began making small changes after I finally understood why it was so critical that I change my life. The principles of the 3LS are not a quick fix, but upon making changes, I did begin to feel better quickly. I feel like I've found access to such great information that I no longer have to settle for accepting my symptoms as common. I've been empowered to take responsibility for myself.   —*C.D., Homemaker, Lawrence, KS*

On the Whole Foods Diet and doing Skilled Relaxation, I continue to feel this amazing sense of energy—of health even! Wow! I have had two to three pretty intense/bad healing crises but keep trying to remind myself that that is most likely what they are—and then take it easy through that time and yes, amazingly, I DO come out the other side feeling even BETTER. It's just a constant effort to remind oneself of these things and NOT get discouraged.

—*Anonymous*

It is amazing how fast my health improved with only three months of practicing the Whole Foods Diet and Candida Diet and Skilled Relaxation. Improvement: severe acne, 90%. Seborrhea, 80%. PMS, 100% (it amazingly became pain free). Thank you, Dr. Stoll!

—*Anonymous*

Sometimes I have fallen down with implementing Wellness in my life, but somehow, I have always picked myself up, dusted myself off, and started the journey again. The longer and longer I continue with Wellness, the fewer falls I seem to have.

—*Maria Keswell, Service Assurance Consultant, Beldon, WA, Australia*

Cheating on the diet is always a dilemma and is a question of your own cost/benefit analysis —what you sacrifice and what you get. Sure, there are friends who do not understand this. But I feel I do not have to have the same way of living as my friends in every aspect of my life to be able to talk to them. Being different does not mean to be lost. And, there are not just known results of leading a different life. You may be surprised to get what you otherwise would not be able to get—finding new people, energy gain causing better, social, personal, and other abilities, etc. People stick to you more if you shine out your health. Friends sometimes change in this process, too. I have noticed some of my friends did not understand my dietary changes at first. Now some of them do as their health deteriorated, or just hear more about various diets.

—*K.M., Europe*

I have a tall 6'3" husband who loves to eat big hearty meals and the longer we were married, the fatter I got. I blossomed to 289 pounds and size 22. One day I got very determined and went to the closet and threw out all my FAT clothes and began a lifestyle change. I walked five miles a day, ate a vegetarian diet sprinkled with protein. I wrote down what I ate every day and drank lots of good spring water. I took green food and psyllium whole husks and attribute most of the weight loss to getting my bowels working regular. Now I weigh 145 lbs and am 5'8" and every area of my body is in good shape. Last spring (2003) I got all new clothes that fit and I have kept the weight off since 1998. All of my life I was active roller blading, walking five miles a day, biking, swimming and loving it.

I fell in 1999 and x-rays showed problems in my knees, back, neck and lower back. I was diagnosed with rheumatoid arthritis. I have a doctor who wants me to see a rheumatologist and take strong medications. I am being pressured to take strong arthritis meds but I won't and can't. They made me so sick. I called my massage therapist and chiropractor and they came and adjusted me. I put them on my calendar not only as my very best friends, but as the number one priority from now on for me and my body. I like positive, good things and I am determined to learn and grow. Do the same and people will stand amazed at your courage to improve. People keep a close eye on you when you can produce a testimony of courage. It is easy to set goals and master them easily when you are young and in perfect health, but producing those results when disease arrives on the scene require a lot more creativity.

— *Judy Hulett, Art Teacher, Mom, and Grandmom, New Oxford, PA*

I recently realized I have a stress/anxiety problem. I think I've had it for quite some time, but it had become such a way of life that I didn't recognize it as that. One thing I am trying to do, that I think helps, is awareness. As my stress/anxiety level has improved, I've been able to notice more when I'm feeling it so I take actions to alleviate it... I take several deep breaths and relax my muscles. I plan to practice this and/or other stress-relieving things from now on because I don't want to feel that way again. I've been working on this for three or four months and am feeling much better.   —*Anonymous*

It's been since November, 2002 (five months) when I was first diagnosed with costochondritis after being in a mild car accident. It was not a pleasant experience at all. I missed almost a month and a half of work, and I thought I was dying. That's when I started experiencing the anxiety/depression/panic. It was horrible. Since then, I have attended physical therapy for eight weeks, massage therapy, done Skilled Relaxation at least three times a day (and still doing it) and started walking on my treadmill for ten minutes a day at a slow rate. Also, I am taking Xanax two times a day for the anxiety. Also, I am practicing stress management. Today, I am TOTALLY pain free. The TMJ [temporo-mandibular joint—jaw] pain has also gone away. I am walking 45 minutes on the treadmill and doing some weight lifting to improve my strength. I am also going back to work, part-time only because my doctor does not want to take a chance on me going back full-time yet. Thanks for all of the great info Dr. Stoll and Jan. It just takes a lot of time and patience!

—*Anonymous*

CHART 5.1:
TWO-WEEK CALENDAR FOR TRACKING THE 3LS

Write in the date below	Write awakening pulse rate*	First daily SR session 20 minutes, check off	Second daily SR session 20 minutes, check off	Followed PWFD perfectly today?	AE–3x/week 20 minutes. Write post-exercise pulse rate	Symptoms, improvements or notes
Sun.						
Mon.						
Tue.						
Wed.						
Thu.						
Fri.						
Sat.						
Sun.						
Mon.						
Tue.						
Wed.						
Thu.						
Fri.						
Sat.						

This calendar may be used for keeping a record of your experience with the 3LS. The last column may be used to note changes and improvements in symptoms, frequency of remissions and exacerbations, or for any notes about your daily practice.

*Check your awakening pulse rate for 10 seconds immediately upon awaking in the morning. Write the number of beats on your calendar. Also, take your pulse in a similar way during and immediately after aerobics to make sure you are reaching and maintaining the correct heart rate for your age (see the Target Heart Rate Chart in Chapter 4). Four to six weeks after starting aerobics, you can expect to see your awakening pulse rate drop about 15% to 25%. This drop is a sign of improved metabolism and enhanced bodily function.

CHART 5.2: SYMPTOM TRACKING CHART

Date(s)	Symptoms	What events, food eaten, or thoughts occurred, etc. Just before symptoms began?	What made it feel better?	What made it feel worse?

This chart is to help you increase your self-awareness and to give you clues as to what might help you create wellness. After it is filled out, you can also take it to your practitioner to help look for patterns in your symptoms.

CHART 5.3: CHART FOR RECORDING RESULTS OF THERAPEUTIC TRIALS

Date(s) of Trial	What was tried (food eaten, modality, supplement, exercise, etc.)	Result

This chart will help you keep track of experimenting with different treatments and their outcomes. Be sure to detail the specifics and variables (e.g., for a supplement, write the exact brand used, quantity, frequency, etc.). By keeping this detailed record, if you decide to try the same treatment again later, you will have a record of exactly what you did and so will know if you are introducing new variables such as different brand, quantity, frequency, etc.

CHART 5.4: BLANK MONTHLY CHART

1					
2					
3					
4					
5					
6					
7					
8					
9					
10					
11					
12					
13					
14					
15					
16					
17					
18					
19					
20					
21					
22					
23					
24					
25					
26					
27					
28					
29					
30					
31					

You may use this monthly chart any way you wish to keep track of your health condition, symptoms, exacerbations, remissions, and treatments, in an easy-to-see full-month format. Fill in the column headings at the top according to what you would like to follow. This was the chart Jan made up for her own use, but you can also devise your own and make something that works for you.

Part II

Getting the Most from the 3LS Wellness Program

Chapter 6

How Did This Happen?— Causes of Illness

With all forms of healing, unless you understand the causes of the imbalance that created your illness and are willing to change those causes, the healing will be temporary. Eventually, the imbalance will return, along with the recurrence of symptoms or related problems. This chapter guides you to understand the causes of illness and how the 3LS lifestyle addresses those causes to improve and maintain health. (Remember, the Glossary is available for determining the meaning of any terms that are unfamiliar to you.)

WHAT ARE THE CAUSES?

Although this discussion relates most directly to the causes of chronic (long-term) illnesses, many or most acute (short-term) conditions have the same contributing factors and root causes. Maintaining health may also be understood through these causes as well.

Three contributing factors affect a person's well-being and cause chronic illness:

1. Genetics
2. Stress

   - Biophysical stress (including physical, electromagnetic, and biochemical)
   - Psychosocial stress
   - Stress-effect

3. Choice (lifestyle choices)

These three contributing factors are not equal in importance in creating health or illness. The last factor, choice, has the greatest effect in determining a person's health condition! Good lifestyle choices can reverse the results of poor genetics and too much stress (both avoidable and unavoidable stress) and can cure illness. Poor lifestyle choices, on the other hand, contribute to illness.

Let's take a look at each of the three categories.

1. Genetics and the Bell Curve

All illnesses are related to, but not totally dependent upon, the hand you were dealt by nature when you were conceived—your genetics. Your genes determine your characteristics, including your physical strengths and weaknesses. Therefore, your genetic inheritance, or the characteristics you were born with, is the baseline that determines what kinds of illness you have a propensity for in this lifetime.

Each characteristic that a person is born with could be represented on a separate chart that compares it to the same trait in a large number of people. Scientists have consistently discovered, when charting a large set of data about people's characteristics (regardless of what the actual data is), that most of the people fall in the middle (as average) and only a few people place at each of the two extremes. For example, if you were going to chart the height of a large random sample of people, you would note a small number of people at both the high and low ends on the graph (i.e., short and tall people) while many people would fall in the middle range (average height). Making a chart that illustrates this would produce a curvy line that looks like a bell. This type of data distribution is so common that such a chart is called a bell curve and is considered a normal result for random samples.

One could make a separate bell curve for all characteristics of a person. Besides charting traits like height, eye color, weight, and skin tone, there could also be bell curves for things like liver function, calcium levels, thyroid function, blood pressure, testosterone production, muscle strength/muscle mass, brain chemistry interaction, etc. Any person's health condition is a combination of at least hundreds of bell curves. Depending upon a person's genetics, a person might have a low, middle, or high position on a bell curve for any particular trait or function. Most people are probably at the top of some bell curves in some aspects, at the bottom of other bell curves in a few other aspects, and in the middle for most aspects.

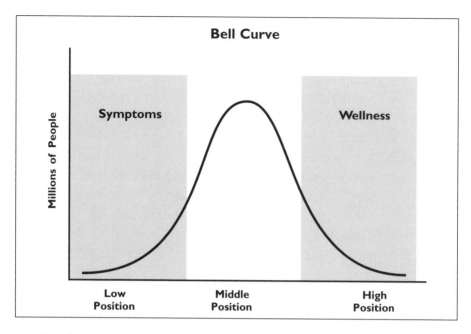

People may be low or at the bottom of a bell curve in a particular genetic characteristic, due to factors such as inborn errors of metabolism, structural deviations, and electromagnetic disturbances. For example, more than 40,000 genetic errors of metabolism are already known, and more are being identified all the time. No one is perfect, and so everybody is genetically low in something.

When it comes to health, the bell curve is a useful concept, because it can help you understand why a particular symptom or illness manifests for you. The combination of low positions on your bell curves gives you specific symptoms. The places where you are low indicate where you will have to strengthen yourself (relieve your symptoms and improve your health) to put you back in the middle of the curve for that characteristic.

2. The "Real" Stress

As we mentioned in the chapter about Skilled Relaxation, a major problem in today's world is chronic stress, and the average person today is exposed to more than 1,000 times as many stresses every day than people were exposed to just 100 years ago; more than 386,000 per day per person.[1] Hans Selye, the father of stress research, showed conclusively that each tiny (and sometimes not so tiny) stressor adds up and contributes to a person's total stress load.[2] At the present time, stress-related chronic conditions make up at least 80% to 90% of office visits to gatekeeper physicians (family practitioners, internists and pediatricians).[3]

At this point, however, we need to redefine stress. Modern stress is more than what most people think of as stress (that is, just psychosocial stress). There is much more to stress than psychosocial influences! Remember, stress in our definition is *anything* that puts the body into the fight or flight (FOF) mode (sympathetic nervous system activation). Countless things can activate the FOF response, including many kinds of biophysical stress, plus the phenomena of stress-effect (both of which we will discuss below). The fact that stress is more than psychosocial phenomena is a new idea for many people. It may take a little while for you to catch this concept, but please follow along.

The truth of the matter is, modern stress consists of about 90% biophysical stressors (including physical, biochemical, electromagnetic smog, and nutritional stressors) and only 10% psychosocial stressors.[4] C. Norman Shealy, M.D. (founder and first president of the American Holistic Medical Association) first published these figures 30 years ago. This percentage might surprise you if you're used to thinking that all stress is psychosocial, but this is the *exact* reason why patients say, "I don't have any stress in my life, so how can I be ill?" They are not aware of the 90% of biophysical stressors that affect their lives.

Why don't most people know about the other stressors besides psycho-social stressors? Physical and biochemical stressors are not always visible. The fact is, we are only aware of those stressors that actually push us over the edge of the cliff, *not* the ones that have been dragging us closer to that edge for years and years.

Here's another way to think about this. If the average American uses 40% of his or her reserves to deal with underlying physical stressors and 50% of his or her reserves to deal with underlying chemical stressors, then only 10% of all potential reserves would be available to deal with emotional stressors, which may simply not be enough. This is the reason emotional crises so often lead to illness and why psychosocial stress gets the attention and blame.

This large percentage of invisible stressors is why the average person in our culture is now operating dangerously close to the edge of his or her cliff[5] and why chronic illness is so prevalent today.

All types of stress have the common effect of decreasing the general vitality of the body. Below we will examine the three categories of stress in greater detail.

What are biophysical stressors?

Biophysical stressors include anything that causes physical or biological stress to the body. A simple example of a biophysical stress is when a person plunges his or her arm into a bucket filled with ice-water, holding it there for a while. The body's response to the physical stressor, of course, is the FOF response (i.e., the heart, respiratory, and blood pressure rates all increase, and blood moves away from the digestive organs and into large muscles). Smaller stressors, like chemical additives in the food you eat, all create the same FOF effect, but usually in a less dramatic way.

The bio*chemical* environment is playing a larger role in the cause of illness, and it is one of the greatest stressors in modern times. There is biochemical stress inside the body (such as nutritional stressors or toxicity) and biochemical stress outside of the body (such as electromagnetic smog). Many stressors are present today that did not exist 150 years ago, partly due to advancements in technology.

Below we have listed some typical biophysical stressors:

Biophysical Stressors
Physical

Physical stressors include:

- Bracing (muscular tension is both a stressor and a response to stress)
- Excessive dampness or dryness
- Excessive exercise
- Extreme temperatures
- Holding the body for a prolonged period of time in one position (as in computer work)
- Illness (this is both a stressor and the body's response to chronic stress)
- Noise
- Obesity
- Repetitive and excess exhaustion
- Repetitive motions
- Severe and incapacitating injury
- Shifting sleep cycles
- Sleep deprivation
- Surgery

Moreover, as an individual ages, the cliff edge automatically gets closer, so age itself is a physical stressor.

Biophysical Stressors
Biochemical

Biochemical stressors include:

- Additives to your tap water
- Chemical additives in personal care products
- Cigarette smoke
- Drugs (both prescription and over the counter)
- Environmental toxins such as all types of pollution
- Household cleaning products
- Insecticides
- Microbiologic contamination
- Plastics
- Pollution
- Synthetic clothing
- Synthetic materials used in household furnishings, paint and other products.

Just think about all the things in your house that are synthetic. Besides in the environment and the home, there are also pollution and chemicals in the workplace. Only 200 years ago, you could count the number of chemicals on your fingers. A mere 10 years ago, the American Society of Chemical Engineers (ASCE) bragged to the media that they had just synthesized the 500,000th chemical available to the world market for commercial use that had never before existed on the planet.[6] Ponder the bombardment on our bodies due to these biochemical stressors.

Biophysical Stressors
Biochemical (Nutritional)

Nutritional stressors (these are a subcategory of biochemical stress) include:

- Deep fried fatty foods
- Deficiencies of trace micronutrients in foods due to soil depletion
- Flavor enhancers
- Food additives
- Food colorings
- Genetically modified foods (GMOs)
- Hormones in animal/meat products
- Irradiation of foods

- Poor or improper preparation of food
- Preservatives
- Refined carbohydrates (which cause deficiencies of micronutrients)

Specific genetic inborn errors of metabolism (at least 40,000 of them already known) also exist. These include those in which the individual needs more than the normal amount of particular nutritional substances to have optimum health. Simply not having enough of the nutrients your body needs, not having enough food to eat, eating a very poor or inappropriate diet for your body, or eating under constant pressure are also nutritional stressors.

Biophysical Stressors
Biochemical (Electromagnetic Smog)

Electromagnetic smog stressors (another subcategory of biochemical stress, in that they can affect the biochemistry of the body) include things like:

- Appliances
- Background radioactivity
- Cellular and cordless phones and other wireless gadgets
- Computers
- Electric wiring in homes
- Energies that occur due to negative thinking or thoughts
- Fluorescent lights
- Geopathic stress (abnormal earth energies)
- Heating elements
- Low-level radiation
- Microwaves
- MRI's
- Palm Pilots
- Radar installations
- Radio waves
- Television
- Towers (high voltage, radio, TV and microwave)
- X-rays

Fifteen years ago there were already more than 200,000 electromagnetic frequencies that have been introduced in our environment whereas, prior to 100 years ago[7] we experienced none of these frequencies for billions of years.

∎ ∎ ∎

An entire book could be written listing all of the biophysical stressors of modern life. Biophysical stressors greatly reduce the body's reserves needed to deal with daily life and are a major demonstrable cause of degenerative disease.

Psychosocial stress

Psychosocial stress is generally caused by social and cultural environments. Some years ago, scientists from the University of Washington developed a scale to help people evaluate the amount of psychosocial stress in their lives. Called the Holmes-Rahe Test, you can find the test on the Internet, at the library, and in the *Relaxation and Stress Reduction Workbook*. The Holmes-Rahe Test assigns numerical values to psychosocial events that impact people's lives, such as loss (death, divorce, etc.), change (health condition, employment, moving, etc.), gain (marriage, pregnancy, etc.), difficulties (in-law trouble, business trouble, etc.), success (praise, etc.). The Holmes-Rahe Test is recognized as the first attempt to quantify or give a rating to stressors and has merit in doing so. However, our estimation is that the items on this list make up only about 20% of all the psychosocial stressors that exist.

The Holmes-Rahe test especially misses chronic psychosocial stressors that exist in the backgrounds of people's lives. Examples include conditions like living in an unsafe neighborhood, experiencing many years of poverty, or being stuck for a long time in a job one is not particularly good at or dislikes. Psychosocial stress also includes things like carrying unexamined emotional issues from early childhood, never emotionally resolving traumatic experiences, and trying to cope in the world with ineffective or inappropriate belief and behavior patterns.

Keep in mind that a reciprocal effect exists between the two types of stressors, biophysical and psychosocial. Biophysical stressors make an individual much more susceptible to the effects of psychosocial stress, and vice versa. Chapter 8 (healing mind, emotions, and spirit) has more information about psychosocial stress, and many books have been written on the topic.

Stress-effect

Knowing the difference between a stressor and stress-effect is helpful. A stressor is a thing or an event that causes stress. Stress-effect is how that stressor affects or impacts an individual. Stress-effect is an individual's interpretation of what is experienced (often a totally unconscious process) and is intensely personal. Stress-effect may be felt inside the bodymind as physical sensations, although many people will not notice any sensations at all.

Here is an example of stress-effect: If you are walking across a field and trip over a rock, you will experience both stressor and stress-effect. The trip over the rock would be called the "stressor," and the effect you would feel inside your bodymind would be called the "stress-effect." Now, trip over that same rock, in exactly the same way, at the edge of a cliff (without falling over the cliff). Tripping over the rock (stressor) is identical in both locations, however, the stress-effect would be dramatically different. The first trip is inconvenient, the second, terrifying. The second describes a much higher level of stress-effect.

So what exactly is stress-effect? It has the physical manifestations of FOF (sympathetic activation). The sensations of stress-effect inside your bodymind are the manifestation of FOF mechanisms controlled by the hypothalamus. Many of these sensations are beyond conscious awareness and cannot be known unless we use something like biofeedback to increase awareness of what is happening inside the body.

As we described in Chapter 2, stress-effect gets stored inside the hypothalamus and builds up to result in a person being constantly in FOF mode. What is stored in the hypothalamus is the effect of the stressor on that individual, not the stressor itself. No one yet knows exactly how it is stored, but Hans Selye, the father of modern stress research, clearly demonstrated that it was.[8]

FOF is also called chronic autonomic arousal and it is measurable in many ways. Just a few examples are blood pressure, pulse, perspiration, cholesterol elevation, clotting speed, muscle tension, breathing rate, and cortisol levels. The accumulation or storage of stress-effect has the effect of decreasing the ability to feel, and there is ample evidence that the worse the stress-effect burden gets, the more "numb" a person becomes.[9] This numbness is an accommodation survival mechanism. The chronic stress of continually being in FOF mode eventually results in chronic illnesses.

Acute stress is different from chronic stress, and a certain amount of acute stress is healthy. Acute stress comes and goes quickly, in contrast to chronic stress, which is long-term. A certain amount of acute stress is good for people, because the bodymind is benefited by responding and acting on a stressor through fighting or fleeing. Actually, the hypothalamus was designed, over at least millions of years, to function most efficiently in the rest mode interspersed with short periods of total and abject terror (when the saber-toothed tiger appears, for example). The human body was not designed to cope with constant low levels of chronic stress and chronic stress-effect (such as being constantly exposed to high levels of pollutants). It is the stress-effect not acted upon and stored in the hypothalamus that creates a constant FOF state, which in turn causes us to over-react to many of the little stressors of daily life.

If you do nothing to discharge your accumulated stress-effect, even if you are not exposed to 386,000 stressors every day, the stress-effect you have already stored in your body will keep you where you are in terms of health and actually get worse as you age. Your systems become less capable as you age and less able to tolerate stressors of any kind.

People often ask if stress-effect is solely personal psychological interpretation of a stressor. In some cases, it is. The illustration of tripping over a rock by the edge of a cliff might be considered psychological interpretation. However, what about invisible biophysical stressors, such as poor nutrition or pollution? They also cause stress-effect no differently than psychosocial stressors.

An example of how invisible stressors cause stress-effect is how people who already have symptoms (are over the edge of their cliff) have a greater stress load than others. Let us explain. When any system of the body is close to its limits (the edge of the cliff), that system becomes hyper-reactive, and if any stressor affects that system thereafter, the effect of that stress—the stress-effect—will be even greater. Thus, people at the cliff edge react much more strongly to any stressor than they do when they are in the middle of the field. The more distance to the edge of our cliff, the less stress-effect occurs with each stressor. This shows that manifestation of stress-effect is not just psychological interpretation.

3. Choice (Lifestyle Choices)

By far the most influential and important of the three causes of illness is choice. Choice either enhances or worsens what genetics has given you. Choice either increases or decreases the amount and effect of stress in your life. By our choices, we all contribute to, or resolve, our own problems. The positive side of this in terms of chronic illness is that most individuals only have to improve a few items to vastly improve function and health.

Lifestyle is an effective place to start making better choices to transform your health. Lifestyle choices dramatically increase (or decrease) enjoyment of life, resistance to disease, length and quality of life, and can even reverse (or accelerate) the progression of chronic disease. The single most effective and dynamic lifestyle choice you can make to improve your genetic potential and overall health is to practice all aspects of the 3LS. The vast majority who Practice Serious Wellness usually also become students of health and start making additional choices for a healthy lifestyle. This gratifying cycle of learning and then feeling more alive *can be irresistible.*

■ ■ ■

The rest of this chapter ties together and integrates many of the important concepts in this book.

Choice makes a difference with regard to stress. Stress can be reduced by anything that increases the distance between you and the edge of your cliff. As we discussed in Chapter 1, there are two ways to distance yourself from the edge. We believe the most effective of these two ways is to move the cliff away from you by practicing the 3LS, which increases the bodymind's resistance to disease. The other way, moving away from the edge of the cliff by reducing the large number of stressors, may be less effective, because stressors are so plentiful. Of course, combining both approaches—reducing stressors plus doing the 3LS—would be an even more effective and prudent choice for achieving optimum health.

Choice also makes a difference with regard to genetics. You cannot get rid of or change your genetic inheritance. Genetic inheritance is called the genome and is the combination of the genes or the entire DNA structure of an individual. However, you still have control over at least 80% of the *expression* of your genes by the choices you make. This control is called the phenome and is the possible health potential for a person. Thus 20% of your genetic factor is unchangeable, and 80% is changeable. This has been proven by the Human Genome Project, which is identifying all the approximately 30,000 genes in human DNA. The Human Genome Project has already established that our choices determine at least 80% of wellness, quality of life, and longevity, and genes only determine 20%.[10] This 80% variable is because the expression of the genes can change depending upon the interaction of the environment with the genes. Our lifestyle choices can change our health condition, such as improving molecular, cellular, and atomic mechanisms.

This is to say that 80% of your health potential is determined by your choice. In terms of genetics, lifestyle choices add another dimension to how a person can realize his or her potential in this world.

GENETICS, STRESS, AND CHOICE INTERACT

The whole health condition of a person is made up of an infinitely complex interaction of all of the factors that we have discussed. Each factor is different within each individual and *each* factor *magnifies* the complexity of the whole, rather than *adds* to its complexity (e.g., 3 x 3 x 3, not 3 + 3 + 3). Just consider the interaction among all of a person's hundreds or thousands of bell curves (genetic traits). The complexity increases as you multiply that by all of the daily biophysical and psychosocial stressors you encounter.

Since there are so many factors that have the potential to contribute to illness and so many interactions among them, there is rarely only one simple cause for a chronic illness. Even just by itself, the human bodymind is so complex that one can only truly understand what is going on by stepping back and looking at the whole person—holistically. It is a mistake to think anything is in isolation in the bodymind. Considering an aspect in isolation makes thinking about it simpler, but this type of thinking ultimately draws us away from healing the whole person.

So what makes illness happen? Normally, our bodies are remarkably able to cope with piles of stressors. However, if the stress is too high for too long, that ability to cope ceases. Prior to becoming ill, the body systems or functions that are in low positions on a bell curve "borrow" functional capacity from the ones that are high or strong. The strong ones help compensate for the weak ones. However, this can only go on so long, and one day the part of the person that is low on the bell curve suddenly collapses with an acute condition (examples are strokes, heart attacks, ulcers, arthritis, etc.) or starts experiencing symptoms of a chronic condition. The causative factors have added up and have finally overwhelmed the bodymind's ability to accommodate them. Such health conditions typically come on suddenly, even though the causes have been accumulating for many years. This simple concept truly describes the origin of most health conditions.

It sometimes takes 30 to 40 years for the accumulation of causative factors to show up as chronic disease or acute illness. The amount of time it takes for symptoms to surface depends upon the condition, the person's genetic susceptibility for that condition, and the lifestyle choices that stressed that particular system. There is now ample evidence that the lifestyle of the mother or father *prior to conception* may be very strongly related to health conditions that eventually occur in an individual's life.

Your life choices matter for years and affect you long before any diagnosable chronic condition becomes apparent. If people are not empowered via wellness education to make good choices early on in their lives, after chronic illness happens, significant lifestyle changes are sometimes required to reverse or overcome that illness.

Our bodies are made to keep us going, without symptoms, even though we may be seriously damaged. That is good, in a way, since that allows us ample leeway to survive. However, the other edge of that double-edged sword is that when the body finally gives up compensating, the collapse is often sudden. All acute conditions work that way: heart attacks start 40 years before the person has any clue.

All your choices determine your level of wellness, which makes you responsible, at least in part, for the illnesses you contract. The most common variables that affect illness are the lifestyle choices of relaxation, diet, and exercise.

THE 3LS TO THE RESCUE

The best approach for working on the cause of most chronic conditions is to fall back on the wisdom of the bodymind and Practice Serious Wellness.

When a person's overall health starts out in life at the lower end of a bell curve, this means that the individual began a little closer to the edge of the symptomatic cliff than others. These people have to work harder to stay away from the cliff edge and get to the middle of the field (the middle of the bell curve), which is where most people live. The lower on the bell curve a person is born, the more changeable their lot is by lifestyle choice. For these individuals, practicing the 3LS Wellness Program may reap vast improvements in health. Genetic potential really is changeable.

The holistic medical philosophy says that the most important factor in health and disease is the amount of reserves presented to the environment by the mind-body-spirit totality of a human. Practicing the 3LS...

- builds those reserves by discharging stored stress-effect, reducing biophysical stress through clearing up addictions, balancing brain and body chemistry, improving the function of the Krebs cycle, reversing metabolic sluggishness, and other things.

- helps your body function in the best way possible by giving nature an opportunity to heal itself. That is why the 3LS will reverse both overactive and underactive problems and bring a system into balance. This balance is called homeodynamic.

- improves your experience of life by working with the phenome—the 80% of genetics that is the expression or potential of your genes. You can expect your quality of life to improve in areas of body, mind, emotions, and spirit.

With wellness, even if stressors are still present, the bodymind functions better. Since the average person in this culture is now operating pretty close to the edge of their cliff[11] you can see how the 3LS would benefit most people.

Practicing Serious Wellness according to the instructions is beneficial for nearly everyone. By practicing all three parts of the 3LS, some people (those who are on a high place on the bell curve) will be exerting more effort than their genes need to make them well. They will experience optimum health. A significant percentage of people who desperately want to be well (those people on the low end of the bell curve) definitely need to do all three aspects of the Wellness Program accurately. By doing so, they will move towards achieving the level of results necessary for basic good health. Individuals in the middle of the bell curve can expect to experience significant improvements and may also reach a level of optimum health.

Regardless of where you are placed on the bell curve, if you only do one aspect of this three-part wellness plan and experience improvement, eventually it will probably not be enough. A Three-Legged Stool really needs all three legs to be permanently stable. The longer one lives, the more obvious this becomes. The synergistic effect of the three aspects gives the greatest benefits. This synergy occurs because every part of your bodymind is connected to all the rest.

How the 3LS Practices Support Each Other

■■■ JAN: **Rest and relaxation** provide energy for the body to heal itself. Skilled Relaxation combines with diet by relaxing the digestive tract so that it can better digest and absorb nutrition. Skilled Relaxation combines with exercise by relaxing tightly bound muscles, thus creating a more mobile and efficient body, which can then exercise more efficiently. Skilled Relaxation in particular helps discharge stored stress-effect from the hypothalamus.

A good diet brings nutrition to the body for repairing damaged structures and functioning efficiently. The Perfect Whole Foods Diet combines with Skilled Relaxation by giving the body the nutrients it needs to repair and heal itself during times of rest and relaxation. The Perfect Whole Foods Diet combines with Exercise by providing micronutrients for good metabolism, which supports the exercise process. The Perfect Whole Foods Diet in particular helps decrease biophysical stress.

Exercise provides strengthening, circulation, and efficiency to all parts of the body. Exercise combines with Skilled Relaxation by discharging tension, which helps the body relax more easily. Exercise combines with the Perfect Whole Foods Diet by circulating nutrients to all parts of the body. Aerobic exercise, in particular, improves metabolism and increases energy, which especially helps decrease all forms of stress. ∎∎∎

Every holistic practitioner we know has noticed the same thing: each aspect of the Wellness Program multiplies the effect of the others.

Through professional experience we see that, in general, dealing with the deepest layer of an illness makes most superficial layers disappear or are easier to treat. Also, resolution of any layer of dysfunction or illness then exposes the next layer to work with for improving health. Holistic practitioners all over the world call this mechanism "peeling the onion." The 3LS works with problems at the center or deepest layer of the onion. That is why the 3LS can be so effective in resolving health problems, or if not, it makes them easier to deal with using other forms of treatment.

"WILL I BE CURED?"

When you are working to reverse your chronic condition, it is important to understand the notion of cure. The strict sense of the word "cure" is a permanent resolution of a health situation or disease without continued use of the therapy that alleviated the symptoms. For chronic conditions, the concept is applied a little differently. Since a chronic condition is nearly always related to the genetic condition or genome a person was born with (which cannot be changed), a person's recovery from chronic illness may require a lifetime attention to lifestyle. For example, one cannot cure an alcoholic since alcoholism is related to genetic inheritance. Therefore, once the diagnosis is made, that person is a recovering alcoholic for the rest of his or her life and needs to pay attention to the on-going healthy lifestyle choice of abstinence from alcohol. The same need for attention to lifestyle is true of many other chronic conditions. Thus, if an individual has a genetic predisposition for a certain functional body system to break down, after that condition occurs, he or she will have to do at least some of the practices that resolved that illness for the rest of their lives or be at risk of recurrence.

As far as curing a condition is concerned, the permanent results of the Wellness Program, or *any* medical or healing treatment, also sometimes depends upon how much damage has occurred prior to starting it. Any condition can become so far gone that even working with the causes will not reverse it. There is a limit to what Wellness, or any medical or healing treatment, can do. However, even if a health condition no longer has the potential to be reversed, terminating the causes of that condition by practicing the 3LS will still help alleviate symptoms or prevent future health problems. For example: if chronic diabetic vascular insufficiency has progressed to amputation of a leg, wellness will not grow back the leg, but the 3LS will likely delay or prevent the amputation of the other leg. Regardless of how far any condition has progressed, taking a Wellness approach improves quality of life.

One additional cause of chronic health conditions is worthy of mention, but it does not need a category or deep discussion. A few chronic illnesses are directly precipitated by injury. Practicing Serious Wellness always gives the best chance for helping chronic health conditions resulting from any type of injury, so the 3LS is the best long-term choice for people who have been injured. For example, people who have been in motor vehicle accidents who have ongoing musculo-skeletal discomfort can help themselves and relieve their symptoms using the 3LS. Those who are injured will have to work harder at wellness than those who have not had such a traumatic experience.

Remember, too, that the 3LS works well for *prevention* of chronic health conditions. We encourage all of you to keep practicing the Wellness Program to prevent chronic conditions from occurring in the first place.

CHOOSING HEALTH

Q: You say that choice is the most important variable in causing chronic illness, and that is where I am having trouble getting started with the practices. I can't do the Wellness Program because I don't believe I have any choice in my life. Should I just give up the idea of ever becoming healthy?

A: ■■■ JAN: This question about your perception that you have no choice is one I know will arise for many people. If you feel you have no choice in your life, I recommend that you work towards changing your limiting view to become the belief that you do have many choices. If you really want to improve your health, you *will* find a way to make the 3LS work for you. First, make a clear and firm decision to commit to becoming healthier, then search for ways to bring fulfillment to your decision.

Enhancing Your Opportunities for Choice

There are levels or layers of choice in each person's life. You may not be able to make changes in all of these levels, but it is more than likely that you can work with at least one or two areas and choose to become healthier. Remember, we keep saying in this book to do what works! Creative choice can help you approach the 3LS in the way that works best for you.

First, there is the choice of your overall life situation. Certain life situations make it easier to practice the Wellness Program than others. If you feel that your overall situation makes it difficult for you to use the 3LS, you might choose to make a change to a better overall life situation when the time is right for you. An example might be, when the time is right, changing from a demanding job that requires a 12-hour shift to an easier 8-hour job with no overtime.

Second, without changing your overall situation, you may choose to improve your existing circumstances. For example, if you wish to practice Skilled Relaxation and exercise, but don't feel you have a place to do these practices, you might consider converting your unfinished basement into a place for home workouts and quiet relaxation. Or, if you are in a relationship with someone who you feel is controlling and you believe that there is no room in that relationship for you to practice the 3LS, you may first wish to improve your circumstances by learning some advanced relationship skills. Chapter 8 has some leads for where to learn such skills. Relationship dynamics *can* be changed, and circumstances *can* be improved.

Third, you can choose to adapt the parts of the Wellness Program creatively as needed in your situation and circumstances. For example, if you have a live-in job or dorm where your meals are provided for you, making it difficult to follow a Whole Food Diet perfectly, choose to start a different aspect of the 3LS, such as Exercise or Skilled Relaxation. You can also make choices to improve your diet as much as possible, such as choosing to eat more vegetables instead of brownies. Another example is an invalid who cannot get up to exercise. This person may choose to learn Skilled Relaxation and make dietary changes. Or, he or she may choose an exercise program to fit the situation, such as lifting very light weights or doing isometric exercises.

Fourth, you can choose your belief system. Choice of belief is often the deciding factor in starting and carrying out the 3LS. This refers to what we mentioned in the introduction about locus of control. The belief that your choices and actions do affect your health (internal locus of control) gives the power and potential for healing *to you*.

If you believe that health occurs totally by destiny or external influence (external locus of control), you may be reluctant to start the Wellness Program. To change, just consider the possibility that your actions can greatly determine your health and start one part of the 3LS as an experiment to find out if it works.

What kind of beliefs slow people down and keep them from making healthy choices for themselves? Actually, it is fear (or beliefs or concerns). If the thought of being healthy makes you feel apprehensive, or panic-stricken, or if you feel that the time is not right for you to improve your health, it may be time to look at exactly what your fears are so you can overcome them. You may also want to explore the idea that your lack of health or illness has a payoff or benefit you may be clinging to at this time.

Replacing Your Limiting Beliefs

Below is a list of some fear-based beliefs followed by some new beliefs (in bold) that might replace them. By the way, if you don't like the new beliefs listed here, make up your own new positive beliefs! Do what works!

1. Some people have a mental block about doing something nice for themselves—they think that spending time to improve or take care of themselves is selfish rather than helpful to others. **Improving your health is the best gift you can give your family and friends.**

2. Some people have no or low self-worth and don't believe they deserve good health. **Everybody deserves good health. It is all right to want good health for yourself and to take the steps to achieve it.**

3. Some people are convinced the 3LS will be difficult or that their quality of life or enjoyment will decrease. **After a period of adjustment, most people who do the 3LS find that their quality of life and enjoyment skyrocket! The 3LS needn't be viewed as a sacrifice because what you are really losing is poor health.**

4. Some people find it easier to blame other people, circumstances, or events for their health problems rather than take responsibility to improve their lives. This is taking the stance of "being a victim," and people do it to avoid taking personal responsibility for the outcome of their own lives. **Each person is responsible for his or her own life, choices, and decisions. You can choose to make your life happy and healthy.**

5. Some people prefer anything that is familiar (even if it is sickness) to what is unknown (health). **Changing a way of life and taking**

calculated risks can lead to great rewards. **Facing the unknown entity of health can be one of the most exhilarating and empowering actions you can take for yourself!**

6. Some people have feelings of "deep loyalty" to their families and won't go beyond or surpass what their parents or other family members have achieved, including areas of life like health condition. **What's best for each family member can be supportive of the entire family. Your health and happiness are important and can help your family in many ways.**

7. Some people who have failed to improve their health condition previously mistakenly believe that the present circumstance is the same as the past. **Each circumstance has its own set of conditions, and there are always new variables. For example, sometimes it takes many attempts under new, differing circumstances before a certain treatment will work. Persist.**

8. Some people do not choose to seek health because they receive some form of psychological payoff from being ill. The payoff may be the sympathy and attention they receive from other people. **Living a life that is exuberantly healthy and filled with well-being is far more enjoyable and wondrous than any amount of sympathy people can give you.**

9. Some people believe that they are healthy as long as they are not in the hospital. **There are levels of wellness. You can expect more from life than being in pain, feeling constantly fatigued, being limited mentally, emotionally, or physically, and having recurrent health problems. By making an effort to pursue wellness, you are likely to experience greater well-being and happiness.**

One way to overcome any fears or concerns you have about improving your health or making changes is by concretely looking at what you are actually afraid of. You might write these things down to help you look at them. Then see if each thing you fear might realistically come to pass, and how bad it would actually be if it did happen. Explore the worst-case scenario that could happen, and also the best-case scenario. Oftentimes by doing this, you will find that your worry is groundless. Often, the worst-case scenario is very unlikely to happen, or wouldn't be that bad, and the best-case scenario is closer to reality. This activity of mentally facing your fears might also help you discover that you are really ready for health.

How to "Choose" Health

What beliefs motivate people to start choosing health and to make healthy choices for themselves?

- Having a positive attitude and the belief that you can be healthy can move you in the direction of health.

- Realizing that there are enormous positive gains to be made from being healthy can inspire you toward health. A sense of internal reward is often helpful in this process. This means there is the expectation that something desirable will result from doing the new behavior. (Read all the positive experiences described by people throughout this book for reminders of some of the rewards of good health.)

- A belief or certainty that a chosen treatment will actually work and the desired outcome is possible can inspire healthy choices.

- A sense of right timing can help initiate a wellness program. When there is so much agreement and synchronicity of events that you know you can do something, the time is right. This knowing is a kind of intuition.

- Determination to restore or achieve health regardless of timing, circumstances, and other factors can overcome many obstacles to reaching wellness.

- Believing that there is a purpose to all events in life, even those that seem difficult, and having the willingness to learn and grow from all experiences, can help you accept, work with, and change your health condition.

The outcome of your life and your wellness depends on what you do and the choices you make daily. If after reading this, you still feel you have no choices, and therefore cannot start any of the aspects of the Wellness Program, it might be best for you to start by doing some personal growth work or psychological counseling described in Chapter 8 (about healing mind, emotions, and spirit). Counseling and/or personal growth work can enable you to understand that you *do* have choices, even if they are not apparent to you at the moment. A good therapist or counselor can help you learn that you have options so that you can and will take steps to create positive choice in your life. ■■■

Another choice you can make is viewing wellness and the process of getting better as enjoyment. Consider the 3LS a hobby. Practicing Serious Wellness is not only one of the most enjoyable hobbies, but it also offers the greatest potential for a happy life. If you don't think you have enough energy to make Serious Wellness your hobby, start small—but do start. Once Wellness, at any level of commitment, has been your hobby for a year, your increased health gives you more time and ability to make even more positive choices in your life. Actually experiencing a wellness lifestyle is the only way to know how happy you can feel. This has been our personal experience as well as that of others who have followed the 3LS.

In the observations section of this chapter, we have included one rather long note for you to read. The individual who wrote it worked to understand the causes of his symptoms, applied the 3LS Wellness Program and other treatments to resolve his condition, and then very beautifully shared some of the things he learned about holistic healing during his journey back to wellness. While his success is not uncommon among those who take this path of healing, we feel his description is exemplary and inspiring.

Chapter 6, CAUSES OF ILLNESS—SUMMING IT UP

Chronic illness has more than one cause. Many or most chronic conditions, and also acute illnesses, have the same contributing factors:

1. Genetics
2. Stress
3. Choice

All three factors interact to cause illness.

1. Genetics determines the health conditions for which you have a propensity. Genetics therefore also determines areas to strengthen to relieve your symptoms and improve your health.

2. Stress is a major factor in illness, and needs to be redefined. Stress includes not only psychosocial stress, but also biophysical stress, including physical, electromagnetic and biochemical stress. Biophysical stressors are increasing in modern times. These less commonly known stressors decrease the general vitality of the body. Psychosocial stress includes chronic and acute stressors. Stress-effect, another aspect of stress, is the way stressors affect an individual. Stress-effect is stored within the body and accumulates. Regardless of type, all stressors move you closer to experiencing symptoms. The body can handle piles of stressors until one day it finally becomes overwhelmed, and symptoms appear.

3. Of the three causes of chronic illness, choice is the most influential and most important. Your choices have the potential to maximize your genetic expression and decrease your stressors, and thus determine your level of wellness. The three most common choices that affect health are lifestyle choices related to relaxation, diet, and exercise.

The 3LS Wellness Program works with the choice variable. The 3LS is the healthiest basic lifestyle choice you can make. The three aspects of this Wellness Program interact in combination to work with the deepest layers of cause. The Program builds your reserves to combat stress and helps your body function in the best way possible. For chronic conditions, constant attention to lifestyle choices is important.

The word reversing, rather than curing, may best describe resolving a chronic illness. If a condition is too advanced to be reversed, the 3LS Wellness Program can still help make the most of your remaining health.

You can make healthy choices in your life. Even if it seems impossible to do so, many variables exist that can be changed or altered so you can move towards health. You can create opportunities for making healthy choices in your overall life situation by adapting the practices in the Wellness Program creatively and/or choosing a belief system that enhances health. Beliefs that limit your movement towards wellness can be replaced by more expansive viewpoints to help you make more healthy choices for yourself.

PEOPLE'S OBSERVATIONS ABOUT THE CAUSES OF ILLNESS

Everyone here is talking about Skilled Relaxation, and let me tell you, it works! However, Skilled Relaxation will have limited effects if you are still living a stressful life and not getting enough sleep. I was living in such a state of stress and sleep deprivation that I was actually unaware that I had either. It wasn't until I quit some of what I was doing and started to get a good eight hours of sleep per night that I realized how I was living for several years. I had to go from a full load at school down to half time. I also quit some volunteer things I was doing and had my daughter go down from four after school activities to only two (this was partly because I didn't want her to be stressed also). I would advise that you sit down and make a list of the most important factors in your life (your health, your relationship with your husband, etc.) and then make changes based on that list.

—*Mary Koehnen, Student/Homemaker, St. Paul, MN*

I learned self-hypnosis from reading the book Dr. Stoll recommended, *The Relaxation and Stress Reduction Workbook.* But first I read *Mind as Healer, Mind as Slayer,* by Kenneth Pelletier, and this really helped me understand the effects of stress on the body and the role of the hypothalamus. I work full time. In the beginning it was a challenge to find the time to do Skilled Relaxation twice a day, but once I developed a routine it became very natural. I do Skilled Relaxation first thing in the morning after I wake up (I had to re-adjust my wake up time to 30 minutes earlier to fit in SR), and then I do Skilled Relaxation as soon as I get home from work. That's the first thing I do when I get in the door. In fact, I just came back from a two-week vacation and was concerned about not finding the time, as we were traveling in a group. However, I managed to do it by making choices. The evenings were tricky, but if the group was going to be somewhere before dinner, then I'd make arrangements to catch up with them in 30 to 40 minutes. I know it's easier said than done, but it's really about putting yourself first, and that's the way I look at it. Doing Skilled Relaxation is important to my well-being and that's important to me, so I find the time. One last thing, I have found myself in situations at work where I know I'll be working really late, which would make it too late to do SR when I get home. So I book 30 minutes with myself in the afternoon and go into a conference room and do SR. It's not ideal, but it works. And it's amazing how much more centered and calm I feel afterwards. —*S. Willers, Communications, Toronto, Ontario, Canada*

Finding the source of my illness was like unraveling a ball of string. It kept reaching back further and further, but honest scrutiny and analysis point to a stress crisis I brought on myself in 1997. That year I was a college senior, and played my last season of Division I water polo with seven and a half hours of training a day. I wanted it so badly I pushed myself far past mere overtraining. That season I ate over 10,000 calories a day and yet could barely maintain four percent body fat. By the end of the season, I had insomnia, a heart condition, constant injuries, and the beginnings of a mental breakdown. I was taking huge amounts of NSAIDs, Percocet, Voltarin, hydrocortisone, and Vicodin for pain, and had what I have seen described as anorexia athletica. Even though I had played my last game, I was obsessed with an unhealthy need to see my body look ferocious. I was, no doubt, nutrient-depleted, overstressed, and perhaps copper toxic from the pool, but I did not stop pushing. I dropped weight as I continued to maintain endorphin highs working out three hours a day— which was a rest for me. When my body would no longer tolerate protein and was in a constant state of gastronomic uncertainty I went from omnivorous, to little meat, to vegetarian. My girlfriend began to distance herself from me as I became more anxious, obsessive, irritable, and depressed.

I graduated and moved to Europe. I made so little money that I was literally starving and ate polenta and sugar every day, all day. Soon I was 6'2" and 140 lbs. That's when my symptoms arrived. At first it was fatigue, deep and heavy, laying over me and keeping me on the couch all day. Then depression set in crushing and endless. I began to suffer from migraine headaches that would last weeks, and later, months. My muscles began to twitch and spasm and I became so uncoordinated that I always had to be cautious of tripping or staggering into traffic. My speech became slurred and people would think I was drunk. But worst of all were the mental symptoms: my mind raced, endlessly obsessing in violent whirlpools such that one day I spent 45 minutes staring at a subway map trying to find the most efficient way home, eventually breaking down and crying with frustration. My concentration was so limited that I was, at times, unable to read, as I could not remember words from the beginning of the sentence. Life was two dimensional, and seemed distant.

I wandered for years with food allergies, unable to function, shuttling between bewildered doctors' offices but unwilling to take the anti-depressants they prescribed me and generally watching my experience of life narrow. One night, using my roommate's computer, I discovered Walt's bulletin board and stayed up all night. I read it for months, and still read it today. There is a collection of angels helping out on that board. Eventually I gathered from what I learned that my hypothalamus had been overwhelmed, my body nutritionally deprived, my soul psychically bankrupt, and my life a mess. I found the most important key to healing was that I had the answers and the responsibility to make it through. Though I know I will not be out of this for a while, each month finds me better than before and finally with absolute faith that I will be well again.

I didn't begin this letter as a testimonial, but I suppose people are going to read it and try to apply it to their predicament. I have learned so much on this healing trip, and while much of it has been individual, there are some points I have found to be universally true:

- To say that healing a chronic ailment is like peeling an onion is an apt, accurate, and useful description. It is good to remember this. When you see a piece of information that you discarded as irrelevant at a certain stage of recovery become relevant again and you go back to it, you understand why: because an onion is spherical.

- Healing is a process of dedicating yourself to unraveling both the causes and the symptoms.

- In healing, one does not actually seek to reverse, but to go through and go forward. Once I realized that I needed to reinvent myself in order to heal, I was at first scared. Then I realized I would most likely retain all my dreams, goals, loves, and ambitions, but that I would have to come at them from another angle—change the process so to speak. I am so much more peaceful after having chosen that new angle and reinventing myself. The useless baggage is sloughed off and that which is true perseveres.

- It is not what you take but what you do that will heal you. Actually, you are not healed by what you take at all; what you take and do allows you to heal yourself.

- The body's capacity to heal itself is nearly without boundary.

- Meditation and personal responsibility for your own health create an internal wellness compass. Before I found Walt, I had to ask a doctor when I was getting well. There have been many blind alleys in my journey, but no wrong turns once I was directing the healing.

- Stop chasing the symptoms—the candida, the hypoglycemia, the depression, the irritability, the food allergies, the metal toxicities, and the gut problems. Treat them, but keep your eyes on the source of the pressures that is causing your body to malfunction in the first place.

- Keep notes, be objective, be truthful, and be brave. These are your only markers to test whether progress is being made.

—Michael Warner Kallus, Attorney, Merry Point, VA

Chapter 7

Adjunct Approaches to the 3LS

This chapter covers:

1. Self-help techniques and treatments that you can use at home alongside your practice of the 3LS
2. Use of practitioner-assisted medicines and modalities, both conventional and "alternative" treatments
3. Selecting and working with health care professionals

STEPS TO HEALING...WHAT WORKS FOR YOU?

Regardless of the chronic condition you wish to overcome, the most efficient use of your time and energy for its resolution occurs by following three steps. *The first step* is learning and study—finding out more about your condition and the health and lifestyle approaches that can help you. *The second step* is implementing some of those lifestyle changes for your improved wellness. *The third step* is adding other treatments. While starting with Step 3 is not the most effective way to go about reversing a chronic condition, we understand that many opt to start here. Our hope is that doing so will create enough benefits for you to become interested in going back to Step 1 and Step 2. Following the order as we listed above gives the quickest, best, and most long-lasting results, but we care that you get better more than we care how you go about it.

Of course, these three steps are very appropriate for use with the 3LS Wellness Program. You can also use this three-step protocol to work on health issues that are not addressed by the 3LS. If, for example, you wish to treat toenail fungus, you would follow the same process: learn about it, make good lifestyle choices that help eliminate it and/or prevent its recurrence, then pursue the best treatments (which might include seeing an appropriate healthcare provider for treatment recommendations).

USING OTHER HEALING METHODS CONCURRENTLY

Why might you want to use additional healing treatments or methods at the same time you're using the 3LS? Doing so is actually quite common. Here are the reasons:

1. For symptomatic relief
2. To speed up or enhance the healing process
3. To address issues the 3LS does not work on specifically

Many who start the 3LS Wellness Program early enough in the progression of their chronic illness find that both their main symptoms and many secondary disorders disappear. Just getting rid of stored stress through the practice of Skilled Relaxation, eliminating a refined carbohydrate addiction through eating a Perfect Whole Foods Diet, and clearing up metabolic sluggishness through doing Aerobic Exercise can often be enough. Some people have health problems, however, that will need to be dealt with *after* resolving the hypothalamic overload, the refined carbohydrate addiction, and improving metabolism. These other conditions are secondary to a functional body system having broken down, and may not resolve without specific treatment. We are referring to conditions like candida, parasitosis, arthritis, colitis, allergies, and endocrinopathies.

If any condition remains after you have followed the 3LS for six to twelve months, specific treatments can be used and have a better chance of being successful since the causes are already being addressed. The advantage of having done the 3LS before using other healing methods is that the Wellness Program makes it much easier to find the source of the still existing secondary problems and resolve them. Your bodymind has used the healthy lifestyle to clear out all of the distracting junk. For those remaining conditions, there are two ways to go forward with additional treatments: using self-help techniques and obtaining the services of one or more appropriate health care practitioners.

The 3LS, when used together with other treatments (either self-help or assisted), typically magnifies the effectiveness and results of any modality used. For example, combining Skilled Relaxation with a treatment such as acupuncture, self-hypnosis, stretching, Rolfing, etc., can greatly enhance the benefits you receive from each. If you are looking for additional ways to help yourself, read on. There are integrative benefits that result from combining approaches to healing a specific condition, so continue using the Wellness Program while you investigate and use other methods.

We encourage you to start by learning. The more you learn, the more likely you will be to find out what treatment will be most effective for you, therefore saving time, money, and effort. Learning and study is also beneficial before beginning any treatment option presented to you by a healthcare provider. With more information, you can make better, informed choices.

Informed choice is based upon access to, and full understanding of, all necessary information regarding potential treatment of your condition. To make an effective choice, you must know the advantages and disadvantages of each treatment option available. Learn both the benefits and possible side effects of any treatment. When selecting practitioners, choose those who educate you and empower you to make your own choices.

This chapter gives you more options so you can make a more informed choice about how to heal.

SELF-HELP

Self-help involves observing yourself, your body, habits, thoughts, feelings, and actions. It is about examining anything that contributes to your health condition and finding lifestyle changes and techniques that will enhance and improve your health and well-being.

Some Self-Help Methods

The following are powerful ways to help yourself and can be learned and practiced to help reverse chronic conditions and increase health:

Acupressure
Affirmations
Alexander technique
Aromatherapy
Art therapy
Breathing practice
Castor oil packs
Color therapy
Detoxification

Educational
  kinesiology
Eliminating or
  decreasing stressors
Feldenkrais
Herbs and herbal
  formulas
Hydration (drinking
  enough water)
Hydrotherapy

Light therapy
Movement therapy
Music therapy
Nutritional supple-
  mentation
Personal growth work
  (Psychological
  self-help)
Play therapy
Qi gong

Reflexology	Stretching	Vision therapy
Self-hypnosis, visual-	Support and self-help	(eyesight
ization, and guided	groups	improvement)
imagery	T'ai chi	Yoga
Self-massage	Toning/chanting/	
Stress management	singing	

Of course, this list only scratches the surface. By doing some research, you may find more self-help ways to improve your health condition. Refer to the Resources Section at the end of the book. Chapter 8 offers self-help approaches for healing mind, emotions, and spirit. Since all is related, working on mental, emotional, and spiritual aspects of yourself may very well bring healing to your physical condition, too.

Here are a few methods we have experienced and are most familiar with as being helpful adjuncts to the 3LS.

Breathing practice: Correct and deep breathing can increase lung capacity and help provide more oxygen to the body. Special breathing practices can alleviate ailments related to the respiratory system and improve other chronic conditions and symptoms. Some ways to increase and control breath include practices like counting or holding the breath, learning to breathe properly (using the muscles appropriately), awareness of breath, and postural improvements that help expansion of the rib cage. Breathing practice may also be helpful for those unable to do aerobics. Consult books or instructors for precise directions for breathing practice.

Detoxification: Several processes and methods of cleansing the body can eliminate metabolic wastes and toxins, strengthen the healing powers of the body, reinvigorate organs, aid circulation, stimulate glands, improve digestion, and heal many disorders or symptoms. Curative fasting, flushes (such as a liver flush), cleanses (such as colon cleansing), herbal detoxification methods, cleaning up one's diet, juicing, saunas, infrared saunas, and drinking adequate water are all methods of detoxification.

Detoxification can be effective in improving health. Methods are chosen according to each individual's health condition. For example, people who are underweight, undernourished, have weak hearts, have blood sugar issues, or are ill should avoid fasting. Be sure to do thorough research before beginning any kind of detox program. Some people go to a healing resort for detoxification because such locales may offer medical supervision and other healing opportunities such as massage, yoga, and mineral baths.

Eliminating or decreasing stressors: Decreasing external stressors in your environment is a good strategy for increasing health. There are two main types of stress to decrease, manage, or eliminate. One is *biophysical* (chemical, electromagnetic, and physical stress). The second source is *psychosocial*. We've included some information on eliminating and decreasing stressors later in this chapter. Chapter 8 (healing mind, emotion, and spirit) particularly addresses psychosocial stress.

Nutritional supplementation: There are nutritional substances essential to human life that the body itself cannot make, therefore these nutrients must be obtained from outside sources. Beyond eating a Whole Foods Diet, nutritional supplementation may be helpful to restore nutrients or micronutrients lacking in the body. Since supplementation is such a popular way of self-help, we have included an entire section about self-help nutritional supplementation later in this chapter.

Personal growth work (psychological self-help): Having an illness or health condition for a long time (especially if it started in childhood) may affect the psychosocial aspect of a person's life. Physical or mental illness may hinder learning skills in the areas of socializing, basic life management, emotional awareness and expression, critical thinking and evaluation, and relationships. Consequently, learning more about and improving your abilities in these areas can greatly enhance your life and relationships. We often call this personal growth work (psychological self-help). See Chapter 8.

As one bulletin board participant aptly described it, "A person can undo a lot of the damage to his system with whole foods and super healthy life choices, but those things cannot make his mental issues (thought patterns or emotional concerns) go away. Those issues will always creep back in some form or another, like a wake-up call saying 'you need to deal with me.' It seems to be the last thing that anyone addresses, though. Some people will go out of their way to pursue a healthy diet, supplements, exercise, etc., even to the point of making their day-to-day life so far removed from anything balanced, but they won't examine the mental side of their illness, and their own responsibility in it. The mental is sometimes what leads the body into a state of 'unhealth.' Perhaps the next step for many people is to address that part which prevents them from being totally alive—the mental or cognitive aspect of life."

Reflexology: Reflexology is the application of pressure to specific points on the body according to the concept (and the reality) that these points relate to specific corresponding parts of the body. You will find a "map" of these points for the entire body on the soles of your feet, the palms of your hands, your ears, your irises, and your teeth. Foot reflexology, for example, uses the map on the soles of your feet. By massaging in a certain way the places on the feet that correspond to the organs in that location of the map, the organs are indirectly stimulated or sedated. Activation of points can be deeply relaxing while simultaneously encouraging healing and balancing of the body. Reflexology may be especially helpful to indirectly help those areas of the body where direct contact must be avoided, such as a burn or open wound. If you are interested in learning reflexology for self-help, you might go to a professional reflexologist for one or several sessions to learn what reflexology is like and how it feels before trying it yourself from a book or a class.

Self-hypnosis, visualization, and guided imagery: These three techniques use the power of the mind to help control symptoms. They are skills that must be learned and practiced regularly to be effective. For bothersome symptoms, do *both* regular practice twice a day *and* practice whenever symptoms appear. What you are doing with these practices may be learning to suppress and ignore symptoms. However, a plethora of research says these exercises actually improve function and speed the healing of areas visualized.[1] ■■■ WALT: In my experience with those who have used these techniques, symptoms tend to disappear suddenly. ■■■

These three techniques are most effective when done in the alpha or theta brainwave. Everyone goes through these brainwaves on the way to sleep, and these rhythms are also reached in Skilled Relaxation sessions. Thus, good times to practice self-hypnosis, visualization, and guided imagery are when in the alpha or theta brainwave just before sleep and during your Skilled Relaxation practice. Thus for even greatest effectiveness, do these practices twice a day during your Skilled Relaxation sessions, whenever symptoms appear, *and* before going to sleep.

Self-hypnosis can consistently and effectively manage many symptoms, including those from hives, hypersensitivities, hypothyroidism, itching, pain, postherpetic neuralgia, recurrent warts, tinnitis, and vitilego. Self-hypnosis uses words to create a suggested outcome. This technique can be learned from an instructor or helper in a few sessions. To find a good self-hypnosis instructor, look in the Yellow Pages. The one who says that she or he can teach you to do this (not the one who says she will "do it for you") is the one from whom to learn. Some people learn self-hypnosis by reading a book about it and making a personal self-hypnosis tape. The wording you use must be precise to achieve the desired result.

Visualization and *guided imagery* are similar to self-hypnosis, but use images instead of words. People can invent their own images (visualization) or listen to a tape that has been created for them (guided imagery). To the bodymind, images created in the mind have a similar effect as actual, external events. Several years ago a book about tennis was written describing how to improve one's game purely by the use of visualization techniques. Because such visualization is so effective, this book is mentioned in the Resource section of Chapter 4 (exercise). Most professional athletes do some kind of visualization to improve physical prowess and give them a winning edge. Visualization can be applied to healing and many other aspects of life, as well as sports, with positive result.

The *Relaxation and Stress Reduction Workbook* has a chapter on self-hypnosis and one on visualization. Other books and audio materials may also be found for these three techniques.

Self-massage: ■■■ JAN: Self-massage can be used for giving yourself a full-body relaxation massage. Although it is not quite as enjoyable as being massaged by someone else, you will find that it can still soothe your tension and be very beneficial for your wellness. To give a relaxation massage to yourself, it can be helpful to consult books on self-massage or any book about massage that includes a section on self-massage.

For this activity, plan to be undisturbed for an hour or longer, and use lotion or vegetable oil. Massage your entire body, or just do part if you don't have time to massage everywhere. For example, massaging just your feet can help relax your entire body or help induce sleep. Face and scalp massage can also be very relaxing.

If you are massaging your whole body, you might start from the feet and work up, or from the head and work down. Do the massage on a carpeted floor (covered with a sheet) or in bed. Adjust your position to be able to reach and massage areas without getting tired. For example, I recline—leaning against the headboard or wall—when I massage my feet. I sit up to focus on my legs, then I lay down on my sides to massage each hip. I sit up again to do my arms, and lay down on my back to massage my neck and face. The back is hard to reach, so just do the best you can. Whatever area you are working with, position yourself in a way that is comfortable for you.

Use easy, non-tiring massage strokes. Slow gliding strokes are for relaxation and calming. Other strokes include gliding, rubbing, grabbing, kneading, pulling, and application of pressure. Applying simple pressure on sore, tender places can often release tight spots.

If you want to use deeper self-massage to heal an area of the body bound up with chronic pain, soreness, tight muscles, or restricted tissues, it's a good idea to first see a professional massage therapist to ask about your specific condition. Your therapist will know if there are any precautions, because a few health conditions can be worsened by deep massage. With the knowledge that it is safe, you can then proceed confidently and effectively to help yourself. Your therapist may even give you some tips on what to do. A good picture anatomy book can be of assistance, because the more you know about the area of the body you are massaging, the more quickly and accurately you can help yourself.

Massage and self-massage are especially helpful for people who are bracing, anyone who has any kind of tension, stress, or mental-emotional distress, and those who engage in lots of exercise (for injury prevention and recovery). It can also enhance self-awareness of your body, giving you clues about your health condition and where to focus your overall healing efforts. ■■■

Stretching: Stretching can be considered a form of exercise, but it is also a self-healing method. Stretching relieves bracing, decreases tension and muscle spasms, restores flexibility, releases connective tissue restrictions, and increases range of motion. What this means is if you stretch regularly, your body will feel more relaxed all the time and you will move more easily with less restriction, stiffness, and fatigue.

Regular stretching can be useful for any specific area of the body, but the greatest benefits come from daily or regular stretching of *all* the major muscle groups (full-body stretching). Full-body stretching relieves tension in the entire nervous system and is great for enhancing self-awareness. Stretching can especially help chronic bracers and individuals with nervous system disorders, since it relieves the load on the nervous system. Stretching can also lessen pain and discomfort resulting from postural or structural problems, or injuries. For best results, stretch daily. Books, videos and classes on flexibility and stretching are readily available. (See Chapter 4 Resources for stretching information.)

Support and self-help groups: Many self-help support groups are accessible for people who have a particular condition or wish to change a lifestyle habit, etc. Twelve-step programs (based on the successful program started by Alcoholics Anonymous) have been created to provide help for a variety of conditions and problems. There are other types of groups.

■■■ WALT: A sound support group helps individuals learn about the causes of their condition and how to resolve those causes. I believe in support groups when they offer real suggestions towards cure, not when they only offer emotional support for keeping and living with a chronic condition. I also think support groups are fine for conditions that truly have no solution. If a group is really interested in teaching people about health/wellness alternatives, it would be a great thing to be associated with them. If a group just focuses on helping people live with any condition that is resolvable, it may not be the best group to join. I used to refer people to support groups a lot when I did not know that so many conditions could be resolved. However, once I learned to teach the person how to be well, I found my patients who wanted to get better had no need for these groups. ■■■

■■■ JAN: I agree totally with Walt: be selective about the group you join. It is important to find a group that has a positive direction and will help you resolve your condition. If you are so inclined, attend a group and see if it is helpful for you. Some support groups may be very helpful for generating new ideas for self-care and treatment, obtaining referrals to good practitioners, and ending the isolation that often comes with having a chronic health condition.

Sometimes people with long-standing chronic illnesses tend to avoid social interactions because they do not feel well enough to be with other people. Joining a support group can be one way to help end loneliness. Consider also sharing this book and the 3LS with your support group as one of the methods for reversing your common illness or problem. ■■■

Q: Dr. Stoll, have you ever owned or used self-help devices like magnets, the zapper, and others? Are these devices something you would recommend?

A: ■■■ WALT: I have experimented with some of them, but it takes consistent use to give them a good trial. I have had patients, who on their own, have used some with success and others for whom these things have not worked at all. In my opinion, these are among the many methods that can only be evaluated after trying it to find out if it works for you. Determine what your own bodymind says about the effectiveness of the product.

My longest experience with such devices was when I bought a conventional isolation tank and used it for about two years of nearly daily Skilled Relaxation sessions in my garage. It was the quickest way into alpha that I have ever experienced.[2] ■■■

The next two sections provide more guidance about two commonly used self-help methods.

Eliminating and Decreasing Stressors

In terms of working with the causes of illness, we encourage people to put their efforts toward the 3LS Wellness Program, since it is usually more effective to strengthen oneself than to try to remove the mountain of stressors that exist in modern times. *Any* aspect of Wellness is usually the most important thing you can do to get better. However, it is also a good idea to see what you can do to decrease external stressors.

Biophysical stress

Some patients have suggested some simple choices and changes as being greatly beneficial for decreasing biophysical stress:

- Adjust your commuting times (go earlier or later) to avoid congested, rush-hour traffic.
- Avoid using chemical-laden personal products such as cosmetics, perfumes, and deodorants.
- Avoid using over-the-counter and/or prescription medications.
- Avoid using plastics.
- Drink purified or spring water, and drink lots of it daily.
- Eat organic foods.
- Make sure that sporting and computer equipment, furniture, shoes, etc. all have proper fit and placement for your body size and type. This is called ergonomics. Incorrectly fitting products can cause mechanical stress.
- Read books about detoxifying the home and remove chemical substances.
- Read labels of everything you eat and drink, and avoid additives.
- Stop smoking and avoid passive smoke.
- Avoid electromagnetic smog by turning off the TV, avoiding using the computer all the time, relying on a day-timer notebook instead of an electronic palm-pilot, and using a land line instead of a cell phone.
- Make sure your head is not next to an electrical outlet as you sleep.
- Use a steamer, toaster oven, or other cooking appliance instead of a microwave.
- Use natural cleaning products instead of chemical cleaning products.
- Avoid synthetics by using natural fiber clothing.
- Visit nature frequently.

Be a Detective to Uncover Harmful Stressors: If you have chronic symptoms, it helps to be a detective. Here are a few examples of how decreasing external stressors resolved some chronic conditions. 1) A patient suffered from recurrent severe headaches, and nothing made them go away. Finally, we figured out that she was taking a prescription medication (Estriol) that had the side effect of causing headaches. As soon as she stopped taking it, the headaches went away. 2) Some people who break out in rashes on their feet learn that the shoes they are wearing are causing an allergic reaction. 3) A woman who worked in a wood stove showroom became fatigued and felt ill shortly after she began her job. Only after she found different employment did her health return. Her problem was due to the smoke from the wood stoves.

Psychosocial stress

Some patients have recommended the following to help reduce or relieve psychosocial stress:

- Read books about communication skills and relationship skills, and practice what you learn.
- Make a plan for resolving one of the problems in your life and follow it.
- Pay your debts; also keep some emergency money in a savings account.
- Learn to say no, comfortably.
- Simplify, simplify, simplify.
- Stop overachieving.
- Take a stress management class, and apply what you learn.
- If you lack social connection in your life, find activities for meeting other people. One strategy is participating in ongoing activities (that do not end, for example, after 8 weeks) where you have an opportunity to get to know the regular attendees over time. Examples are volunteering, taking an ongoing yoga or meditation class, or joining a self-help group.
- Identify areas of life where you are imbalanced (do not do enough of something or do too much) and make a conscious effort to bring more balance to that area.
- Tell the truth under all circumstances.
- Watch less news on TV (or none at all).

- Get a massage every two weeks or once a month.
- Get more rest and relaxation.
- Go dancing (or take lessons).
- Clean and organize your closets.
- Limit the number of hours spent working each day.
- Engage in a hobby that allows your self-expression and the utilization of your talents.
- Find a less stressful job.
- Join Toastmasters and learn more effective communication and leadership skills.
- Make sure to get seven to eight hours of sleep every night.
- Make sure your job is appropriate for your personality and physical characteristics.
- Plan and go on a relaxing trip.
- Play with pets or children.
- Proactively find positive ways of changing or improving difficult circumstances.
- Spend more time in nature.
- Stay home more often (reading, bubble-bathing, relaxing, puttering around the house).
- Stop doing the work of two to three people by telling the boss you have more than you can handle.
- Take an extra half-hour to lie in bed in the morning, or go to bed 30 minutes earlier.
- Talk to friends.

This list is just the tip of the iceberg. There are many ways to decrease the level of psychosocial stress in your life.

Addressing psychosocial stress: Here are real-life examples: two patients improved their health by decreasing psychosocial stress. They both disliked their stressful jobs. One suffered from fatigue, depression, and an aching feeling all over. The other experienced muscular pain in a different place in his body each week. Both finally made a decision to quit their jobs and found less stressful employment that they enjoyed more. Consequently, their symptoms disappeared—with no further treatment. Another patient was confined to a wheelchair. When she became aware that she simply could not *stand* (tolerate) how her family treated her, she was able to stand and gave up her wheelchair.

There is an entire science of how the mind can restrict the body. For a literal interpretation of psychosocial situations and specific physical symptoms, you might read *The Symbolic Message of Illness,* by Calin V. Pop, M.D. (Sunstar, 1998).

Many books, materials, classes, etc., are available in the marketplace that cover the topics of reducing, managing, and controlling external stressors. We encourage you to search for them and grasp any good advice you find. *The Relaxation and Stress Reduction Workbook* is one of our favorites. Also read Chapter 8 (about healing mind, emotions, and spirit).

Nutritional Supplementation

Most of us would benefit from nutritional supplements, and in some cases, a lot of supplements. There are three reasons why nutritional supplementation can be useful in a healing approach that includes the 3LS.

First, the body cannot produce certain substances, and these must be obtained from sources outside the body. With only a few exceptions, the body cannot make vitamins, minerals, phytochemicals, essential fatty acids (EFA's), or essential amino acids,[3] and there surely are other micronutrients not produced by the body that are still undiscovered. Therefore, taking supplements helps ensure that your body is getting what it needs for normal function and ordinary health. While the Perfect Whole Foods Diet is best for obtaining these nutrients, due to modern farming practices (which deplete nutrients, etc.), most people on the Perfect Whole Foods Diet would benefit from supplementation as well.

Second, some supplements can help speed up results while the 3LS is giving the bodymind an opportunity to heal itself. Some examples include eczema, seborrheic dermatitis, recurrent sebaceous cysts, psoriasis, arthritis, colitis—all of which may be helped by the use of Essential Fatty Acids (Omega 3 and 6 oils.) There are already more than 40 chronic conditions known to be improved by simply taking omega 3 oils.

Supplementation for general nutrition (nutritional doses) is very safe and can be very beneficial to many individuals for balancing bodymind chemistry. Here are some self-help guidelines for taking ordinary nutritional amounts of supplements.

General guidelines for taking supplements

Although all ʻsupplements work in synergy, if you want to find out if supplements will do you some good, test them one at a time. That way, you will be sure exactly which ones give results. In the absence of helpful laboratory tests, often the best way to determine which supplements you need, and the exact dosage that is right for you, is by trial and error.

The average or "nutritional" dose for each dietary supplement is marked on the package label. The standard dosage—just like for medications—is traditionally based upon the body weight of an average human. Average is considered 150 pounds. Therefore, when giving supplements to children or to much larger or smaller people, use a ratio. For example, a 15-pound child would take 10% of an adult dose, and a 100-pound person would take 66%. This is just a guideline, because everyone's needs are different.

Once you know that you have a connection with a particular nutritional substance, you may need to experiment to establish how much of that substance you require for optimal functioning. This can be very individual.

To determine a nutritional or maintenance dose, start by taking the dosage recommended on the label (or the quantity suggested by your health care provider). Try it for a few days, weeks, or months, or until you know you have a beneficial connection with that substance. Then determine that you have achieved the full benefit from that supplement. You know you've reached the full benefit because you stop improving for a period of time, which could range from a few weeks to a few months (depending on your unique situation). After you have achieved the full benefit, determine a correct dosage by cutting the dose in half for a few months. See if you maintain your progress. If your symptoms do not return, cut the dosage in half again. Continue cutting in half, until your symptom starts to come back again, and at that point you will know you have cut the dose too much. When this happens, go back to the previous dose and continue it indefinitely, as that is likely the amount your bodymind needs for most efficient function. Once you determine the dosage, you take that much for as long as necessary, whether a few weeks or forever.

If you ever have a flare-up of your symptoms, go back to the maximum dosage until you are better again. Although larger doses of many supplements will not harm you, some become toxic if taken in larger quantities over time, so it is wise not to take more than you need. Consult practitioners and books for assistance and knowledge.

Taking a pharmacological dosage (therapeutic, large, or megadose) to cure a specific condition can be very individual and is beyond the scope of this book. We recommend that you read books about orthomolecular therapy (nutritional therapy) and consult a qualified orthomolecular practitioner for guidance if you are interested in doing this. Read more about orthomolecular therapy in Chapter 8 and see the Resources for that chapter.

If trial and error seems difficult, chancy, or complicated to you, or if you are not doing well with trial and error, consult an appropriate health care practitioner. Naturopaths, certain kinds of nutritionists, orthomolecular specialists, and a variety of holistic practitioners are the ones most likely to be able to assist you with nutritional supplementation.

Specific supplements

The following section provides general information about a few basic dietary supplements that are essential for healthy function but cannot be produced by the body. The supplements we discuss below tend to be beneficial and often quickly provide health benefits for almost everyone. The suggested doses are amounts that help most people and are safe to take. However, you may need to experiment to find your optimal dose using the instructions above or consult a health care practitioner. Remember to read labels of all supplements carefully, especially if you are following the Perfect Whole Foods Diet, because they may contain additives.

■■■ WALT: **1. Vitamins, minerals, phytochemicals, and micronutrients**—The word "vitamin" refers to substances that generally cannot be produced by the body. Minerals, phytochemicals, and micronutrients are also needed by the body and must be obtained from outside sources. Some people, especially after their health has been restored, may obtain enough of these substances through eating a highly nutritious diet. The substances listed below are commonly found to be deficient, though.

> **Whole foods concentrates:** Whole foods concentrates fall into the category of recommended supplements to boost your recovery after years of eating a less-than-perfect diet. Select a supplement that provides concentrates from a wide variety of whole foods. Please note that if you are starting with the Skilled Relaxation or Exercise aspects of the Program, taking whole food supplements can begin to restore the missing micronutrients to your body right away, even before you begin the Perfect Whole Foods Diet. Some individuals see dramatic health improvements just by taking whole food supplements. Read more about whole foods concentrates on page 95.

> **Magnesium:** Magnesium is a mineral that helps most people who take it. Magnesium may be the most important mineral as far

as the function of the entire body is concerned and is also one of the most common minerals lost in the refinement of foods. A high percentage of US citizens are magnesium deficient. Its ingestion can usually relax muscle tension and decrease bracing. The best and most absorbable kinds of magnesium are orotate, aspartate, or glycinate. You might start by taking a trial dose of 2,000 mgs (two grams) twice a day. Make sure that you are taking the correct amount of magnesium in terms of its elemental weight. Only a few brands list the elemental weight on the label. Benefits are usually seen within a couple of weeks. Then, you can start reducing the dosage until the maintenance dose is found. Magnesium is a co-factor with B vitamin complex, so it can be helpful to take the two supplements together.

Vitamin C: Most people would benefit healthwise from taking extra esterified vitamin C. The average maintenance dose of vitamin C for adults in this country is 5,000 mg. (five grams) a day. Taking 5,000 mg. of vitamin C is safe and fairly inexpensive, but experiment to find out what the correct dose is for you. I recommend that you take esterified C because it is twice as absorbable and four times as available to the intracellular environment where it does most of its boosting of immunity.

Vitamin E: Most people would benefit healthwise by taking extra vitamin E. The vitamin E should say "mixed tocopherols" (or "d-tocopherols") on the label; if not, it is probably synthetic (or "dl-tocopherols"). Take a trial dose of 400 IUs of vitamin E each day or according to package directions. Knowledgeable manufacturers add selenium to their Vitamin E since it enhances the effectiveness of the E.

Balanced B Complex: A therapeutic trial would be taking 100 mg of balanced B Complex two to three times a day. If it is helpful, you should start seeing benefits in a month and full benefits in six months. It is normal for the urine to turn bright yellow when taking B complex. B complex and magnesium are both co-factors for many different metabolic reactions in the body, which means they work efficiently together.

2. Essential fatty acids (EFAs)—The body is unable to make certain oils that are necessary for healthy function in many areas of metabolism.

These oils are called EFAs, or Omega 3 and Omega 6 oils. Nearly all people are deficient in Omega 3 oils and a small percentage are deficient in Omega 6 oils. Most US citizens who started taking EFA supplements would notice improvements in areas they were unaware were "wrong" with them.

Omega 3 Oils: The Omega 3 oils you need are Docosahexaenoic acid (DHA) and Eicosapentaenoic acid (EPA). They are both found together in fish oils, flaxseed oils, and hemp oils. The average 150-pound person will need at *least* 2000 mg (2 grams) of fish oil, flaxseed oil, or hemp oil, daily. It is best taken in two divided doses. Note that some people cannot convert the type of oils in flaxseed to the proper EPA and DHA molecule. Therefore if flaxseed does not seem to be helping you, try fish oil or hemp oil instead.

Omega 6 Oils: *Most* who take extra Omega 6 oils will get *no* benefit from them since they were not deficient in them in the beginning. Some are genetically deficient, however, and require more than others, even though conventional tests for these substances would show normal results. You won't hurt anything but your pocketbook by trying a high dose of Omega 6 oils for a few months. The main Omega 6 oils you need are gamma linolenic acid and linoleic acid. They are both found together in evening primrose oil, black currant oil, or borage oil. Try at least nine grams of any one of these oils daily (best taken in two divided doses) to give this substance a fair trial.[4] Many—not most—people will notice improvements within a few days if they are going to get any results, but you really need to give it a few months to see to what extent it can help. The least expensive source of Omega 6 oil is fine.

3. Essential amino acids—"Essential" means they cannot be produced by the body and must be provided by food. Generally, only strict vegetarians (especially those who have not studied how to get adequate nutrition while eating a vegetarian diet) or people on a prolonged fast need to take essential amino acid supplements. However, taking a recommended nutritional dose (listed on the bottle) of predigested essential amino acids cannot harm anyone, and for some, predigested amino acids can be helpful in supporting the restoration of health. Look on the label or the advertising for the words "predigested essential amino acids." ■■■

■■■

There is one more thing to consider about supplements. Be aware that since no standards have been set for supplements, there is a wide variety of quality variations in nutritional products. Research the reputation of companies before selecting products. Higher quality products are more likely to be found in health food stores.

Supplements Q & A

Q: I began taking a new multivitamin, which includes superfoods, minerals, and herbs. The tablets are food-based and designed for easy digestion and absorption. It says to take one to six tablets as desired immediately after a meal. How do I know how many to take?

A: When you are trying to discover whether or not something is going to help you, it is a good idea to take the maximum dose for a while to find out if you feel better (although some sensitive individuals will want to start oppositely, with the smallest dose and work up). Once you have a positive result, you can always reduce it gradually until the good effect stops. Then you will know you have bypassed your maintenance level and need to raise your dose back to the previous level.

Q: I've been using different kinds of vitamins and supplements, and while they worked at the beginning, now I'm feeling like they cause exacerbations in my health condition.

A: Try less supplementation. Generally it is our experience that anything that makes you feel worse (and the feeling worse goes away when you stop it) should not be taken at that stage of healing. That means that it might have been good for you before, or may be good for you later, but not at this time.

It is worthwhile to occasionally retest foods and supplements you have been using regularly to see if those items are now unnecessary or have become harmful. If one is really changing things and getting better, there actually is change in the bodymind, which then changes the requirements for external support. Thus it is a good idea to re-test your use of supplements periodically (such as every six months or once a year) to be sure they are still helping you. Retest the supplements you normally take by going off of them and, after a period of time, see if taking them once again still makes a positive difference. Balance is everything, and too much of anything can be toxic. This process of testing supplements may be a lifetime process. The same is true of food.

When you take supplements, also remember, if you have a reaction, it may be a healing crisis as your bodymind adjusts to a higher level of function. Thus, several trials may be necessary to obtain accurate results.

Q: My vitamins make me feel sick. Why? Should I keep taking them?

A: A good general rule is to stop doing whatever is causing you to feel worse. The cheaper vitamins have an average of 35 additives in them that the manufacturers are not required to list on the label (preservatives, colorings, binders, bulking agents, etc.), and nearly every so-called reaction to multivitamins is a reaction to one or many of these. The quality companies list everything on the label and include statements like, "This product contains no artificial preservatives, color, dairy, sweeteners, starch, wheat, or yeast." In general, health food stores tend to carry higher quality supplements than regular grocery, drug, or discount stores, but be sure to read the labels anywhere you purchase supplements.

Q: Is there anything good to take for general inflammation that is occurring throughout the body while I'm waiting for Skilled Relaxation to work?

A: Many people do well with esterified Vitamin C to tolerance and at least 3000 mgs of Omega 3 oils twice a day. Other herbal supplements are available to reduce inflammation; consult a qualified practitioner.

USING THE SERVICES OF PHYSICIANS AND PRACTITIONERS

Some people, when practicing the 3LS, will find that self-help is not enough. Self-help has its limitations. There is only so much that a person can do by oneself. To totally resolve symptoms, certain individuals will need to work with health care professionals and use other healing methods. Some may also want to have the reassurance and support of someone knowledgeable while practicing the Wellness Program. If at any time during the process of healing you feel the need, do not hesitate to seek appropriate professional help.

The key is finding someone you feel comfortable with and can communicate with easily. Because the health care world can be confusing, we would like to discuss the kinds of help available and most useful for healing a chronic condition.

Allopathic Medicine

■■■ WALT: Allopathic medicine is the dominant form of medicine practiced in the United States. All medical doctors in the United States are trained in allopathic methods, and that was my original medical training, too. The term allopathic medicine, coined by Samuel Hahnemann, M.D. in the late seventeenth century, is derived from Greek roots and refers to the use of modalities based on the assumption that symptoms need to be treated. Allopathic medicine claims a scientific basis, and the main treatments are pharmaceutical medications and surgery.

Conventional allopathic medicine is useful for and is still the best choice for acute conditions like broken bones, gunshot wounds, acute infections, and management of trauma. We need conventional (allopathic) medicine, and it's useful for what it does best—work with acute conditions. However, for chronic illnesses, standard allopathic treatments may not always be the optimum choice. They may produce temporary results in a short time, but along with this, there is commonly a high price in complications. Since only symptoms are dealt with, not causes, the problem will surely recur because unresolved causes will just move deeper into functional body systems. In my opinion, allopathy is incomplete when it comes to healing chronic conditions.

Many times in this book we have mentioned using holistic medicine and holistic healing for resolving chronic conditions. Lets go into more detail.

Holistic Medicine

In its broadest sense, holistic medicine could include all of the healing philosophies and modalities that exist in the world. There may be other ways of defining holistic medicine (for example, some people do not consider certain allopathic methods as part of holistic medicine), but the following is the definition we will be using in this book.

Holistic medicine encompasses all safe modalities of diagnosis and treatment, emphasizing the necessity of looking at the whole person, including analysis of physical, nutritional, environmental, emotional, spiritual, and lifestyle values. Holistic medicine searches for the root cause of illness in consideration of the whole person and the whole situation. It particularly focuses upon patient education and the patient's personal efforts to achieve balance. Medicine that is holistic has an emphasis on health and individualized care, rather than on disease and high technology. Ideally, the best form of holistic medicine matches the best modality to the individual problem.

Holistic medicine has a broader philosophy than just disease-crisis management. It includes the science and art of preventing, curing, or alleviating ill health. C. Norman Shealy, M.D., Ph.D., wrote this description: "Holistic medicine has been defined by the American Holistic Medical Association as 'a system of health-care that emphasizes personal responsibility and fosters a cooperative relationship among all those involved, leading toward optimal attunement of body, mind, emotions, and spirit.'"[5]

The name used for holistic medicine is currently in flux in the United States, which means that many names are being used to describe it. Some of those names are functional medicine, integrative medicine, complementary medicine, alternative medicine, or natural medicine. The term CAM, short for Complementary and Alternative Medicine, is a popular term being used by the National Institutes of Health to describe all methods that are not drugs or surgery. We do not think this term is very accurate, because many of these approaches have a totally different function than drugs and surgery. Therefore, they are not really complementary (done alongside), nor are they alternative (done instead of). The term complementary seems to give conventional medicine the upper hand. The term alternative tends to give the connotation of rejecting conventional medicine.

To describe all of the world's healing modalities, including allopathy, we would use the terms "Holistic Medicine" or "Functional Medicine." To describe all the healing approaches that are not allopathic, we could just use the term "healing methods." All approaches are a co-equal part of a comprehensive health care approach. I believe, more and more, that allopathy does not deserve the pre-eminence it receives in the United States, and I look forward to the day when the safer, more effective, and less expensive approaches are the *first* things attempted for healing, rather than the last. ■■■

The foundation of holistic healing

The word "holistic" comes from the same root as "whole," "health," and "holy." The goal of holistic healing is to achieve maximum well-being, where everything is functioning the very best that is possible.

Here are some of the principles of theory and practice of the holistic approach outlined by the Association for Holistic Health.

1. Holistic health is wellness-oriented.
2. Health is a holistic process of balancing body, mind, and spirit.
3. Environment, lifestyle, and relationships are taken into consideration when creating optimum health. This includes social responsibility.
4. The result of holistic health is optimum health. It concerns itself with prevention, with growth and change, and with healing and restoration to a state of balance.
5. There are a variety of methods for attaining balance. Holistic health recognizes what works and utilizes traditional and nontraditional resources. Preference is given to the more natural and gentle forms of healing available.

6. Holistic health acknowledges the immediate problem but emphasizes correcting the cause(s) of the imbalance.

7. The primary role of the holistic health practitioner is to provide information and experiences for clients, enabling them to take responsibility and to make decisions that will optimize health.

8. Holistic health respects the right of the individuals to make their own choices, be they enhancing or not, and to assume responsibility for those choices.

9. Holistic health respects individuality: the right of the individual to grow at one's own pace and to have one's own awareness, values, attitudes, and behaviors.

10. Positive attitudes, including love, harmony, responsibility for one's own actions, self-acceptance, forgiveness, and a sense of purpose are promoted.

11. The practice of holistic health includes a comprehensive assessment and diagnosis of states of balance and imbalance in the body, a goal-oriented plan, and evaluation of results in terms of effectiveness.

12. Holistic health is democratic and tolerant, rather than authoritarian.

13. The basis of delivering holistic health is the giving of loving care and concern.

14. The result of holistic health is an ever-higher expression of potential, fulfillment, and joy.[6]

Holistic health and healing sees illness as a creative opportunity for a person to learn more about oneself and one's fundamental values. When following the holistic model, everyday choices are used to take charge of, improve, and maintain one's own health.

Below are some of the systems of medicine and variety of modalities in the broad spectrum of healing methods and approaches available to assist your health and healing.

Systems of medicine include allopathy, anthroposophic medicine, Ayurvedic medicine, chiropractic, homeopathy, Native American healing, naturopathy, osteopathy, Tibetan medicine, and traditional Chinese medicine.

Bodywork techniques include acupressure, Alexander Technique, Aston Patterning, bioenergetics, Bowen Technique, Breema Bodywork, craniosacral therapy, deep tissue bodywork, Feldenkrais, Haelan Work, healing touch,

Hellerwork, Jin Shin Ji Tsu, kinesiology, manual lymph drainage, massage, myofascial release, neuromuscular therapy, physical therapy, polarity therapy, rebirthing, reflexology, reiki, Rolfing, Rosen Method, shiatsu, sports massage, therapeutic touch, touch for health, Tragerwork, trigger point therapy, tuina, watsu, and zero balancing.

Mental-emotional health approaches include addictions counseling, art therapy, behavioral kinesiology, biofeedback, body-centered psycho-therapy, coaching, cognitive-behavioral therapy, eating disorders counseling, emotional (anxiety, depression, grief, mood, self-esteem, stress) counseling, family counseling, Hakomi or sensorimotor psychotherapy, hypnotherapy, marriage or relationship counseling, movement or dance therapy, music therapy, neuropsychology, psychiatry, psychotherapy for adults, children, teenagers, elders, men, or women, somatic (body) psychology, sexual abuse therapy, transactional analysis, transpersonal psychotherapy, and trauma therapy.

Nutritional therapy includes dietary therapy, herbology, nutritional therapy, and orthomolecular approaches.

Other approaches include applied clinical ecology, energy healing modalities, kinesiology, holistic dentistry, holistic nursing, physical fitness, qi gong, religious and spiritual approaches, sports medicine, t'ai chi chuan, and yoga.

■ ■ ■

This is not a complete list of all the current modalities or methods that are available.

Each approach, paradigm, or philosophy has areas of strength and weakness. Also, no one approach to healing works for everyone, because chronic problems are too complex, plus we are all so very different. Eastern approaches can be very effective when Western approaches have not worked. Of course, the opposite is also true. One can even be healed by what some people call the Grace of God. There are thousands of documented cases of spontaneous remissions of incurable conditions following devout prayer or through faith healers.

With such a large number of healing options, it may be hard to know which one to choose first. Research and study, and hearing other people's experiences, may give you clues. Often, the best way to see if something works for you is just to try it.

We hope this discussion has helped you understand the difference between allopathic and holistic medicine. Another way of looking at the difference between the two medicines is to consider the difference between atomism (allopathy) and vitalism (holistic medicine).

Atomism holds that the human bodymind is nothing more than tiny particles that get combined and recombined. That means eventually, by breaking things down into small enough pieces, we would be able to explain and control everything.[7]

Vitalism is a healing principle which holds that the human bodymind has the capacity to protect itself from the ravages of the environment and aging, and healers should focus on helping the bodymind use its own resources for healing. All the healing traditions in the world, except allopathy and osteopathy, are purely vitalistic.

Using the Allopathic Approach for Chronic Illness

If you have a chronic condition, giving conventional medicine one good chance to come up with a diagnosis that can be resolved by allopathic precepts may be worthwhile, since about 10% to 15% of conditions are best approached allopathically. If you have one of those conditions, it can be resolved by that allopathic approach forthwith. However, by definition, except for acute conditions, allopathic approaches are not "healing." Drugs and surgery are usually designed for treating the symptoms of chronic illness and can be effective for that result, but do not resolve the causes of the illness.

Examples of conditions that are best approached allopathically are broken bones, acute or life-threatening infections, end-stage hypertension, heart disease, diabetes, heart failure, and poisoning. The point is that anything that gets bad enough may be helped allopathically, but the idea is to do all the holistic things earlier so that point is not reached so soon or so chronically.

■■■ WALT: Let me explain why medications and surgery often do not resolve the causes of chronic illness. As we mentioned in Chapter 6, chronic health problems are caused by an accumulation of factors (genetics, stress, and choices) that finally push an individual over the edge of the cliff, to the point where symptoms become visible. Symptoms are only made apparent by the "straw that breaks the camel's back"—the last small thing that made the problem apparent. Allopathic medicine tends to focus on getting rid of the straw (by making the symptoms disappear with drugs or surgery), and unfortunately, does not even look at the rest of the underlying load that caused the symptoms.

Using allopathic medicine for conditions that have been building up for a long time can be initially helpful, or help for a while. The problem with short-term and long-term medications, surgery, or even taking something essentially nontoxic such as herbs is they often temporarily work to relieve chronic symptoms. Consequently, the person who has the problem thinks she is cured and puts off doing something about the real problem until it evolves into something worse. In the end, the medications and herbs you take, or the surgery you have had, may eventually stop working—if that is all you do to try to improve your condition.

I see no problem with using conventional medicine as long as you have also started dealing with the causes of your chronic condition by using the 3LS or other lifestyle approaches. Unfortunately, as I mentioned, once a person uses conventional medicine and the symptoms are better, human nature is to ignore the cause and just go on with the same lifestyle. Focusing on the straw or symptoms using allopathic medications practically guarantees that a condition will continue to become more serious the longer you live.

Although we would all like to finally have a magic pill, there is not one out there yet. When something is not a true cure and has significant risk to taking it (such as drugs with all their side effects, or surgery, which is mostly irreversible), why bother, except for temporary relief? Many people get along (some for a long time) with covering up their symptoms, but this does not resolve what is causing the symptoms. If that is their choice, it is all right as long as they truly understand what they are doing.

About using prescription medications and surgery

Prescription medications: When it comes to taking prescription drugs for chronic illness, if it is true that the average prescription drug is only 66% effective with a 30% rate of side effects, what are you getting?[8] Sometimes the treatment complications of taking medications are worse than the disease they are meant to treat. To find out how safe any medication you are taking is, go to the library and have the reference librarian show you how to look up each of your drugs in the *Physician's Desk Reference* (PDR). Also, read the entire package insert first before taking any medication.

One of the first things that medical students are taught is that anyone placed on three or more drugs at the same time will always get better if all the medications are stopped. This is because the side effects of one, combined with the side effects of each of the others, along with the more serious interactions of all the drugs, causes more symptoms than any illness can cause. With three or more drugs, there is no way any doctor can possibly have any idea what they are causing. In my practice, I frequently (at least several times a year for 30 years) saw patients who were on 20 to 25 different medications from their previous doctors, incredible as it may seem.

However, here is an important caution. One should never discontinue any medication or treatment without consulting the professional managing that treatment. Remember, there are medications that cannot be stopped. Examples are insulin for diabetes, and the prescription drug digitalis, which is for congestive heart failure. Of course, if the cause of the congestive heart failure, such as low magnesium, myocarditis, atherosclerosis, hypertension, or other factor, can be addressed, the digitalis becomes a burden rather than an essential support.

Surgery: If you are contemplating surgery for a chronic condition, reflect on this. Surgery is irreversible and does not always bring the desired results. Therefore, if your problem is not urgent, I would Practice Serious Wellness for a year first and see what happens before considering surgery.

In many cases, after a patient practices Serious Wellness for a year, the physician, upon observing that the condition has improved (without the drugs and surgery previously recommended), would start a wait-and-see approach. Further improvement might finally convince the physician of a so-called misdiagnosis and he would drop the suggestion of surgery. Few physicians would recommend their original approach in light of the fact that a patient was on the way to getting well.

However, if after you have done the Skilled Relaxation, Perfect Whole Foods Diet, and Exercise program for a year, and also looked into other healing methods, if you still have symptoms you would be willing to undergo surgery for, I think you should consider it. Sometimes so much damage has occurred over the years that structural changes require surgery. This is a minority of cases, though. None-the-less, if nature has handed you a lemon, the more knowledge you can amass *before* doing anything irreversible, the better chance you have. You need to sit down with your surgeon and not budge until he has fully explained all of your options to your satisfaction and not just to his. Then obtain similar opinions from other kinds of practitioners. Surgery may be only one of many viable options for you, and the other possibilities may have less chance of damage and be more effective.

In the end, if you do choose surgery, I still recommend that you practice the 3LS before your operation. After all, the healthier you are from practicing the Wellness Program, the less damage there will be, and the better you will do following surgery. ■■■

Using the Holistic Approach for Chronic Illness

If you have a chronic illness, the vitalistic or holistic approach is frequently the most effective way of addressing your condition. The goal is to relieve symptoms by supporting the body's own self-healing mechanisms.

Ideally, when addressing your symptoms, you would consult a holistic physician who is very knowledgeable about many healing methods and who can point you in the direction of the options most helpful for you. Another approach would be to first see an allopathic physician for a diagnosis or to rule out any acute or life-threatening conditions. Then, do enough research and study on your own to learn about a variety of healing methods, and then make your own choice about which lifestyle choices to make and which healing modalities and practitioners to try. Generally, unless a condition needs urgent care, start by using less invasive and less expensive modalities before choosing those that have side effects, are irreversible, or are expensive.

With holistic medicine, many techniques recommended to diffuse any symptom or condition often help a person's *entire* health condition. This has lead to the descriptive statement about holistic medicine that "doing anything good may help everything." This does not mean we are saying that anything cures everything. It means that all parts of a person are connected to each other, and each thing influences the other. Since everything works together and is interconnected like a spider's web, anything that helps any part also helps the whole. Because of this, when you are on a path of holistic healing, pleasant and unexpected surprises in healing often occur along your way.

Since holistic health and healing emphasize the body's innate ability to heal itself, your relationship with your holistic practitioner or physician is not one in which you put your life into the hands of an "all-powerful" doctor. Instead, it is more a relationship of mentor and disciple, or a partnership.

The number of holistic physicians and practitioners is increasing, but there are many places where they are not yet available. Statistically, more people are looking for other healing methods than are going to conventional physicians. They have been doing so for at least a decade, and the ratio is increasing every year.[9]

How to find a practitioner or physician

As you become knowledgeable from your study of available alternatives, you can find and choose the best professional to serve as a consultant to you. You choice will range between appropriate conventional (allopathic) physicians, holistic physicians, and practitioners of other healing methods. See the Resources for this chapter and Chapter 8 for referral sources.

We want to be straightforward with you. One of the reasons we have written this as a self-help book is because in the United States, at the time of writing this book, holistic physicians/practitioners and practitioners of other modalities can still be hard to find or expensive to see. See the Afterword to this book for the reasons why. We are happy to say that more than ever before, larger numbers of qualified and skilled holistic physicians and practitioners are available. However, there are still not enough of them, and most other healing methods are still inaccessible to many people. Thus, we have attempted to infuse this book with as much self-help information as possible. We've given you clues, ideas, and leads for ways to do as much as possible yourself in the event that you cannot locate practitioners or modalities in your area to help you.

We also wish to make you aware that you may encounter other difficulties in your search for the right physician or practitioner to help you. Some professionals who call themselves holistic do not accurately subscribe to holistic principles. We have summarized these principles on pages 263–264 of this chapter and in the Appendix for Health Care Practitioners. Moreover, professionals in any field have varying levels of skill and expertise. Each practitioner has areas of strength and weakness, too. Therefore, you might first interview physicians or practitioners to find out their level of training and scope of practice, and obtain word of mouth opinions from your colleagues and friends, to help you make an evaluation before you choose one. This is a good policy for any service or goods you choose in any realm of life.

Since the current state of technology is still rather primitive (compared to what we may wish for in terms of specificity and depth of accurate information), tests and laboratories do not always provide reliable or useful information. Sometimes, therefore, self-help (and trial and error) may be the best choice for trying to resolve certain health issues where laboratory tests are not useful.

Remember, when you go through the process of choosing a holistic practitioner or doctor, that professional has the same option of choosing you as a patient. Beginning this relationship means that you are both accepting responsibility for each other and giving each other rights that need to be honored throughout your relationship. Once you've selected your practitioner, and he or she has selected you as well, then you both need to work on making the relationship mutually beneficial.

The following contains information about preparing yourself for your appointment with a physician or practitioner.

Your Medical Records
and Health History

Keeping medical records: Obtain copies of all your medical records to keep at home. The records belong to you, and the doctors only keep them in trust for you. It is illegal for any doctor to refuse to give you copies of all of your records (although some may charge a fee for this). If any of them refuse, you have recourse to call the county medical society where the physician practices and make an official complaint. Usually, all it takes is the threat to do so before the doc is eager to give you your records.

Compile a lifetime health history: List the episodes and age at the time, but no details. If the physician or practitioner wants details, he or she will ask. Put in your list the following data:

- List as many things as you can recall, in chronological order, whether or not they were considered serious enough at the time to require medical consultation. The more things you list, the more likely a pattern will be revealed. It is important to know that it existed and when, but specific details about those things are not needed.
- Describe your lifestyle: diet, exercise, practice of Skilled Relaxation, medications, alcohol, drugs, exposure to tobacco smoke, etc. Again, list everything but not much detail.
- List any and all treatments you had, how well you did them, and for how long. Describe the effect they had on you (good or bad).

It is much better to list something that does *not* seem to be helpful than to miss something that might have helped fill in the pattern of causation—but be brief.

Taking copies of your medical records with you may save repeating any tests. When you see a new physician, take both medical records and health history. Any physician who ignores this information should be replaced with one more caring and competent.

Never give the originals of your records or health history to anyone. The originals are best kept at home or in a safe-deposit box. Your physician can make copies if desired, or you can make a complete set of copies for the doctor to avoid any chance of losing any of your own information.

WORKING WITH PRACTITIONERS Q & A

Q: Why do holistic practitioners say that working with them is a partnership?

A: In the holistic healing model, each person is responsible for his or her own health and makes his or her own choices in healing. Therefore, you are the most important member of your own health team, and for the most effective healing, you and your practitioners must work together. The healer's job is to facilitate healing and to show the way to individual change toward health. Your job is to decide which course of treatment you will follow and, when you are ready to make lifestyle and other changes, to make them. Open and clear communication with your practitioner is very important. There is no way a practitioner can make good decisions if you withhold the facts. The reverse is also true—there is no way you can make good decisions if a practitioner withholds information.

Your efforts at studying and learning to become an expert about your own condition will make you a very powerful member or partner with a practitioner or competent team of professionals. Your knowledge will help you make better decisions and do more to assist your own recovery. At some point, many of you will become healthy enough and no longer need professional help because you are able to draw upon your own resources.

Reading Appendix A, "For Practitioners," may also give you some more insight about working effectively with a professional.

Q: Patient A: I hate doctors, so I have yet to make an appointment. But I may have to since my problem isn't going away. Patient B: My doctors tell me nothing is wrong with me.

A: If your doctors have stopped taking you seriously, you need to be seen by one who cares and who will give you an honest evaluation. My suggestion for both of you would be to see an honestly concerned and competent holistic physician. Take your health history and medical records with you. If you reject any professional help due to past experiences with conventional doctors, you are "throwing out the baby with the bathwater." It's important to have some of your faith in healing professionals restored.

If your health problem is not one of those conditions that is best approached allopathically, or if you can't find a holistic physician, you may do well to see another type of practitioner. Much of the healing that needs to be done does not require a medical license, and many types of holistic or other practitioners may be able to help you.

Q: I've tried allopathic medicine, and it hasn't helped my chronic condition. But my insurance doesn't cover other healing methods, so what else can I do?

A: You can continue to go for "free" treatment paid by your insurance that has not worked for you, *or* you can pay out of your pocket for other healing treatments that have a better chance of effectively treating your condition. It is your decision whether you want to be well and whether you are willing to do what it takes to get there or not. The real cost of illness is not usually the money; it is how you feel and the reduction in productivity and enjoyment of life.

Keep in mind that by using as much knowledge as you can gain about your condition, together with your no-cost or low-cost 3LS Wellness Program, you may not even need other healing methods.

Q: I have three different practitioners, each telling me to use totally different approaches to improve my condition. What should I do?

A: At a time of very rapidly developing knowledge, you are bound to find differing opinions. Learn as much as you can about each one, and then choose what you think will work best for you. Having to make such choices is one reason why it is so helpful that you become self-aware and attuned to your own bodymind, in addition to learning as much as you can about your condition. Combining self-awareness and self-knowledge with the cutting edge of new breakthroughs and discoveries in healing will help you make the best decision about which one to choose.

It may be quite fine to try any or all three approaches. If one is less expensive, you might try that one first. They might also work well together synchronistically if you do all of them.

Q: Massage, Rolfing, Hellerwork, Alexander Technique, and Feldenkrais are recommended in this book to help bracing. What about other forms of bodywork such as Tragerwork, Aston Patterning, etc.?

A: When one is bracing, any of these approaches can be considered, although they differ in exactly what they do. You can try different techniques and methods to find what works for you. We are hoping that just by opening the door to the concept of bodywork that people will seek out what works best for them. Chapter 8 (about healing mind, emotions, and spirit) has additional discussion about bodywork.

Q: Have you ever used energy work for healing, and do you think it is effective?

A: ■■■ WALT: Electromagnetic medicine, and other approaches, can be a solution for those persons for whom the 3LS Wellness Program is not the final answer. If a person uses electromagnetic or energy medicine, however, using the 3LS and working with causes is still an essential part of reversing any condition. Even though I have healed patients by the laying on of hands and by doing energy work, I found that most of those healings were not permanent unless the individual *also* began to deal with the reasons they got sick and started the 3LS. Since the Wellness Program makes any other approach work better, the synchronistic combination of the two healing methods can be an advantage. Again, see Chapter 8 and the Resources section for more information about electromagnetic medicine and other energy medicines.

Q: What do you think of using a combination of different approaches in one healing session?

A: I could write an entire chapter just about the effectiveness of combining many alternative approaches in one session. I once had a therapeutic intuitive working in my center who used a variety of alternative methods. She helped us all see how Bach Flower Remedies, detox sessions, aromatherapy, and other modalities could fit together to form a whole for those complex patients none of the rest of us could do anything about. In the beginning, we only sent her patients whom we could not work with successfully, but eventually we included her as a front line referral for the most complex and advanced cases. We were never sorry.

She decided which modalities to use for each individual and had them all ready to use before she started a session. An average of four to six professionals participated, including her. I have taken part in a few of these types of sessions and can tell you that miracles do happen, even though I cannot explain them. ■■■

TROUBLESHOOTING CHECKLIST FOR DIFFERENT TREATMENTS AND PRACTITIONERS

✓ Have you researched your particular symptoms, condition, or illness?

✓ Have you studied and learned about the self-help technique, medicine, or modality you wish to use? Do you fully understand its advantages and disadvantages?

✓ Have you worked with your physician or practitioner long enough to give their treatment or modality a chance to work?

✓ Have you talked to one, or better yet, several practitioners about your issue or problem to get different opinions?

✓ Have you communicated honestly and clearly with your practitioner or physician about how things are going?

✓ Are you keeping track of what changes occur after you try a new modality, treatment, supplement, etc? (Helpful charts are in Chapter 5.)

✓ Have you continued looking for all possibilities, including trying new practitioners or modalities?

✓ Have you looked into all possible options before doing anything that is irreversible?

THE AUTHORS' EXPERIENCES

■■■ WALT: Only after I had been in practice for a few years did I begin to question the allopathic paradigm. I had swallowed it whole. Actually, that is how my own health got in such a fix. However, if I had not had so many problems that all cleared up when I began the 3LS, and learned from it what I had *not* been taught in medical school—holistic healing—I probably would still believe the allopathic paradigm. Seeing everything by the allopathic paradigm alone was like trying to see and understand the world through a pinhole. Seeing healing through a holistic approach removed the restriction and cleared my vision.

Applied kinesiology was what first totally changed my perception of reality and put me on the path to wellness. I used to have sciatica, but Skilled Relaxation and Rolfing resolved it. I have had no symptoms from it for the past 20-plus years.

After experiencing so many improvements to my health, I soon found that I didn't know enough to tell my patients about what had helped me get better, so I went back for additional training in as many alternative approaches to healing as I could learn. I developed a Holistic Medical Center with a team of six practitioners who specialized in a variety of alternative disciplines.

I became knowledgeable in many healing philosophies and was able to coordinate the talents of the entire staff for the benefit of the patients.

I personally tried other modalities so I could know better which of my patients might benefit from each of them. That way I'd be able to share my experiences with them if they asked. I tried every modality I offered at my center before I looked for a practitioner with that expertise. After all, my reputation, as well as the welfare of the patient, would depend upon their effectiveness thereafter.

I certainly had no trouble finding complementary practitioners in and around Lexington, Kentucky, to work with me. Over the years, my wellness center employed a holistic dentist who was an expert in TMJ syndrome, electromagnetic medical diagnosis and therapy, electro-acupuncture, and homeopathy; a minister with a master's degree in counseling, who was also an expert in biofeedback and Skilled Relaxation techniques; a Chinese medicine practitioner who was also an expert in macrobiotics, several forms of therapeutic massage, acupressure, and reflexology; a practitioner of applied kinesiology who also used herbology and aromatherapy; a chiropractor; and a certified physician's assistant. We also offered behavioral kinesiology, science of breath, self-hypnosis, and other modalities. The result of this combination of approaches was considerably more effective than what I had experienced when I was limited to allopathic medical options alone. I was astounded. ■■■

■■■ JAN: In seeking my own health improvements over a period of 20-plus years, I have experimented with a wide variety of modalities, treatments, and supplements. Each healing method I tried helped add one piece of the puzzle and was useful. I saw any difficulty that arose in my healing journey not as a setback, but as a pointer towards the next steps in getting better. The 3LS, plus increased self-care and self-awareness, were actually the most effective parts of my health recovery. For several years, I spent at least three hours a day working on my body (in addition to the time I spent learning and cooking, and yes, I was working, too). I realized that it would take that kind of commitment to restore my health, and I was willing to do it. I am happy to say that I am reaping the vast rewards of that faithful dedication to my health improvement.

Dr. Stoll told me I'd still experience improvements 10 years after starting the 3LS since my condition was so deeply rooted. He's been right so far. Four years into the program, I'm still improving and feeling better and better. I've found that I had to add some other modalities to continue peeling the layers of my chronic illness. Interestingly, even four years after starting the 3LS, I discovered that 3LS still enhances any new treatments I try by making them work more effectively.

Presently, along with the 3LS, I use the following: I receive massage on a regular basis, stretch regularly, and take several nutritional supplements. I've done some detoxification practices and found them to be very helpful. I learned to breathe diaphragmatically (belly breathing) which decreased my upper body tension. A yoga class once a week also helps strengthen and align me, which decreases my physical stress. I have recently consulted with holistic practitioners for specific advice about which nutritional supplements would be optimal for me. All of these, along with the Wellness Program, combine to keep my bodymind in the healthiest state I have ever known. I continue to learn and experiment with new self-help techniques and practitioner-assisted modalities to further my improvement. As far as I'm concerned, my health improvements can always continue! Why stop here? ■■■

Chapter 7, ADJUNCT APROACHES—SUMMING IT UP

There are three steps to follow for the most effective approach to healing.

- Learning and study
- Lifestyle choices
- Additional treatments

Learning can come from reading this book and doing research. Lifestyle choices may be made by beginning the 3LS. Additional treatments may also be beneficial.

For some people and conditions, the 3LS Wellness Program will be enough. Others will need additional treatment after six to twelve months, either self-help methods or professionally assisted treatments.

Why use other healing methods along with the 3LS?

1. For symptomatic relief
2. To speed up or enhance the healing process
3. To deal with conditions the Wellness Program does not address

Informed choice means knowing the advantages and disadvantages of each potential treatment method for making an effective selection.

Some self-help techniques that complement the 3LS include: breathing practice, detoxification, eliminating and decreasing stressors, nutritional supplementation, personal growth work (psychological self-help), reflexology, self-hypnosis, visualization and guided imagery, self-massage, stretching, support and self-help groups. There are many other self-help methods.

External stressors can be the main cause of a chronic condition, and removal of the stressor can resolve some illnesses or symptoms. Generally, for healing most chronic illnesses, it is more effective to strengthen oneself than try to remove the mountain of stressors that exist in modern times.

Nutritional supplementation can help your health. Some supplements help speed up the healing results of the 3LS. Also, the body cannot produce certain substances that are required for its function, and these substances must be obtained from outside sources such as food or supplements. Some people need more of certain substances for their specific metabolism than others, so taking supplements is individual. It is safe to take nutritional doses of supplements, but pharmaceutical doses (large doses) are best taken under supervision of a qualified practitioner. Nutritional supplements that help many people include whole foods concentrates, magnesium, vitamin C, vitamin E, vitamin B complex, essential fatty acids (omega oils), and essential amino acids.

Physicians and practitioners can provide reassurance, support, and additional healing opportunities. Allopathic medicine is the main system of medicine in the United States and has a scientific basis. Its main treatments are pharmaceuticals and surgery, which are very effective for acute conditions. Conventional medicine is useful for chronic conditions as long as a person is also working on the causes by using a method such as the 3LS Wellness Program. If taking medications, study available information about them, including learning about side effects. If considering surgery, investigate other options before making an irreversible choice.

Holistic medicine is a phrase that covers all healing philosophies and modalities. Ideally it matches the best modality to the individual problem and takes into consideration the whole person and his or her lifestyle. Holistic healing is known as the science and art of prevention, curing, or alleviating ill health. Each individual is responsible for his level of well-being, and everyday choices are used to improve and maintain health.

Before working with a health-care practitioner, prepare a lifetime health history and take it with you for the first visit. Keep copies of your medical records at home.

PEOPLE'S ACCOUNTS OF USING ADDITIONAL TREATMENTS

I had a sudden onset of symptoms in January 2000 and was diagnosed with rheumatoid arthritis in April 2000. I went from a VERY active person to an invalid in a matter of days. We were (finally) able to slow the disease down with methotrexate, and my symptoms did decrease. I then started worrying about what all these drugs were doing to my body! Over the past year I did the E-diet (still NO grains, dairy, sugar) and am following the 3LS Walt preaches. I've been able to come off ALL medication (methotrexate, prednisone, NSAID's) with no signs of increased disease activity. I can't say that this approach will stop the disease in its tracks for everyone, but what can it hurt? I feel like I've taken charge of my health.   —*Donna W., Austin, TX*

I used to get bronchitis several times a year—sometimes pneumonia. This was the first year I haven't been that sick. In fact, I have yet to get a cold or the flu. Here is what I've done differently: 1) Monitor humidity so that it's above 40% in the house. 2) Take 2,000 mg of esterified-C three times per day (I take a good amount of other vitamins too). 3) Exercise every day. I love to run. 4) Eat no sugar or refined carbohydrates. (Sugar inhibits your immune system a lot.) I follow Beth Loiselle's Whole Foods diet. She has an excellent book. Walt's first book is excellent, too. 5) Drink 64 ounces of water each day. 6) Practice Skilled Relaxation twice a day for 20 minutes. 7) Get enough rest. I have a 5-year-old at home and am around other sniffly, sneezy, runny-nosed children several times per week, so something good is going on for me!   —*Anonymous*

I have had PVC's [palpitations], anxiety and other symptoms for years and never had any relief. I didn't realize it, but stress and constant self-talk (mostly running business scenarios) dominated my days and nights. When the symptoms showed up, it was devastating. I was in excellent shape on the outside, so I never considered anything other than it being an unfortunate condition that no doctor could explain. Up until I read what Dr. Stoll was saying, I simply thought I was one of the unlucky people who was afflicted with something I could do little about. Then it became clear that I was often in this state of readiness, often tense, often bracing, and thinking negative thoughts. Taking the correct form of magnesium and doing skilled relaxation daily along with exercise has made a big difference. I would encourage anyone who has this condition to consider a commitment to regular aerobic exercise, maintaining a healthy diet, supplementing with magnesium, and practicing skilled relaxation techniques daily. This combination has made my symptoms almost non-existent.   —*Doug K., Financial Consultant, Santa Barbara, CA*

At age 38 I was diagnosed with stage four cervical cancer and a cancerous lump in my right breast. I refused allopathic treatment and began my search for ways to clean, heal, and maintain my body using only natural, non-toxic protocols. I got rid of all pre-packaged (dead), chemical-laden food products from my pantry. My body responded quickly to the change of diet and supplements. Within six months, I was declared cancer-free by the same doctor of gynecology that initially examined me and who had previously wanted to perform a complete hysterectomy and mastectomy. She was shocked by my complete reversal. I am 54 years old now and the cancer has never come back. I took no drugs, had no surgery or radiation, yet the cancer was eliminated from my body.

—*Deborah Sage, Health Professional (Herbalist, Iridologist, Kinesiologist),*
Alpharetta, GA

I have a small bunion on each foot that would periodically erupt in painful jabs that would wake me and make sleeping impossible. The affected area would be red and swollen and sometimes hot to the touch. The only available remedy, according to my podiatrist, were cortisone shots in each foot, which I reluctantly agreed to have. Although my doctor warned me about the harmful effects of cortisone on the liver, I knew of no alternative that would eliminate the pain. But I was concerned about the detrimental effects that cortisone would have on my health. However, I decided to stop all cortisone shots, and started taking emulsified cod liver oil. Within weeks my shooting pains had practically disappeared and the reddened areas and swelling were almost non-existent. Today, after several months of taking the cod liver oil, I have no redness on my feet, there is no swelling and the pains are rare, if any. All that remains are two small bunions that are barely noticeable.

—*M.M., Philadelphia, PA*

My friend Janet had arthroscopic shoulder surgery a week and a half ago to correct a swollen bursa and pinched nerve that happened during an old injury. To give you a little background, she had been practicing Skilled Relaxation for two and a half years, once a day. She has many health problems, including fibromyalgia (FMS), chronic fatigue, IBS, etc. She has had surgery in the past and she has found that because of her FMS she has taken twice as long to recover from surgery as other people usually do. Two weeks before her surgery, I told her about Dr. Stoll. She began doing Skilled Relaxation twice a day or more. After the surgery she continued to do the extra Skilled Relaxation. Today she went to the doctor and he said she was recovering TWICE AS FAST as his normal patients. ... For myself, I can tell you that after two weeks of doing Skilled Relaxation twice daily, my interstitial cystitis started improving. It's been a month now, and it's definitely not gone, but it's much more manageable.   —*Anonymous*

I'm a 26-year old male who has been clinically diagnosed with interstitial cystitis (IC). I have been practicing Skilled Relaxation for three and a half months. Basically, my symptoms came on last summer, which were frequency and pain in the prostate area. For my IC, I take Algonot Plus, which has been helpful and side-effect free, and also 50 mg of hydroxyzine (antihistamine—also side-effect free) at night. And while I am pretty sure both of those have helped, the Skilled Relaxation I have learned from this site has helped *tremendously,* far more than either of the medicines. My overall symptoms are greatly decreased. I am generally pain free (at least 90% less pain than I had) now in my pelvic regions. I still have some frequency, but I think that is reduced as well. So three and a half months into this, I am not cured of IC, but I am getting much better, have much more control over IC, and I'm basically living life freely again. I am no longer a prisoner of my own body!! Since Dr. Stoll says it takes six to twelve months to truly be effective for IC, the future looks bright.   —*Anonymous*

I cured my major depression 90% with many miles of exercise a week; one to two hours of sunlight a day; consistent water intake; a high raw nutritional diet; strict avoidance of refined foods, gluten, and dairy, chocolate, sugar; relaxation and therapy, and a whole heck of a lot of motivation. My depression began as a child; I was on three heavy-duty medications due to severity and history of attempt. I have genetic history as well as a history of extensive trauma. I decided I did not want to be dependent on medicines for the rest of my life. I decided that I wanted to be well. I decided to take full responsibility for all my actions, thoughts, words, beliefs, my life. With Walt's ideas, I kicked depression. My physician of several years was stunned and ultimately deeply supportive. As Walt says, it won't be something you take, it will be something you do. Keep trying, these are all healthy ways of living, you have everything to gain.   —*Anonymous*

Chapter 8

Health for the Complete You: Mind, Emotions, and Spirit, Too

In this chapter, we will look at the mental and emotional aspects of life and the growth of one's spirit, and discuss their healing and integration when practicing the 3LS. If you think you don't have difficulties in these areas, we recommend that you read this chapter anyway to learn more. Since all is related, what is written in this chapter is actually another resource for improving overall physical health, and for reaching a state of optimum health or high-level wellness. Thus, this chapter is relevant for *all* readers.

WELLNESS IS MORE THAN JUST PHYSICAL HEALTH

The general area of "mental or emotional problems" is one of the most poorly managed and least understood classes of chronic medical ailments in this country. This type of diagnosis may also be the most feared, perhaps only after cancer. Therefore, we have included a separate chapter to specifically address mental and emotional health in this book—not because it is so different from any other type of chronic health problem, but because mental-emotional health is so misunderstood. Since current treatments often miss the mark, we want to clarify causes and suggest treatments that might be more effective, thus giving hope and guidance to individuals experiencing this type of health concern.

After this discussion, we include a short section about how the Wellness Program helps your spirit grow, which will complete the picture of the 3LS as a holistic modality enhancing every part of life. The growth of spirit is not separate or different from improving health, but each person approaches this aspect of life in his or her own time and way.

Note that this chapter addresses chronic mental-emotional conditions, not acute or emergency situations. If an emergency occurs, e.g., if a person is suicidal, violent, experiences visual or auditory hallucinations, or is showing signs of having a "nervous breakdown" (when anxiety or depression escalates to the degree that a person is unable to perform normal functions), seek emergency help. Dial 9–1–1 or call your local mental health department's crisis hotline. National hotline numbers and websites are listed in the Resources at the end of this book.

BODY, MIND, AND SPIRIT ARE ALL RELATED

Forty years ago, everybody was taught that mind, body and spirit were best treated as three separate entities. M.D.s and D.O.s took care of the body, psychiatrists or psychologists cared for the mind and emotions, and ministers, rabbis, or priests, etc. took care of the spirit. Woe be to the practitioner who encroached upon the other's territory. We now know that every aspect of a person is connected and related to the rest. *Every* function of a person—mental, spiritual, or physical—influences everything else about that person. We divide up our world in order to make sense of it, but we must not divide it so much that we forget about the wholeness of it all.

Especially in terms of health, the body and mind cannot be separated. Throughout this book, to indicate the connection between body and mind, we have been using the term "bodymind." It may be even more accurate to say bodymindspirit. An example of how the body and mind are connected is that emotions are called "feelings." We feel something in our bodies as a response to something that goes on in our minds, a kind of tangling together of thought and physical feeling or sensation. These sensations are all processed through the hypothalamus—a part of the brain—further evidence that the mind and body are one. The brain is actually the major "switchboard" of the entire bodymind.

Because of the connection between mind and body, when a person has what seems to be a physical malady, this does not mean it is unrelated to the mind. When one suffers with mental or emotional distress, this does not mean that it has nothing to do with the body. Your life experiences (psychology) interact with your body (physiology) to affect the functions of both. ■■■ WALT: I have been convinced that all is related, since in my practice I have routinely seen everything in a person's health improve when one part is properly treated. ■■■

To understand more about conditions that have mental or emotional symptoms, let us first look at the causes of such conditions.

HEALING MIND AND EMOTIONS

Causes of Mental-Emotional Difficulty

What our society commonly calls mental or emotional problems or illnesses are not due to a character flaw nor are they a sign of personal weakness. Like all chronic conditions, mental-emotional difficulties are caused by the same three basic factors, the combination of:

Genetics: Genetics determines the *specific* type of biochemical or chemistry imbalance that occurs, such as anxiety, depression, and schizophrenia.

Stress: The biophysical influences and psychological factors in your past and present (psychosocial environment) can cause stress. The *stress* aspect of mental-emotional difficulties has two main components: biochemical imbalance of brain and/or body, and psychological or psychosocial stress. Both components are inextricably connected.

Lifestyle choices: These are choices you make, which will either improve or worsen your condition.

All three factors interact to cause conditions with mental-emotional symptoms. Here is a typical scenario of how genetics and the two components of stress (biochemical imbalance and psychosocial influence) interplay to become pathological mechanisms, causing mental-emotional symptoms.

1. Genetically, some individuals are born with disadvantaged metabolic function or have a tendency towards biochemical imbalances.

2. Psychological trauma and psychosocial circumstances, especially in childhood, affect the individual by upsetting brain chemistry and making it more difficult to function. Early trauma and stress have been shown to "permanently" change brain chemistry—and even brain structure—for life.

3. Biophysical stressors in the environment continue to accumulate, contributing to most chemical imbalances. The two most common biophysical stressors include *poor diet* (which plays a larger role than

most people realize) and *stored stress-effect* in the hypothalamus. In addition to causing bracing and gastrointestinal weakness, the stored stress-effect in the hypothalamus also throws off a person's chemistry via the endocrine system. Increasing amounts of chronic stress-effect magnify borderline chemistry.

4. Leaky gut syndrome and candida-related syndrome result from those two stressors (poor diet and stored stress-effect) and continue to interact to create an even greater imbalance in brain chemistry. Nearly all people with brain chemistry problems have and must resolve LGS and C-RS.[1]

5. Environmental stressors, such as environmental toxins and pollution, can also affect chemical balance within the body. There is good evidence that even short-term use of either pharmaceutical or recreational drugs or use of electronic equipment like cell phones can permanently alter brain chemistry.

6. Insufficient nutrition and stress of all kinds continue to deplete the bodymind of specific nutrients. Without sufficient nutrients to function correctly, chemistry becomes further imbalanced, and problems in function become visible. The brain, nervous system, and endocrine system are the first and hardest hit of all by insufficient nutrition.

7. Psychological symptoms such as anxiety and depression, along with any or all of the above mentioned changes in brain chemistry produce deleterious effects. Psychological symptoms originate in the psychosocial stress experienced while trying to function in social situations with abnormal brain chemistry.[2] As symptoms appear, the abnormal brain chemistry worsens the individual's ability to cope with the psychosocial climate.

   Often, when emotional symptoms become visible, other people start to react and the psychosocial climate worsens. Perhaps the boss is agitated, the spouse is upset, friends are concerned, and/or trouble has occurred.

8. Psychosocial stress causes biochemical imbalance, and biochemical imbalance causes psychosocial stress. This pattern becomes a vicious cycle.

9. The key to healing is finding a way to break the cycle.

This scenario illustrating how factors accumulate to cause chronic mental-emotional difficulties is also true of chronic physical conditions.

Conventional Treatments

Current conventional treatment for mental-emotional issues usually consists of drugs to deal with chemical imbalances and counseling for psychosocial difficulties.

The approach of using drugs has an appeal because it actually works for a certain period in many people, and so a market for drugs is created. However, pharmaceuticals have limitations. Besides their cost, pharmaceuticals are relatively ineffective and can have many negative side effects. Many are even seriously addictive. Using drugs to try to force the brain to work differently is like throwing sand into Big Ben to keep it from gaining time—too simplistic and destructive. The idea of working with chemistry is a good one, but drugs are in many cases not always the best way to achieve health. For that reason, many psychoactive drugs are only recommended for a few months' use and are not considered a long-term solution. (Note: If you are using any kind of medication, do not discontinue use without first consulting the professional managing your treatment.)

Psychological counseling or therapy helps psychological difficulties, and just about everyone (including people who do not have a diagnosis) would benefit from appropriate psychological counseling with the right person. However, counseling is often used as a singular approach to mental-emotional difficulties, and often nothing else is done. With most mental-emotional difficulties, the psychological part is *not* the whole problem, so with counseling alone, fewer than half of those who started with counseling would succeed at resolving their condition.[3]

Sometimes conventional approaches are the best option for certain individuals. However, for many people, other solutions are more effective. Thus, we recommend the following as an effective method of treating mental-emotional difficulties. Individual variations may be needed. ■■■ WALT: As a clinician, I always strive to find the treatment that best matches the individual's need. When writing a book to be read by many, however, I must provide recommendations that will work for the largest percentage of people.■■■

A Holistic Approach

The type of chronic illness bundled into the category of "mental-emotional conditions" is best treated using a holistic approach that addresses different aspects of a person. This approach works because multiple causes and mechanisms usually create such conditions. A wide variety of methods, techniques, and treatments can work synchronistically to enhance the specific health needs that resolve mental or emotional symptoms.

A Holistic Approach May Help These Conditions

Alcoholism	Memory loss
Agoraphobia	Nervousness
Anxiety	Neuroses
Attention deficit disorder	Panic attacks
(ADD)	Phobias
Autism	Psychoses
Chronic fatigue	Schizophrenia
Depression	Post-traumatic stress disorder
Drug addiction	(PTSD)
Learning disabilities	and others.
Manic-depression (bipolar)	

Since one of the major causes or components of mental-emotional difficulties is imbalanced chemistry, the next section focuses and acquaints you with the subject.

Understanding Brain and Body Chemistry

If you are suffering from any kind of chronic mental-emotional difficulty or distress, you may find part of the solution in chemistry improvements. If you have physical symptoms such as fatigue or general malaise, you may also benefit from balancing brain/body chemistry.

Before discussing what balancing chemistry means, let us be clear about the following: brain and body chemistry imbalance, in many cases, do not require pharmaceutical treatment. (If you are already taking prescription medications, do not discontinue their use without consulting a trained professional.)

Improving your chemistry

Balancing or improving chemistry means giving the brain and body everything needed for healthy function, and removing what harms or impairs function. An imbalance in chemistry is usually caused by the deficiency of one or several specific *nutrients* such as vitamins or minerals or by too much or too little of *naturally occurring chemicals* such as hormones in the body.

Imbalance may also be caused by *an excess of substances harmful to the body* such as refined carbohydrates or other toxins.

When mental-emotional symptoms exist, it's often not just brain chemistry that is involved, but also body chemistry. There is actually no separation between the two, and each influences the other. Dysfunctional chemistry can be improved in various ways. One way is through improved diet.

Diet

■■■ WALT: I have routinely seen great beneficial results from altering the diets of my young patients with learning disabilities and behavioral problems, including hyperactivity, increased aggressive tendencies, and delinquency. The behavior changes that occur in these children after correctly making certain dietary changes are both dramatic and immediate—within a week or two. This result is without the use of either drugs or counseling.

The same results hold true with the adult population, but since adults have more self-control, they instead tend to have symptoms like chronic fatigue, panic attacks, free-floating anxiety, depression, and increased aggression. The changes that occur from dietary improvements in adults are similarly impressive, but sometimes take a little longer to see (a couple of months). This is due to the years of psychological overlay (the repetition of life experience, which deepens the groove like a record that is played over and over) that has been a lifelong habit. Nevertheless, diet is one of the important ways to improve brain and body chemistry. ■■■

Another important way to improve chemistry is orthomolecular therapy.

Orthomolecular therapy

Specific nutritional therapy is one of the most useful approaches to healing imbalanced chemistry causing mental-emotional difficulties. Called orthomolecular therapy, it is the practice of preventing and treating disease by providing the body with optimal amounts of substances that are natural to the body. This type of nutritional therapy provides specific vitamins, amino acids, trace elements, fatty acids, or other substances in therapeutic amounts sufficient to correct biochemical abnormalities. Ortho means "right" and molecular means "molecules," so the term describes getting the correct kind and amount of molecules to the body. It is now known that some people, because of their genetic makeup, need as much as 1,000 times as much of a specific nutrient as someone else just to be healthy. Thus, it may be necessary for an individual to take very high doses of some nutrients to resolve a physical or mental-emotional problem. Orthomolecular nutrition makes use of foods or change of diet, and orthomolecular medicine uses pharmaceutical doses of supplements.

Orthomolecular psychiatrists believe that, in some cases, the so-called mental illnesses that are said to run in the family are intolerances to certain foods or chemicals. It's often an overall unhealthy diet shared through family habit, tendencies to develop specific vitamin deficiencies, or dependencies that cause mental or emotional symptoms that get handed down from generation to generation. These are nutritional issues that can be corrected.

Taking therapeutic (pharmaceutical or large) doses of substances to balance brain or body chemistry is best done under the supervision and guidance of an orthomolecular specialist (see the Resources for this chapter). Orthomolecular therapy can be very powerful in treating mental-emotional conditions, especially those that seem severe. Sometimes just taking high doses of one or two vitamins or minerals is all that is needed to restore a person to normal function. Abram Hoffer, M.D., a pioneer in orthomolecular nutrition, has written several books describing his clinicial experience of totally reversing schizophrenia in many individuals within five years just by using large doses of Vitamin B3 (niacin).[4] Researchers and practitioners who have followed in Dr. Hoffer's footsteps have contributed further knowledge about working with schizophrenia and other biochemical imbalances.

As chemistry improves with a better diet or orthomolecular therapy, an individual restores or develops better mental, emotional, physical, and other capabilities. With this increased energy and strength, the person has more attention for working on psychosocial issues, such as changing the habits and repetitive thinking of years. Improving chemistry also increases an individual's ability to cope with psychosocial conditions. Thus, we recommend chemistry improvement along with or even before starting psychological counseling.

■■■ WALT: When I practiced in Lexington, Kentucky, I worked closely with one of the founders of the Orthomolecular Psychiatric Association. I saw some pretty amazing changes in patients who, after many psychiatrists had given up on them, sought him for orthomolecular treatment. ■■■

Knowing that your chemistry needs balancing

How do you know if you have a chemical imbalance in body or brain and you need to rebalance that chemistry? There are several ways to this awareness.

1. One way to tell if your chemistry is off is by a diagnosis.

2. Another way to know is if you have any bothersome mental-emotional distress patterns (even though you may not have an official diagnosis), such as experiencing symptoms of panic attacks, unexplained mood swings, lack of concentration, poor memory, brain fog (sluggish thinking or difficulty concentrating), anxiety, nervousness, fatigue or malaise.

3. You may know if you have imbalanced chemistry by simply seeing if you make any improvement by doing trial and error experiments with different nutritional approaches.

4. Also, a family member having a mental-emotional condition or diagnosis is a clue. You may have a similar chemical imbalance to a greater or lesser degree.

An Experience with Chemistry

◼◼◼ JAN: While healing through my practice of the 3LS, I noticed the following:

Brain chemistry: After one year of following the 3LS and six months of the Perfect Whole Foods Diet with no fruit, I reintroduced fruit into my diet. I got a bit carried away and ate a lot of fruit in a short time (this is not recommended!). To my surprise, I could actually feel the effects of eating the fruit from the sensations in my brain that occurred after eating it. Eating fruit caused my thinking to become cloudy, and my concentration worsened. I could actually feel a physical sensation like congestion in my brain, in addition to a slowdown in thought. I noted another change on a day that I ate a mango; I was very emotionally reactive. Before I started the 3LS, certain foods caused allergic reactions including brain fog and poor concentration. Now, I understand that all of these reactions were chemistry imbalances caused by what I was eating.

Body chemistry: I became aware of a body chemistry imbalance by close observation of myself in various activities like exercise. For a long time, I had suffered from fatigue, and at one point I began to do trial and error experiments with a few supplements to see if I could improve my condition. After reading many books and researching to learn my best treatment options, my solution appeared to be taking Vitamin B3. I started by taking three grams of B3 and right away noticed that I was less fatigued. Every other day I increased one half gram until I was taking ten grams a day.

The B3 made me a little spacy, but I could tell it was helping my body. For a few nights when I was asleep, I was awakened by the need to make shifts in my body position due to the changes that were happening in my nervous system. From taking the vitamin, my body was relaxing deeply and slightly elongating, especially along the spine, requiring me to shift my position. I could actually feel the change in the body structures brought about by improved chemistry. I took ten grams for only a few days, then suddenly I could tell I needed to stop. I'm pretty sensitive to my body and what helps it and what doesn't, so I went off all the B3 at that point. I tried taking smaller doses (one to three grams), but it was clear that my body had already gotten what it needed and didn't want any more concentrated B3. I then switched to taking B 100 complex, and learned over time through trial and error (like with the B3) that I generally need to take some B100 complex each day.

A year later, after a stressful period, I needed to take high doses of B3 again. I also began experimenting with other vitamin and mineral supplements and found some others to be helpful. At this point, I realized the potential benefit from working with someone more knowledgeable, so I found an orthomo-lecular practitioner whom I consulted to fine-tune my supplement program. It was a wise decision to obtain professional help since successful nutritional therapy can be rather complex.

If you read this and are thinking of experimenting with nutritional supplements, I strongly urge you to study a number of books about orthomolecular medicine (see Resources) and/or obtain professional help. Some vitamins and other nutritional substances can be harmful if taken in large doses, and there are interactions between nutrients. Before I did the experiment described above, I studied about six books on the topic. I was glad I did it, because my fatigue was much improved after I worked my way through this process. I have also consulted several practitioners for advice, which has been useful.

Since I had already been practicing the 3LS for one and a half years before these nutritional experiments, this is also an example of how becoming healthier increases self-awareness and sensitivity to what happens in one's own body. ■■■

Some people have the awareness and sensitivity to experience such changes, but others do not. For many people, chemical changes happen below conscious awareness. These individuals might experience slow gradual improvement rather than a sudden and dramatic change. Whether you are physically aware of changes or not, chemistry and nutrition can still be an important factor in your healing. Usually it is wise to work with a practitioner for nutritional therapy.

Now let us move on to the self-help protocols for the mental-emotional aspect of life.

WHAT YOU CAN DO TO IMPROVE MIND AND EMOTIONS

Here are three approaches for improving mental-emotional issues.

1. Improve your chemistry by following the pattern of the 3LS.
2. Implement psychological and personal growth approaches to improve your relationship with yourself and others.
3. Use other healing approaches including bodywork, certain modalities that promote the growth of spirit, vibrational or energy medicine, and combination techniques.

There is overlap in what each of these approaches accomplishes. For example, using the 3LS will help balance chemistry, and both psychosocial and physical functions will improve as well. Working with psychosocial approaches will do more than just improve your social relationships; it will also help balance body and brain chemistry. Everything helps everything else, although it may take a combination of all three approaches to fully resolve mental-emotional symptoms.

1. Use the Pattern of the 3LS

The basic program for working with mental and emotional difficulties and balancing chemistry follows the same format as the 3LS Wellness Program, with just a few variations. Regardless of the type or severity of your health issue, the 3LS Wellness Program is still the foundation for health and the best tool for improving your well-being. Thus the 3LS may best be used first for mental-emotional difficulties, even before trying other approaches.

Relaxation

- *Practice effective Skilled Relaxation regularly.* (An aroused hypo-thalamus leads to heightened emotional states and chemical/hormonal imbalances. Reducing the total stress-effect load through practicing Skilled Relaxation enables the hypothalamus to recover its healthy function and rebalance chemistry and hormones. Correct Skilled Relaxation practice also results in improved digestive tract function. Thus chemical imbalances due to leaky gut syndrome, dysbiosis, candida-related syndrome, and food hypersensitivities may also be corrected.)

Diet and nutrition

- *Follow the Perfect Whole Foods Diet* in Chapter 3 to balance blood sugar, end the addiction to refined carbohydrates, and remove stimulants from the diet such as caffeine. All of these actions will help restore chemical balance to the body and brain.

- Elimination/provocation dietary testing (eliminating foods for a period of time and then reintroducing them) can be done with foods that are suspect as causing hypersensitivities or allergies. (See the Resources of this chapter, Chapter 3, and the Glossary for more information).

- Have digestive function checked for malabsorption, insufficient hydrocholoric acid, inflammation, leaky gut syndrome, heavy metal toxicity, or other gastrointestinal problems that might be interfering with healthy digestive function or brain function.

- Nutritional supplementation of substances essential for normal healthy function (such as certain vitamins and minerals) can be very beneficial for balancing chemistry. Here we are talking about nutritional doses for ordinary daily living. This has been described in detail in Chapter 7, on pages 255–261.

- Orthomolecular therapy (pharmacological doses) may also be beneficial for chemistry balancing or neurotransmitter production. (Under certain circumstances, high doses of specific supplements may be the best nutrients to take to help restore chemical balance to brain and body tissues. More approaches are being discovered regularly, but right now the most common supplements are balanced B complex, individual B vitamins such as B1, B3, B6, or B12, vitamin C, magnesium, essential fatty acids, whole food concentrates, CoQ10, and the like. If you manage to choose exactly the right supplement, at exactly the effective dose, improvements can happen in as soon as a day.[5] Relatively large doses may be used as a therapeutic trial to establish whether a particular supplement is going to help.) The best type of practitioner to assist with this is an orthomolecular psychiatrist, although any orthomolecular practitioner can help you get started (see the Resources for books and practitioners).

Exercise

- *Exercise,* especially aerobics (see Chapter 4), helps mental-emotional issues by increasing the percentage of oxygen and improving metabolism (chemical reactions) in the entire body and the brain. (Your metabolism is the interactive combination of the multitude of chemical reactions that have to work in a certain way in your body and brain, as well as all of the electromagnetic and structural reactions. Aerobics and, to a certain extent, any form of exercise, create healthy effects by enhancing these thousands of chemical reactions towards optimal function. Anything that is really healthy for any individual will tend to bring his or her metabolism back towards wellness; exercise, especially aerobics, is one of those healthy things.)

Most, if not all, mental-emotional problems improve when an individual starts putting effort into improving the quality of his or her body. Practicing any part of the 3LS (or better yet, all of it), is usually enough to bring benefits by altering chemistry toward optimal function. Some people's mental-emotional problems can be cleared up by using the Wellness Program alone—many within six months.

2. Employ Psychosocial Approaches to Healing

The second part of healing mental-emotional difficulties is working on the psychosocial aspect of life. Improving the psychosocial or nurture part of the wellness equation through appropriate counseling can make a significant difference in healing mental-emotional difficulties. This is especially true if you have had any condition for a long time resulting in undesired behavior patterns that you want and need to change.

Psychosocial approaches to healing can teach new skills to replace thoughts and behaviors that have been used as coping mechanisms that originally started from having less-than-adequate brain function. The sooner this therapeutic process is begun, the better—before unproductive habits are solidified.

Healthy habits and healthy social relationships support life, and unhealthy habits and unhealthy relationships are detrimental to happiness and health. This may seem obvious, but many people do not realize that behavior and habits can be changed and improved. Typically, such changes are made after receiving constructive input from an outside source providing a new, objective viewpoint. The services of a counselor or therapist can be invaluable in this process, but much of this learning can also be done on your own through self-help, such as reading books.

Psychologically, what runs in the family and gets handed down from generation to generation (besides the dietary habits mentioned earlier) includes relationship styles, communication habits, beliefs and attitudes, personal hygiene habits, and many of the unique characteristics found in any given family. These can be changed or improved through counseling or personal growth work.

Psychological counseling

A wide variety of approaches is available for healing psychological difficulties and reducing psychosocial stress. Practitioners range from psychiatrists, who can prescribe medications, to licensed therapists and counselors of all types. Patients who have more serious disorders or problems are usually best served by highly trained professionals. Orthomolecular psychiatrists can help with both chemistry and psychological issues.

We recommend balancing brain chemistry before getting counseling help, or doing them simultaneously. Doing counseling before making chemistry changes is like running a race with a 100-pound weight on your shoulders. With enough effort and determination, some can accomplish the psychosocial work first, but it is usually not the easiest way to make progress. When brain chemistry is balanced first, followed by counseling, the success rate goes up about 50% to 75% with the same amount of effort.[6]

Social influences on healing are very important. If the influence of unhealthy people is too strong in a person's life, progress in healing can be impeded. Because other people can be such a strong influence, some individuals may be helped by obtaining psychological assistance for improving relationships or life conditions before being able to embark on the 3LS Program to enhance health.

Some professionally assisted approaches to working with psychosocial difficulties include:

Addiction counseling
Anger management
Art therapy
Behavioral kinesiology
Bioenergetics
Biofeedback
Body-centered
  psychotherapies
Coaching
Cognitive Behavioral
  Therapy
Eating disorders
  counseling
Emotional (anxiety,
  depression, grief,
  mood, self-esteem,
  stress) counseling
Emotional Freedom
  Technique

EMDR (for trauma
  resolution)
Family therapy
Focusing
Gestalt Therapy
Grief therapy
Hakomi method
Hypnotherapy
Inner child work
Life coaching
Marriage or
  relationship
  counseling
Movement or dance
  therapy
Music therapy
Neuro-Emotional
  Technique

Neuro-Linguistic
  Programming
Neuropsychology
Play therapy
Psychiatry
Psychosynthesis
Psychotherapy for
  adults, children,
  teenagers, elders,
  men, or women
Rapid Eye Movement
  Therapy (EMDR)
Sensori-Motor Method
Sexual abuse therapy
Somatic approaches
Somatic Experiencing
Transactional Analysis
Trauma therapy

When choosing professional help, interview therapists or counselors until you find someone you feel comfortable with and who charges reasonably. You want someone who will help you grow and not foster a dependency. Finding just the right therapist for you, someone you feel happy to work with, may make all the difference.

Sometimes, after brain chemistry has been improved through the 3LS or orthomolecular approaches, one's health condition is so much better that psychosocial therapies are not even needed. But if psychosocial issues need addressing, any of the above practitioner-assisted approaches could help, as can individual efforts for personal growth described below.

Personal growth work (self-help psychological work)

If you wish to work through specific life challenges or issues, or want to change and improve your personality or character, you may be interested in self-help personal growth work. Taking this path helps you develop yourself as a whole person and can greatly enhance your life, bringing you greater fulfillment. Personal growth may help you more easily reach the top of the mountain of wellness.

■■■ JAN: Personal growth work is about improving your character, personality, and skills. Working on and improving yourself is a key to reducing psychosocial stress and increasing happiness. You can use it to:

- Improve the quality of your mind and emotions
- Set and achieve goals
- Resolve stressful life situations
- Manage challenging life events
- Gain knowledge of advanced relationship skills
- Become more skilled at communication
- Improve your emotional awareness and expression
- Learn conflict resolution
- Develop negotiation skills

Healthy patterns of thought, skillful understanding of emotions, and fulfilling relationships are all an important part of the journey to optimum health and wholeness. For some people, one aspect of personal growth work may be learning basic life skills that were not taught in childhood, including things like successful financial management (getting out of debt, managing money, etc.), housecleaning, and cooking skills.

Doing personal growth work does not mean that something is wrong with you. On the contrary, it means that you have awareness and courage to learn about and master your life and yourself, as well as wisdom to face and overcome challenges. Working on yourself increases your personal skills, decreases stress, and increases enjoyment of life.

Much personal growth work can be done through self-help. Some self-help methods include:

- Journaling (writing in a notebook)
- Attending a 12-step or other support group
- Reading books or Internet sites about relationships and emotional skills
- Taking a class in peer counseling and forming counseling relationships with others also interested in personal growth
- Reading books about psychology
- Writing letters (that you don't send) to discharge old emotions
- Attending personal growth workshops

Much can be accomplished for little or no cost. The interesting thing about personal growth work is that once the emotional or relationship problems that had your attention are resolved or healed, if you continue to work on yourself, you can further enhance your personality, and the quality of your life will continue to improve exponentially and wonderfully.

There is, however, a limit to how much personal growth work can be done on your own. You will eventually reach a place where it is more effective to work with someone more experienced and knowledgeable who has been down this path of healing. Your work can also be greatly enhanced by the assistance of a helpful, caring person, such as a counselor, psychotherapist, mentor, or even a mature friend. ■■■

3. Use Holistic and Body-Mind-Spirit Therapies

A variety of treatments exist for healing a person on multiple levels. These techniques may reconnect mind and body or relieve stress that has become embedded in the structure and function of the body. Such methods often have a foundation in bodywork or body awareness and may be combined with psychotherapy or energy therapy. Below we have described some of these approaches.

- **Bodywork:** The term "bodywork" is used to describe methods of manipulating the physical body. Bodywork can restore freedom of movement. It may also relieve memories of stresses and traumas imprinted and stored in the muscle structures of the body in certain patterned ways, called (among other names) bracing, engrams, cellular memory, or armoring. We recommend using bodywork in addition to balancing chemistry and doing psychosocial work for resolving mental-emotional difficulties. Since bodywork is often passively received, it can often be accomplished without making any extra effort while you are improving chemistry and practicing the 3LS Wellness Program.

- **Spiritual or religious approaches:** Some spiritual or religious approaches may be helpful for mental-emotional difficulties and health on all levels of life. There is something to be said for adding prayer and healing intentions to a medical program, no matter what the illness. Scientific studies on the effect of prayer and healing intention on various illnesses have statistically shown that these activities create positive improvements in health.[7] More discussion about spirit follows in the next section of this chapter.

- **Vibrational or energy medicine:** Healing approaches known as vibrational, electromagnetic, or energy medicine involve balancing and enhancing the energy field or vibrational frequency of the bodymind. These approaches focus on non-physical methods of working with health and illness. Actually, whenever either healing or illness occurs, changes in the a person's energy field happen first, then biochemical changes occur, and lastly structural changes occur. Thus, these methods work at a deep level.

- **Combination or integrative approaches:** Some techniques blend any of a number of methods (bodywork, spiritual or religious approaches, vibrational or energy medicine, personal growth work or psychology, relaxation techniques, or exercise) to heal and reconnect mind, body, and spirit. This is a very creative arena of therapy that can be very helpful. The effectiveness of any technique generally depends upon the skill of the individual practitioner as well as the receptivity of the client.

Here is a partial list of mind-body-spirit techniques or methods:

Acupuncture	Hellerwork	Prayer
Alexander Technique	Homeopathy	Psychic healing
Bach flower remedies	Jin Shin Jyutsu	Psychic surgery
Chakra balancing	Laying on of hands	Reiki
Color therapy	Light therapy	Rosen Method
Crystals	Magnetic healing	Sensory-Motor
Detox sessions	Massage	Therapies
Energy field balancing	Neuromuscular	Shiatsu
Feldenkrais	Therapy	Somatic therapies
Flower essences	Polarity Therapy	Therapeutic Touch
Harmonic chanting		

Note: One other approach is clinical ecology. Some mental-emotional symptoms can arise from biochemical origins, such as chemicals, allergenic substances, or other substances in the environment. See a clinical ecologist if environmental influences are suspect.

See the Resources at the end of this book for how to locate practitioners.

HEALING MIND AND EMOTIONS Q & A

Q: I am a healthy 40-year old female. I do suffer with extreme anxiety at times. I started taking Xanax everyday. I notice lately upon awakening my heart is fluttering, just for a few moments. Could the Xanax be causing this? I did have this symptom occasionally upon awakening long before I started this med. This is the only med I'm on. It is too late for home remedies, have had anxiety all my life, need the meds.

A: Your current symptoms are an indication that it is either time for you to increase your dosage or change to another. However, think about what you are doing. If you keep following the medication road, there is no solution to your problem. However, this does not mean that you are doomed. Remember, the human genome project has shown that only 20% of chronic conditions is genetic (the unchangeable genome or genetic structure) and the other 80% is due to what we decide to do with the genes we were dealt (the phenome, the changeable expression of the genome). Therefore, your anxiety is only incurable as long as you think it is so and fail to start working to improve it.

When you get serious about changing your life, start with brain chemistry and the 3LS, and then use any psychosocial approaches you need. Use other holistic treatments if necessary. After you start to do this, you will begin to understand exactly what your drug has been covering up, and you will begin to see a resolution of your anxiety.

Q: Can I do all the treatments at once that you mentioned, or do I have to do them one at a time? I mean, can I do psychological counseling at the same time I am practicing the 3LS and seeing an orthomolecular specialist to balance chemistry?

A: Certainly, doing as much as possible synchronistically can expedite healing. While theoretically all the approaches could all be done at the same time, it may be too much for a person to make that many lifestyle changes simultaneously. A person can only do so much at once and maintain balance. Plus, the bodymind needs a certain amount of time and space for healing. When a person is nearly crippled by illness (particularly by what is called mental illness), they are even less able. How many people have the wherewithal (monetarily or energetically) to do everything at once? Therefore, usually it is more beneficial for a person to pick one approach and do it for a while before adding another.

The best thing is to first get going on the right track, and add more as you are feeling better. Figure out what will give the greatest benefit in the shortest time with the least output of energy. Each step makes the next step easier and more effective. Improving brain chemistry is a good place to start, because it usually brings immediate results.

TROUBLESHOOTING CHECKLIST FOR IMPROVING MIND AND EMOTIONS

✓ Are you doing all three parts of the Wellness Program before or with other treatments?

✓ Have you tried dietary elimination-provocation testing?

✓ Have you used nutritional supplementation of essential nutritional substances?

✓ Have you read books about orthomolecular nutrition and consulted with an orthomolecular specialist?

✓ Have you looked for possible environmental toxins, including chemicals and pharmaceutical drugs?

✓ Have you done personal growth work to become aware of effective ways to resolve relationship conflicts, improve thought patterns, express emotions, and decrease psychosocial stress?

✓ Are you facing your life challenges with the help of a therapist or counselor?

✓ Are you using self-awareness of body, emotions, thoughts, and spirit all day long, every day, to give you clues as to what might be the next best healing approach for you?

✓ Have you tried therapies that integrate body and mind, such as bodywork, vibrational or energy medicine, or combination/integrative approaches?

✓ Have you considered approaches that bring growth to your spirit?

THE SPIRIT OF LIFE AND THE 3LS

Spirit Is a Part of Life

An important aspect of health is a person's spirit. For the purpose of this book, we will define spirit as the non-physical aspect of life, but the meaning of the term "spirit" is subject to individual interpretation. Some people consider the spirit of life on a larger scale to be a majestic sense of beauty and order. Others use names to describe it such as God, Allah, Buddha, Cosmic Consciousness, Great Spirit, Tao, Soul, or Higher Power. On a personal level, the growth of a person's spirit may involve becoming aware of a higher meaning to life and life's experiences. Some people consider the growth of spirit as developing a sense of connection with life itself or with something greater, wiser, and more powerful than an individual's sense of self. Such growth usually includes a movement towards a more positive and mature personal expression.

Taking a world view that acknowledges spirit as a part of human existence will help you see how a chronic illness is a purposeful and meaningful part of the flow of life. Our health problems can show us where we are not balanced in our lives and lifestyles. Illness may be seen as a useful catalyst for growth and self-improvement or an opportunity for reaching a level of healing that goes beyond the physical sphere of life.

A person with such a world view may also use religious or spiritual approaches as a means of healing illness. As mentioned earlier, numerous cases of spontaneous remission of incurable conditions following devout prayer have been documented. Studies have even been done that demonstrate the effectiveness of using healing intention and prayer in improving health conditions.

Spirit is an important part of life. If the Three-Legged Wellness Stool had four legs, the fourth leg would be spirit. Since everything is connected, improving the physical, mental, and emotional areas of life also create the potential for changes in the non-physical aspect of life. Just from practicing the 3LS—going no further than the standard practices of Skilled Relaxation, Diet, and Exercise—one's spirit is likely to develop from the increased health. As people become healthier, they tend to find a sense of meaning or connection to life in their own time and way. In our experience, a sense of greater connection with life is inevitable for anyone who persists for even just a year with the 3LS.

The bodymind is the physical "temple of the soul." No matter where people start to get their temple in order, it always leads them to being interested in other healthy things. Typically, by doing any part of the Wellness Program, a person starts to grow in the direction of some kind of higher consciousness. Theoretically and practically, anything that improves the quality of the bodymind helps one get back in touch with the spirit.

After practicing Wellness for some time, patients would often make statements such as, "I am grateful for my chronic condition for giving me this opportunity to learn." Their world view has shifted from their experience.

For those who are interested in personal spiritual evolution and wish to know how to enhance their relationship to spirit on a deeper level, we offer this understanding. The finer the tuning of your bodymind, and the more you take care of it (i.e., the healthier you are), the closer you will be to the Cosmic Consciousness (or whatever name you use to describe the non-physical depth of life). Since the body is the temple of the soul, the higher the attunement of the body, the more the soul can be experienced. It is basically an inner connection.

In terms of spirit, we are in favor of you doing whatever is appropriate for your current level of development and understanding.

THE AUTHORS' EXPERIENCES

■■■ WALT: I had none of the above understanding about mental-emotional difficulties or growth of spirit when I started learning about the 3LS Wellness Program and holistic medicine. I was just interested in what I could do to be healthier. However, the longer I did Skilled Relaxation, which I started for health reasons, the more I found the benefits far surpassed just physical health. I can say the 3LS broadened my appreciation of the spirit of life. As I got healthier, I found that I wanted to know how far I could go, and that is when I began to learn more about spirit. I also have seen this exact process of evolving from greater health to growth of spirit in a number of my patients who have practiced wellness by doing the 3LS. It has been described almost universally by many evolved beings and my holistic colleagues as well. ■■■

■■■ JAN: My healing journey has been long and filled with growth, and it has enriched my life in many ways. The personal growth work I have done over the years has greatly enhanced my life and has brought me fulfillment and joy. The 3LS has now become a lifelong friend, and the longer I practice it, the more I benefit and learn from it. Orthomolecular nutrition has helped me feel better on all levels of life, including improved concentration and more energy. And, my path towards developing my spirit is one of the most rewarding parts of my life.

Continuing to work with various forms of relaxation, different aspects of diet, and a variety of exercise methods along with ongoing psychosocial work continues to further my ascent towards the top of the mountain. Through doing all of this, I have become happy and healthy. I have discovered that healing is infinite, which means there is always room for improvement and growth. My learning becomes more and more subtle and refined, and is far greater and more wonderful than I ever could have imagined! With this continued healing, my life keeps getting better and better, deeper and fuller, more interesting, and more filled with love. ■■■

Chapter 8, MIND, EMOTIONS, AND SPIRIT—SUMMING IT UP

Learning about mind, emotions, and spirit is beneficial for people, whether they are healing any kind of chronic illness (physical, mental, or emotional) or just managing daily life. Body, mind, and spirit are all related, and cannot be separated. Thus, mind affects body and body affects mind in daily life and in healing.

The general area of mental-emotional difficulties is one of the least understood classes of chronic medical problems. Mental or emotional difficulties are not character flaws or signs of personal weakness. They have the same causes as do all chronic illnesses:

1) Genetics
2) Stress
3) Choice

These three causes interact to become pathological mechanisms which cause symptoms to appear. Conventional treatments for mental-emotional difficulties are medications and psychological counseling. It is a good approach for some, but since chronic illnesses usually have more than one cause or contributing factor, these treatments do not usually address all causative factors involved in mental or emotional difficulties.

A holistic approach considers imbalances in brain and body chemistry as one of the causative factors in mental or emotional difficulties and seeks to restore balance through proper nutrition. Balance is achieved by giving the brain and body all the nutrients needed for healthy function in correct amounts, and removing substances that harm or impair function. The branch of medicine that works with balancing chemistry is called orthomolecular therapy. Orthomolecular therapy may involve taking high doses (megadoses) of nutrients, which is best done under the supervision of an orthomolecular specialist.

What You Can Do to Improve Mental-Emotional Difficulties

1) Follow the pattern of the 3LS Wellness Program (Skilled Relaxation, Whole Foods Diet, and Right Exercise) and consider some additional variations to the approach that may be specifically applied to the mental or emotional realm.

continued on next page

continued from previous page

2) Employ some of the many psychosocial approaches to healing. Professional assistance is available from psychiatrists, psychotherapists, and counselors for working with a variety of issues and concerns. Personal growth work, called working on yourself or inner work, is what you do by yourself or with the help of others to improve your mind and emotions, resolve stressful life situations or events, and learn advanced relationship or life skills.

3) Use holistic approaches and other types of body-mind-spirit therapies including bodywork, spiritual or religious approaches, vibrational or energy medicine, and combination or integrative approaches.

Spirit, an important part of life, may have different meanings to different people. One is becoming aware of a higher meaning to life or moving towards a more positive and mature personal expression. It may also mean connecting with what is greater, wiser, and more powerful than an individual person. Practicing the 3LS can also enhance your relationship to your own spirit of life.

REAL LIFE EXPERIENCES TOLD

I was on Zoloft for 9 years. I decided I was tired of being drugged and of the feelings I got when I missed a dose. My whole family has depression and alcoholism. I made my choice that my life was going to be different. I think because I am so adamant not to be on antidepressants any more is the reason everything else I do works for my depression, i.e., exercise especially, magnesium, Skilled Relaxation, and wellness. It took me three months to wean myself off the Zoloft, one half every other day for a week, then every two days etc. until I was up to a week. And they say Zoloft isn't addictive, HA! Good luck in making the right choice.

—Jennifer Boals, Veterinary Technician, Boise, ID

I have two grown children who are schizophrenic and manic-depressive. They are successful people. My daughter works for a stockbroker firm. She loves her job and they enjoy her. She has one son. My son works as a computer programmer designing and troubleshooting a program for computer aided design. He does very well and enjoys his work. Life is difficult for both of them. But they persevered and they won. Most of the time they handle their life problems very well. I read about the problem, and we used niacin therapy (Vitamin B3). Life for us has not been a bed of roses, but we have made it so far. I am proud of both of them and thankful that I found information that was helpful. My best suggestion for anyone dealing with this problem is search, search, search. And pray a lot and often.   *—Coleen Beason*

I suffered from panic attacks. I first took control of my own health by researching and trying to find out first if I had a nutritional deficiency. I discovered the importance of being pH balanced. I was very acid (used pH paper to monitor daily) and dehydrated. I took Perfect Food, Primal Defense, Coral Calcium (above sea), Vitamin B Complex, and magnesium lactate (from whey). Within two months, no panic attacks. Doctors prescribed anti-depressants, which I took for three days and stopped. I know drugs were only a bandaid, and I wanted a "cure." I found it in nutrition and whole food products. I also exercise on my rebounder to keep my circulation (brain included) going good, and I know it is important for my continued good health.

—Deborah Sage, Health Professional (herbalist, iridologist, kinesiologist),
Alpharetta, GA

I suffered with severe depression last year, the worst I have ever suffered. But there were some very understanding people around me at that time. I was able to take time off work, and just recover as best I could, but still the depression continued. Somehow I had to pull myself out of it. It was tough! I remember my M.D. at the time recommending I go onto anti-depressants, but I was very much against that. I knew that was just going to be a temporary band-aid measure. I know that since I changed my diet, I can honestly say that I no longer suffer with depression. I saw a naturopath a few months ago, who helped me, and I have been following the board and receiving help there. Plus, meditation is the GEM that has been helping to heal me on all levels, along with diet and antifungals. I have also been adhering to the anti-candida diet in Beth Loiselle's book and just doing my own research instead of having to solely rely on other people (my naturopath) to give me the absolute correct information. They sometimes don't know the accurate information, and I prefer getting it right myself. It's my health after all, and I am the one responsible for it! And now after following the diet for over two months, I am so much better! I hardly recognize the person I was last year. My life just keeps getting better and better. My optimism and excitement for life is 100% to what it was. I sometimes can't believe I am so changed, and how small things don't get me down as much. It's like life has taken on a whole new meaning for me.   —*Maria Keswell, Service Assurance Consultant, Beldon, WA, Australia*

I had lifelong major depression, and this is now resolved 95%. It WAS necessary for me to work through deep, unresolved grief. I value inner work and think it is an ESSENTIAL piece of the puzzle. However, nutritional wellness is what healed me enough to stop ALL medications. An hour a day of exercise in sunlight and fresh air (critical for depression), and relaxation are key. My eating disorders have virtually resolved with whole foods (actually, I eat 90%+ raw foods). Am I healed of depression? I believe I am, as long as I continue with wellness.   —*Anonymous*

The relaxation techniques will be a lifelong practice for me. I don't do a session every day now, but I have made a remarkable discovery. I am a Bible study teacher, and I was finding it difficult to make the time for my relaxation techniques and my prayer/study time. I knew the Skilled Relaxation time was not a negotiable, and one day after I finished my Skilled Relaxation session I went directly into prayer. I could monitor my level of relaxation with a "stress thermometer" which measured the temperature in my finger with a probe taped to the finger. My goal was always to get the temp to 98+ when meditating. As I went from my meditation tape into my prayer time the finger temp rose *even higher!* As a result of that discovery, now I spend about an average of 45 minutes each morning by starting my Skilled Relaxation time with deep breathing to center down and focus. Then I go directly into prayer, and the temp in my fingers goes up very naturally. Through this discovery my prayer life has grown by leaps and bounds, my relaxation techniques have been consolidated into my spirituality, and I have also noticed my creativity has increased immensely. I led a seminar about this discovery at my church, which I entitled "Closer Walk." It was very well received.

—*Johnelle Donnell, Wichita Falls, TX*

My son had many behavioral issues, learning disabilities, Attention Deficit Disorder, and more. When the brain requires specific vitamins, minerals, amino acids and enzymes to make it work (make it's own neurotransmitters) it just makes sense that vitamins can help heal the brain like they can heal other organs. In my opinion that is why malabsorption (digestive issues) are at the core of the cause of many behavioral problems, many learning disabilities, etc. Vitamin supplements and correcting malabsorption definitely has helped my child. You should see his teacher comments from summer school! Awesome! And on no medication! Of course, it took many years for us to get this far. It isn't an overnight cure ... So I'm not sure if he would need as many vitamins if the malabsorption was corrected (leaky gut, food allergies, yeast, celiac, etc), or the food supply and preparation was also better ... but I do think you have to get the correct vitamins in there one way or another.

—*Angela Roberson, Financial Industry, Dallas, TX*

I have had dermatographia for about two years. It took me about one and a half years to get it under control. The things that have helped and continue to help me are Skilled Relaxation, massages, exercise, and magnesium glycinate supplements. Surprisingly, I now am thankful that I have chronic hives as it made me aware of slowing down, relaxing, exercising, and the magnesium deficiency before I had more serious problems from stress build-up. I can immediately tell if I need to get back on track because the dermatographia will then rear its ugly head again.   —*Anonymous*

I have been pretty depressed for the last two years because of my marriage going sour, and I just felt sorry for myself and eating anything I could, getting bigger and crying all the time. Then I finally decided that I didn't want to be depressed any more. I figured I could not change my husband, so I decided to change myself. I started eating only the healthiest foods I could find, a lot of whole grains, lean protein, loads of produce and nonfat dairy. I joined a gym and have been working out three hours a day. I already lost 20 pounds, gained a lot of energy, and have a very different outlook on life. I don't feel so depressed any more. I feel better about myself, and it will be my way of living for the rest of my life. I think depression is a state of the mind most of the time, and changing lifestyle and feeling more confident will help it more than drugs which are not a real solution.

—Luba M., Yarn Business, San Francisco Bay Area

I had my first blood clot when I was in my mid-thirties. I was diagnosed as Heterozygous (two recessive genes) with both Protein C and Protein S Deficiencies (PCD, PSD). For many years I suffered the side effects of blood thinners. Deep vein thromboses are extremely painful. I had to use a walking stick, as I could not put weight on the affected leg. Eventually the Wafarin sodium I was on resulted in my developing skin necrosis and other side effects. Skin necrosis is not very painful, but is a very ugly sight to behold, with raw flesh wherever the skin dies. I had to take a Low Molecular Weight Heparin (LMWH) injection every 12 hours. I had lost all quality of life. The hospital counseled my father and husband that my condition was life threatening and that there was nothing more they could do for me. In 1996 I began research on the internet finding sites like Dr. Stoll's and various others. I began experimenting in alternative medicine. I discovered that Vitamin E acts the same way as Wafarin sodium. I was told to include a magnesium supplement to heal my pancreas. I have been on alternative medicine for four years now and remain free of symptoms. I am fifty-one now.

—Zarin Steven-Johan, Remisier (Stock Broker)
and Author of Life is a Leaky Bucket, *Malaysia*

Conclusion

DEFINING WELLNESS...

■■■ WALT: As we have discussed, there are many paths to the top of the mountain! There are many degrees of wellness, just as there are many degrees of illness. Wellness can be much more than the absence of pain. Being well is exuberant life, creativity, and energy. It is happiness every day. Wellness is the infinite capacity for forgiveness and loving support of others.

With wellness, you become more complete in spirit—after all, the bodymind is the temple of the spirit. Few people experience the pinnacle of spiritual and bodily wellness. However, wellness inevitably results in higher consciousness, and which inevitably takes you closer to wholeness, healthiness, holiness, holism, by anyone's definition.

The top of the mountain is a phrase used in the East to describe enlightenment. I have borrowed and adapted it to mean "perfect wellness." Like enlightenment, it is a goal to strive for that is difficult to reach.

Perfect wellness is a state that is still evolving (read *Cosmic Consciousness*, by Richard Maurice Bucke, M.D.), and reaching it would be a significant challenge. Thus, I tend to resist trying to define it. Only when human potential is studied in much greater detail will we have any idea what perfect wellness is. I do not think that anyone, yet, has plumbed the fullest depths of human potential.

Here are several examples. One is the type of documented super-human feat such as those instances when a frantic 100-pound woman lifts an auto off her trapped baby and then does not remember doing it. This gives just an inkling of the physical potential of the human frame. Here is another: the spontaneous resolution of far-advanced, terminal cancers (more than 1,000 documented worldwide already) gives some inkling of the potential of the human immune system. Still another is the documentation of people with multiple personalities, in which a serious chronic disease is present in one personality and wellness is present in another. This testifies as to how little is known about human potential. If one of the multiple personalities has diabetes and another does not, if one personality needs thick glasses and another has perfect vision, if one personality has arthritis and another does not, what does this mean about the permanence of any chronic condition? How about the savant or eidetic memory (extraordinarily accurate and vivid), which is already known to be trainable in many people? Those are daily reminders of the potential we do not yet recognize as the heritage of humankind. "The appearance of one sparrow proves the existence of birds!"

These examples, plus the fact that many brain physiologists and psychologists agree that humans use less than 10% (I think 1%) of their brain potential, and the fact that we do not really know what the frontal lobes (the largest and newest part of the brain) even do, says that we still do not know what the potential for true wellness really is.

The book, *The Awakened Mind*, by Maxwell Cade and Nona Coxhead, (Harper Collins, 1991) proves that many of these potentials are sleeping within each of us. Already, the insight exists to bring our potential to fruition in those who wish to take the time to develop it. How about the biofeedback documentation (at Menninger Clinic) of Jack Schwartz's abilities of nearly instantaneous healing of wounds while in the alpha state (with increased amplitude).[1] Such abilities are inherently possible within anyone willing to put in the time and effort and training.

All of these examples could extend the prudent person's perception of what wellness might be. The best book I know that even tries to document this potential is Michael Murphy's classic: *The Future of the Body*, published by Tarcher/Putnam in 1992 (nearly 800 pages of fascinating reading with more than 2,000 references). If you want to delve seriously into this, you might ask your library to find you a copy. ■■■

■■■ JAN: What Walt describes is an amazing aspect of wellness. When I think of perfect wellness, I usually think about "being fully functional as a human being in all aspects of life" and/or "a person reaching their maximum potential in this lifetime." That would include achievements like being able to live life in a state of constant balance and centeredness, being fully differentiated (which means having knowledge of all the parts of one's own self as well as being able to distinguish self from others), reaching higher levels of human potential such as being of service to others, and achieving a state of unity with the "cosmic consciousness." ■■■

■■■ WALT: Jan, all that you mention is a part of being a fully functional person. I think few of us could understand even the high level of function you describe. It might take an individual who was a lot healthier than what we now define or accept as healthy to be able to understand what it means to be a fully functional person. At this time in our evolution, all we can do is just accept that the path to the top of the wellness mountain is a lifetime journey with pleasant surprises along the way. The fact is, the farther we progress, the easier the journey becomes and the grander and more profound the surprises get. No one really knows the capabilities of a truly healthy human. ■■■

■■■ JAN: When I think about wellness, I also ponder, 'How can we encourage people to strive for the highest level of wellness possible?' So many people stop short of that, because they think that just being out of pain is as good as it gets. I know too many people who settle for living with mental, emotional, or physical pain. They think it is old age or some type of unresolvable physical problem. Often people believe that it is the nature of relationships to be unfulfilling and unhappy. Consequently, I see so many individuals who don't do anything to improve their condition. I would like to encourage people to continue to work on themselves and to always seek greater health of body, mind, emotions, and spirit. ■■■

■■■ WALT: Anything that moves one closer to wellness, health, wholeness, or holiness is a small step in the right direction. Just by taking that small first step, the easier it becomes to approach the top of the mountain. The 3LS Wellness Program is a great tool for doing just that, and people can keep learning, looking for, and using other approaches that complement the 3LS Program. Wellness is the most fascinating and productive of hobbies and is self-perpetuating. ■■■

■■■ JAN: As you move towards a healthy future …

Take one step at a time to make choices that create wellness in your life. The journey of a thousand miles begins with a single step.

Consciously form good habits. It is through helping yourself with good life habits that you have your best chance to overcome your ill health. If you take the time to make healthier changes, it will be well worth it for you now and in the future.

Face your life challenges. The life challenge for some of us is regaining or recapturing health. As you pursue wellness, you may need to organize your life a little differently than other people and find your own personal enjoyment. Accept what you have been given and work with it creatively. Even with a chronic condition, you can have a beautiful, fulfilling life (even more so if you use it as an opportunity to learn and grow).

Keep moving forward. If you stumble on your path of healing, the most important thing is to pick yourself up as soon as you are able and keep going forward in your quest for health. Always return to your wellness practice without browbeating yourself for missing a step. We all make mistakes. Don't let a mistake be an excuse to give up or stop moving forward.

Always keep looking for the solution to your chronic condition. Don't ever give up. Don't be defeated—chances are that what you need is out there somewhere. Continue to learn. The secret to success is to keep trying.

Stay in the present. It is the things you do and think today that will bring about a rosy future. Do as much as you can to help yourself. ■■■

■■■ WALT: Remember, the most important thing is for you to get started by choosing one leg of the Wellness Program. As you heal and move towards wellness by using the 3LS, we invite you to participate in the Bulletin Board on my website, www.askwaltstollmd.com. Post a message telling others how the 3LS improved your health condition. Your testimonial will help inspire others who are just starting to learn. We all need to support each other on this path of healing. Let us know what you learn, and we will grow right along with you. ■■■

We wish you health and wellness!

Afterword
By Walt Stoll, M.D.

THOUGHTS ON THE ISSUES OF
MODERN-DAY MEDICINE

■■■ WALT: Well, dear reader, now that you have read this far, it is time to share with you another reason why I have participated in the writing of this book.

The word "doctor" means "teacher," and I took that to heart when I decided to become one. In my 30+ years of practice, I have discovered that people mostly learn by personal experience. This book is designed to give you that firsthand experience by helping you understand some basic mechanisms of how your bodymind works better when you improve your condition through following the 3LS Wellness Program.

I firmly believe once you experience an improvement in your condition from practicing this Wellness Program, you will begin to believe what it took me more than 20 years (including medical school and internship) to *begin* to understand: Your doctors are not always telling you what will help you the most. This is *not* because individual docs are evil, but because of the political and economic structure of the American Medical Association (AMA)/pharmaceutical/government/insurance/big business system that directly influences medical education and medical practice.

When I entered pre-med, I believed the "party line" that only conventional medicine (allopathy) was valid and that all other philosophies of healing were quackery. It took me about 15 years of practicing exclusively conventional medicine before I became suspicious that this might not be completely true. It took me another 20 years after that to *fully* understand that we were taught this because of political and economic rather than scientific reasons (i.e., what works best for the patients). Now, another ten years later, I'm still not sure I understand completely how the profession I trusted and idolized could have gone so far astray from the healing principles that I believe in so ardently.

My first clue as to this truth actually came when I was taking my boards immediately following graduation. We had to have our licenses before we could even be interns. The young man sitting next to me for the two days of tests (I got to know him a little in breaks between individual tests) was not even an M.D. He was a D.O. (Doctor of Osteopathy). I was amazed since we had been taught that D.O.'s were "M.D. pretenders" and had an inferior education. Yet, here he was taking the same tests as I was. I learned that not only did he have to pass the same tests I passed, but the day after I went home, he had to stay for an extra day of testing for skills in practical manipulation. In essence, he took a whole day of tests that I could not have passed at all. This D.O. had had a much better education than I.

But I was so full of myself, having just graduated and on my way into practice, that I was able to put this experience behind me and go ahead and practice allopathic medicine strictly and whole-heartedly for years. However, as I began to realize the truth that the current health care system in the United States is also an economic and political system, and not always fully functioning for the health benefit of the patient, this early experience came back to me more and more strongly.

Most doctors go into medicine for the altruistic reasons of helping people. By the time we graduate, however, most of that idealism has been drummed out of us by our *beginning* to see what the health care system really is. Then, in practice, we become entrenched in the system and are told to not do anything that might threaten it, at the risk of losing our licenses.

I believe that most people in the profession recognize that conventional medicine does not have all the answers to the chronic conditions that make up the vast majority of problems facing patients today. So many of the other healing paradigms in the world do a much better job at this, but they are legally or politically prevented from operating in this country by the power of the AMA and the political/economic system that largely influences how health care is provided. I sometimes call this system the "allopathic monopoly."

I want you to have the freedom of choice for whatever approach to health works best for you. Thus, I would like to see all healing philosophies having equal access to insurance coverage, public education via the media, health education programs in colleges, and governmental support. In that way, all modalities—conventional and others—could be utilized for what they do best, and you could choose whatever works best for you.

No complementary or alternative health care provider or modality *should* be hard for you to find. The basic reason they are hard to find is due to the opposition by the AMA as a deliberate national policy.[1] The AMA continues to say that different methods are not proven, and therefore so far it has been able to prevent other healing professions from being licensed or even certified in their professions in nearly every state.[2] They have also been able to prevent insurance coverage for most other healing modalities, and governmental agencies (Medicaid/Medicare/retirement plans, etc.) rarely pays for them either. Consequently, since other healing methods are denied insurance coverage, etc., this continues the public misperception of their "illegitimacy." This is starting to improve, but there is still a long way to go. All practitioners should have exactly the same rights and stature in the health care system as any M.D. or D.O.

The chiropractors were the only ones who had enough money and organization to beat the AMA in court in the 1980's and can now legally prevent the AMA from overtly attacking their very existence. However, the AMA continues to attack them covertly.[3] Other healing modalities have not had the resources to fight the AMA nor conduct the expensive scientific studies needed to prove their own legitimacy. The Flexner Report (sponsored by the AMA in 1911) legally keeps governmental money away from proving the effectiveness of other healing methods, and the movement toward providing research funding for alternative methods is being fought tooth and nail by the AMA.[4]

By all of this, the public continues to be guided into thinking that many or even most "competing systems" or ways of providing health care other than allopathic medicine are quackery. This is one of the reasons why the United States system of health care is in its present quandary and is one of the less effective systems of health care in the world. The health care problem in the US is revealed in many statistics: lower longevity, more time spent in hospitals, higher rates of drug abuse, more time spent off work for illness, higher incidence of chronic illness, higher fetal and maternal mortality rates, more ADD and hyperactivity than in other countries. The United States has the largest percentage of our population in jail of any nation in the world, including many who would not be in jail had they been able to have their psychosocial and related medical issues addressed adequately. As compared with the other industrialized nations in the world, all of this is in spite of spending much more per individual on so-called "health care."[5] This health-care crisis is well known to anyone who reads the newspaper in this country. That is why my first book was called *Saving Yourself from the Disease-Care Crisis.*

The fact is, *for chronic conditions,* other healing methods should be tried first with allopathy used as a last resort. The way things are now in the United States, even though the allopathic paradigm fails miserably for chronic conditions, allopathy is the method most often used. This is especially unfortunate because it is typically only the most highly educated, wealthy, open-minded, and desperately sick people who can fully access other forms of health care. I tell you all of this so that you can understand how far-reaching this situation is and how slowly it is changing, and so that you can help influence positive changes to occur.

So as to not be misunderstood, I reiterate here: conventional medicine is needed for what it *does best,* which is work with acute conditions. It is just *not* best for chronic conditions. Where I part ways with the allopathic monopoly is in its insistence that allopathy is the *only* way, even when it does not work.

There are many allopaths, dissatisfied and disillusioned with the health care system, who retire early in increasing numbers (as soon as they have made enough money to retire gracefully). After all, they no longer enjoy the way medicine is practiced. But, at *holistic* medical meetings, I have always seen excitement and enthusiasm for practicing medicine, and none of the holistic physicians were talking about retiring. I have yet to see one holistic practitioner who retired before age—or before the AMA retired them forcibly, as it did in my case and with many others who were making a difference. The joy of helping people had come back into their lives. They were working for the "treasures more precious than gold," witnessing lives restored to health, rather than having their practices consist of revolving door patients and an unrelenting monetary stream.

It has now become clear to me that expecting change from an entrenched and monopolistic medical system is practically hopeless. There are too many non-medical (political and economic) reasons for continuing the current system. With the political environment as it is, sometimes I despair that all I seem to have accomplished by trying to educate the public about holistic medicine is to be forcibly retired by the AMA (the details of how this came about are on my website), and not allowed to do what I loved above all else—practice medicine holistically. However, I see my role as a public educator as even *more* important than I did when I was practicing. Only an educated and aroused public can bring about change, since they are the ones who are being harmed by the current system and will benefit most by that change. I have come to the conclusion that it will take educating thousands of people to make a difference in the present political/economic system and create a level playing field for all healing paradigms.

Most physicians, including myself, who have converted to holistic medicine did so by personally experiencing its benefits on their own health. The same is true for patients. Personal experience is the springboard that changes and empowers individuals. They become "disciples" of holistic healing, and if they wish to "convert" others, are effective at it simply by being shining personal examples of how well it works. It is plain, to those who know them, that something good is working in their lives, and so others would like to have a part of it as well.

So, through this book, and on my website and Jan's, we offer the 3LS Wellness Program to you so that you have the opportunity to try it and experience its health benefits. When you find that your own health problems are dramatically improved, it is my hope that you will take and continue to use the principles of holistic healing to make better-informed decisions about your own health and that of your family and friends. If this book can help enough people obtain that personal proof of the effectiveness of the holistic paradigm, the world will change for the better.

Unfortunately, in the present environment, the TV floods us all with "Take this or that pill" to fix or suppress our symptoms. Moreover, so many allopaths still promote, shamelessly, the idea that everyone can live any way they want, and "If you just pay me enough, I can take care of you." The influence of the system is everywhere. However, despite this overriding influence, I am gratified to see that public change is coming into being. But it is glacial slow-going against the tidal wave of advertising for fast foods and the miracle pills of the day.

After you start practicing the 3LS Wellness Program and experiencing its benefits on your health, consider the many actions you can take to encourage change in the allopathic health care monopoly and help bring about more options in the system. Here are some ideas:

- Share this book with your friends, family, coworkers, and health care practitioners.
- Talk to your physician repeatedly about needing alternatives to drugs and surgery.
- Spend your "voting" dollars on other healing modalities and holistic physicians/practitioners.

- Communicate with your insurance companies about lack of coverage for other healing methods—ones that work.
- Contact your politicians and share your experience of the ineffectiveness of the entire health care system in this country.
- Write letters to the editors of your local newspapers about your experience of how the allopathic monopoly did not help you and how simple alternatives did.
- Teach the members of your support group about the 3LS.
- Write your local hospital administrators and request other healing modalities be made available to patients.
- Shop at health food stores and high quality grocers.
- Let your school administrators know your concern about the lack of nutritional quality in our children's school lunches.
- Communicate with your grocery store about the unavailability of organic and whole foods. Buy organic and whole foods when the grocers do carry them. Send in customer comment cards asking for a whole foods section.
- Ask for whole foods meals in restaurants and restaurant chains.
- Form and support food co-ops and farmers' markets in your community.
- Support political efforts to safeguard our rights to purchase nutritional supplements.
- Sponsor political efforts to safeguard the rights of practitioners using other healing methods.
- Mention what you have learned about the 3LS and holistic health on call-in radio shows, Internet chat rooms, blogs, and other media to help get the word out.
- There are many other things you could do, based on your positive experiences changing your life for the better with the lessons learned from daily implementation of the 3LS.
- Health care practitioners can also find ways to help such as giving community service talks about health improvement and the 3LS. They can also offer special programs for helping people who have no health insurance.
- Visit the website of Sunrise Health Coach Publications at http://www.sunrisehealthcoach.com/howyoucanhelp.shtml for more ideas.

As you personally witness the benefits of a union between holistic and allopathic medicine, I do hope you will make your voice heard, demanding change in how medicine is practiced—a change that will benefit all of us and generations to come. I wish you access to a truly effective system of health care, and above all, good health and happiness. ■■■

For Health Care Practitioners

This section is addressed to health care professionals, however, all readers are invited to peruse it for their learning. In this section, the term patient refers to all people receiving services, whether patient, client, student, etc. We explore the 3LS as part of a health care practice, the nature of holistic healing, and further opportunities for practitioners to learn.

WHY A SECTION FOR PRACTITIONERS?

There are several reasons why a health care practitioner would be interested in learning, using, and offering the 3LS to patients.

First, practitioners who read this book will better understand the goals and process of patients using the 3LS Wellness Program, and thus can harmonize their healing approaches with it. For example, patients on the Perfect Whole Foods Diet needing nutritional supplements will wish to avoid alcohol-based tinctures and supplements containing sugars or starches, including certain prescription or over-the-counter medications.

Second, patients who do not reverse their condition using the approaches or modalities you usually provide may benefit by your offering this program to them. Some patients simply will not recover without making the lifestyle changes of the 3LS. You may recommend that they read and follow the advice in this book and start them on their path to wellness. Thus, patients who do not respond to any treatment will still have a chance to get well.

Third, any treatment or modality you already provide will work better if your patients also practice the 3LS Wellness Program simultaneously. The 3LS does not rule out using other treatments. The synchronistic effect of using the 3LS along with other methods can be powerful.

Fourth, adding the 3LS Wellness Program to your medical or other type of practice will help make you more holistic in scope. Continuing your professional development by learning the 3LS and the holistic approach to health will broaden you as a practitioner, increasing your professionalism and skill, while making you more effective in helping others.

Fifth, if you use the 3LS yourself, you will set a good example to your patients for improving and maintaining health. There is nothing like personal example. Don't forget the old paraphrased saying, "Healer, heal thyself."

Sixth, by being a healthier person from your own practice of the 3LS, you will be a more effective and responsive practitioner. The healthier you are, the greater effect you can provide as a healer.

This is the health care of the future!

PRACTITIONER Q & A

Q: What type of health care professionals can introduce people to the 3LS and support them to follow it?
A: All types of practitioners can guide patients to improve their health using the 3LS. A few professions that come to mind are:

Physicians: Ayurvedic physicians, chiropractors, cranial osteopaths, dentists, doctors of oriental medicine, medical doctors, Native American healers, naturopathic physicians, and osteopathic physicians.

Bodyworkers: Alexander Technique practitioners, craniosacral therapists, Feldenkrais practitioners, Hellerworkers, massage therapists, physical therapists, polarity therapy practitioners, reflexologists, reiki practitioners, Rolfers, and therapeutic touch practitioners.

Mental health professionals: Behavioral kinesiologists, biofeedback practitioners, coaches, counselors, family therapists, hypnotherapists, psychiatrists, psychotherapists, psychologists, and trauma therapists.

Nutritional counselors: Dietitians, health food store owners and employees, herbalists, nutritionists, and orthomolecular specialists.

Other practitioners: Applied kinesiologists, clinical ecologists, coaches, energy healing practitioners, health and fitness instructors, holistic nurses, homeopaths, independent nurse practitioners, meditation instructors, occupational therapists, orthomolecular specialists, personal trainers, physical fitness trainers, physician's assistants, religious and spiritual leaders, shamans, sports medicine specialists, yoga teachers, and others.

This is not a complete list. If your specialty or modality is not on this list, it probably should be! All professionals can work together and should not hesitate to refer patients to other practitioners who have more expertise in a particular area. Especially given the vast amount of information now available, none of us can know everything, and we need to be humble enough to accept that. "Everybody is smarter than anybody."

Q: How can secondary or tertiary health care providers (i.e., practitioners who are not physicians) offer information about the 3LS Wellness Program legally and safely to patients? For example, for some practitioners, nutritional guidance may not be included in the description of their scope of practice.

A: One way is to call what you do "education" and not "medical advice." As long as you plainly state that you are offering information "for educational purposes only," there is little you cannot do. This is adequate protection, even in the most conservative and restrictive states. However, since every state is different and some modalities are regulated by municipality, be sure you know the laws that affect your practice.

Note that the claimer/disclaimer in this book follows the same precept by saying, "The information in this book is for educational purposes only. It is not medical advice."

Some practitioners can prescribe the 3LS to patients. Others with less education and training can simply offer this book as a self-help program and share their personal experience of the 3LS as an inspiring testimonial of its effectiveness. (You are planning on practicing the Wellness Program yourself, aren't you?)

Anyone can offer a book to patients, friends, colleagues, and family members.

Q: Must a health care professional be a "holistic practitioner" to promote the 3LS Wellness Program?

A: Any practitioner can guide patients to read our book.

Q: What exactly makes a practitioner "holistic" in scope?
A: The American Holistic Healing Association (AHHA) says, "For a health-care career, it is helpful to address two aspects separately. First, you must be trained in a specific modality or method of delivering health care (such as acupuncture, chiropractic, psychology) that can be licensed or certified and gives you the right to deal with patients or clients. Thereafter, you add on the holistic principles and philosophy. Be aware that the term holistic is commonly used in two different ways. We prefer the meaning that includes consideration of the whole person and whole situation, searching for the root cause, and encouraging a partnership between patient and practitioner. Some people use the term *holistic* interchangeably with *alternative medicine.* This latter can be misleading, as not every alternative modality practitioner operates in a holistic manner."[1]

■■■ WALT: Holistic is a concept, not a discipline. It is an attitude and a philosophy. My experience becoming a holistic practitioner is that it takes an open mind, putting the patient first, and courage. As a member of the board of trustees of the American Holistic Medical Association for about 10 years, I had the opportunity to travel the country and meet many holistic physicians who had started as allopaths. They all met the exact criteria of having courageous, open-minded regard for their patients. Also, one of the most universal characteristics of every practitioner of the new paradigm of health is having experienced the effectiveness of alternative or comple-mentary medicines in our own bodies (or witnessed such experiences with close family, neighbors, or friends).

The more healing methods and modalities practitioners are knowledgeable about, the more they can be considered holistic. They do not have to know how to practice them all, but must know enough about different methods to be able to refer patients to a practitioner using other healing approaches. ■■■

Q: Quite frankly, if my patients practice the 3LS Wellness Program and all get better, I'll lose a lot of income because they won't come for office visits anymore. So why should I show them this book and introduce them to the 3LS Wellness Program?
A: ■■■ WALT: This is the unspoken question of many practitioners and I think, one reason why many do not always follow what is best for their patients. It really depends upon why a practitioner goes into business. If it is to help patients, by offering the 3LS, they will be successful, a lot happier, and still make enough money to be comfortable.

I personally had to take a cut of nearly 80% of my income to become a holistic practitioner, and I did it for the sake of my patients. This type of dramatic income change is a lot truer of physicians than other practitioners since we have had an unopposed monopoly for about 100 years to hone our system of making money. Practitioners of other healing methods working with me did not experience the same reduction in income. They did fine, since they kept 50% of what they charged with no expense, although later, when they were practicing on their own, they had financial considerations. In my case, I could give up 80% of what I made and still have a roof over my head and food to eat. I never have been interested in consumerism. I still made a good living and have had a lot more fun and satisfaction. All of us made enough to live on, and we all mainly worked for those "treasures more precious than gold."

If the patient actually did what we recommended (the 3LS) that first visit, many of them never had to come back. In reality, however, my patient load did not decrease, because once they saw how much better they were doing, my happy patients referred many of their family, friends, and neighbors to me. What happened then was most of our office visits were new patient visits, and those take a lot more time than routine follow-up visits, which is where a doctor makes most of his easy money. We still had to spend a certain amount of time with each new patient, for which none of us could justify charging like we would have done for the conventional approach.

My holistic colleagues across the country have not been able to figure out a way to keep the same very high income either. They all seem to have decided, as I did, that money was a secondary concern and the primary consideration was the welfare of the patients. We chose to continue this way because the rewards of the treasures more precious than gold made it all worthwhile. Until one experiences that feeling, it seems insane to take a lot of extra training, while working longer hours and risking the censure of one's colleagues, just to make a lot less money. Our patients were empowered and were healing their chronic conditions. I am sure that many of you who read this would like to give better service because of the enjoyment of seeing your patients get well, and then have them tell others about "this great practitioner."

Now you have the advantage of this book, which just might make the difference in the time you need to spend with each patient. With this book, patient education will most likely take less time so you might be able to maintain your schedule. Also, you might offer adjunctive services, classes, and products to assist patients with the 3LS, which can help with cash flow. These variables may make the difference so that you don't experience as much of a change in income as I did. ■■■

■■■ JAN: I would like to share my experience becoming a holistic practitioner with a smaller, simpler practice than an M.D. For me, adding the 3LS to my massage practice was a great start for calling my practice holistic. Later, having experience healing my own chronic illness and knowing a few other modalities (stretching, psychotherapy, Polarity Therapy, and personal training) made me feel even more qualified to be a holistic practitioner.

From offering the 3LS Wellness Program, both my client load and cash flow have increased. I charge for most educational consultations to cover the time spent teaching new clients. Those who practice the 3LS and get better typically continue to come in for regular massages, plus they are eager to refer new clients. They understand the health-enhancing benefits of massage and trust my integrity as a practitioner. Some clients become so pleased with how much better they feel and how empowered they are, they increase the frequency of massages so their health can improve faster. Also, some take months or years of hearing about the 3LS before they finally catch on to the fact that they really need to begin the practices.

If, like me, you have a smaller practice with much less formal education than any kind of doctor, the goal of working with clients holistically is simple. Just try to interest your clients in practicing the Wellness Program by themselves. Thus, if they have complex health problems or conditions generally considered outside your scope of practice, you are not diagnosing, treating their condition, or giving them advice. You are educating them to consider lifestyle changes to improve their general health—changes that just might help their chronic health problem.

I have found it important to clearly promote my massage practice as holistic, so people would not be surprised to find me talking about lifestyle changes and health-care options. To cover the holistic education part of my practice, I hang a disclaimer sign in my office that says: "I treat musculoskeletal disorders and offer holistic health information, education, and products for general health and optimum wellness. I am not a doctor and I do not diagnose or prescribe. For specific medical advice or treatment for your condition, please consult a physician, physical therapist, chiropractor, nutritional counselor, licensed psychotherapist, or appropriate practitioner." My health history form contains the same wording, and all new clients fill it out and sign it.

When speaking with clients about other aspects of health care besides massage, I frequently remind them of the limits of my education and refer people to other practitioners for further expertise and perspective. Even if my clients consult with other practitioners, usually they continue seeing me because they appreciate the great results of the common-sense wellness approach. This is especially true if they've spent a lot of time and money elsewhere with no improvement.

As a holistic practitioner, I consider it important to stay open-minded and be resourceful. I try to guide people to find whatever they need from a variety of sources and encourage them to do whatever works to increase their health.

In my experience the two greatest assets of a good holistic practitioner are 1) continually doing your own personal growth work and 2) continually learning more skills and developing yourself as a practitioner. By becoming stronger in body, mind, and spirit, and by being more knowledgeable as a professional, you will be the most inspiring example for your patients. Having a clinical supervisor with whom to discuss problems and questions that arise in your practice can also be very helpful.

All in all, offering the Wellness Program complements massage and bodywork very well, and has made me a better practitioner with more to offer. The 3LS truly helps people get better. To be able to genuinely serve others by providing useful information is a treasure. ■■■

Q: For patients covered by insurance, can practitioners bill insurance for patient education related to the 3LS?

A: Yes, in many cases. Refer to the CPT codes or perhaps the new ABC code book if it is now being used, and find what most closely approximates what is done. Books and supplements are probably not billable to insurance.

Q: Is it legal or moral to sell books and/or supplements in a professional office?

A: ■■■ WALT: I found that having books and supplements available in my center was preferred by patients who decided to try the 3LS and holistic healing. My allopathic colleagues thought I was running a store, but my patients really approved of my making the supplies conveniently available to them.

Prior to practicing holistically, I had always believed that a physician should not sell things he or she recommended. For example, it is considered a conflict of interest for a physician to own a drug store. However, when I began to promote wellness and to use complementary approaches to medical care, I spent several years trying to get local bookstores and health food outlets to carry the books, supplements, glandulars, homeopathic remedies, etc., that we were learning to use. And then, since we were learning so fast, we frequently graduated to different books, supplements, etc., and the stores were frequently left with unsold merchandise. I really couldn't blame them for not wanting to carry the items. We were the only primary care holistic medical facility in the area, so it didn't pay them to go to all the extra bother, and we eventually found it necessary to provide items as a service for our patients.

Actually, even getting local stores to carry the goods was still not ideal, because the client was inconvenienced having to go to a second location to get what they needed (and then, more often than not, was unable to get what we had recommended). Even worse than just not having the items in stock, patients need to obtain products right at the time they are interested and motivated to use them. If they have to go to several places, order things, run out, wait two weeks to get started, etc., their motivation and interest wane and they are unlikely to follow up on their health program.

Finally, after having all these difficulties working with patients and local merchants, I realized that my idealism in trying to avoid a conflict of interest was getting in the way of what I was trying to accomplish: *helping people get well and stay well.* Therefore, we started to carry books at the Holistic Health Centre and finally carried the highest quality supplements, glandulars, homeopathic remedies, and other items that were not available elsewhere. The patients greatly appreciated it. ■■■

■■■ JAN: In my office, I sell items that can be helpful to patients wishing to start the 3LS. I also give them the option of borrowing some of the books or videos from my lending library. Otherwise, these items may be difficult to find locally or cost more for the patient to obtain from other places. ■■■

WAYS TO EMPOWER A PATIENT

■■■ WALT: I would like to share some of my experience as a holistic physician/practitioner to guide you to work with the 3LS and make your practice holistic. To heal a chronic condition, your patient needs to be empowered to take responsibility for his or her own health. As health care practitioners, our function is to open doors that may not have been opened before and invite people to walk through. It is they who are suffering and the ones who really have to take the time and responsibility for walking through the door.

The patient is the most important member of the health care team, and to accept this status requires the professional to give both permission and tools for the patient to participate as such. Given permission and tools for wellness, the individual can then choose to become involved to the limits of his desire and ability.

Below are some ideas for empowering patients. These suggestions may be used by any kind of practitioner. In addition, use your imagination and expertise to generate other ways of facilitating patients' success in their quest for health. To obtain ideas, some practitioners provide means for patient input into the organization of the health-care delivery system. Some examples include suggestion boxes in the waiting areas and open invitations to make recommendations and give criticism at any time.

Create a Healing Relationship: In my office, I found that I received more honest sharing from patients by refusing to wear a white coat, refusing to have a desk to sit behind, and encouraging people to call me Walt. Those who were more comfortable calling me doc or Doctor Stoll were not discouraged to do so, though. This is an example of eliminating formalities that get in the way, as well as opening the door to any possibility of what works for the patient.

Another action we took to create a healing relationship for our patients was our all-day Thursday clinic. On that day, we had each of the professional and support office staff bring a whole foods dish for lunch and shared a healthy potluck with all the patients we saw that Thursday. We did this in part to show that nobody has to give up tasty foods in order to have a perfect diet. The other reason was to bring patients and clinicians to the same level—an essential part of the healing relationship, in our opinion.

Each patient was seen and interviewed by a team of practitioners of different healing methods in our Holistic Centre that day. After the interview with the patient, our entire team of professionals would later converge and discuss which modalities might be most useful, and then plan the best course of action to facilitate that patient's healing.

I also developed a New Patient Handbook for all my new patients. This handbook started at about 10 pages but gradually grew to be 80 pages in length. It covered treatment options, prices for individual services, biographies of staff members, how to get service during off hours, and other topics. Since all patients received one of these at the first visit, they knew that they were welcome to discuss anything with us at any time.

Provide Patient Education: People are more likely to actually do something if they understand why it needs to be done. Thus, patient education is the most powerful medication or treatment available in the practitioner's office, assuming patients comply with the instructions given. Health-care providers who do not use this most important tool simply cannot deliver the highest quality care. As a practitioner, the best way to help your patients is to offer resources for them to educate themselves. If the patient gains enough understanding of his problem to at least partially follow what you believe to be the most advantageous action, then the practitioner and the motivated, well-informed patient can work together. Some physicians set up a room in their office for client education and self-involvement in health care. This room may be furnished with equipment and supplies, otoscopes, stethoscopes, study carrels, tapes, and projectors. There is practically no limit to what is available and can be done to empower and educate patients.

Statistics then, and now, show that patients remember only 30% of what the doctor said in exit interviews from the office. If interviewed the next day, they only recall 10%. In other words, they paid for 100% and only use 10%. I was not willing to live with those statistics. I had about 300 handouts and I tried my best to limit each subject to one page. The longest was less than two full pages. In my waiting room, I kept a bound copy of all the handouts that I had available so interested people might request what they needed. Thus, the time spent by patients in the waiting room or examination room could be used profitably to read or view educational material. I also insisted that the patient bring a blank cassette to each visit so everything I shared was recorded. I then had a typist record my message and give it to the patient as she or he left. It was typed as it was dictated in front of the patient, thus, the patient got both a cassette and a typed transcript. I did this with every single patient.

We also began using educational posters describing the 3LS in our waiting room. We found there was always someone standing in front of at least one poster. There was one about exercise, one about Skilled Relaxation, one about nutrition, one about reflexology, one about acupuncture, and others. Some posters showed picture explanations, and others had a list of information. We changed them every few weeks, and then after a few months would rotate them through again.

Some patients will do what you tell them without needing to understand it. I personally think it is better to understand, but I care more that people get well and less how they accomplish it.

Teach the Patient Self-Awareness and How the Process of Holistic Healing Works: Most patients want their physician or practitioner to tell them what to do. They want a quick remedy or to be given concrete answers, even if there are none. Often we cannot tell them for sure, just point them in a fruitful direction and give them helpful hints.

At the beginning of learning to listen to and be aware of their bodymind, and use the bodymind laboratory, sometimes you must provide patients with a concrete answer just to meet the simple goal of helping them get started with something that will show them results. After they have had some experiences and have heard your feedback about what happened, they begin to understand the basics of listening to the bodymind, and then they can better choose what to try and for how long. They will eventually learn that healing is not so black and white, and they will start to do their own thinking.

Every bit of knowledge obtained by you and the patient is useful, whether it brings improvement to their condition at the time or not. If a person has tried something correctly and it does not produce expected results, both of you have learned that it was not a helpful method for this individual. It will provide a wider context and make future learning more meaningful. It is important for people to understand that even what seems like failures are useful learning tools.

Show Patients All Their Options and Honor Their Choices: Do your best to educate your patients to understand *all* of their options and the likely consequences. Even if someone is not interested in putting in the effort needed to help himself or herself, he or she deserves to at least know what the options are. If a patient is satisfied with the conventional approach—fine. When symptoms come back, at least the patient will know that there are other options.

After you are satisfied that you have done your best to help the patient really understand available options, then honor the patient's choice, even if you think it is wrong. Since your patients are likely not functioning very well (the reason they have come to us in nearly every case), they may choose poorly, but it has to be their choice. People have the right to choose their own way, right or wrong. We can gently try to guide them to what would bring them the quickest results with the least effort, but the best way for a patient to proceed is always with what they will actually do. Physicians and practitioners are consultants, not gods.

Validate Their Efforts: Patients need encouragement and support so that they do not become discouraged, when for the first time in their life, they are finally on the right path. Exacerbations and healing crises can be misinterpreted by patients, and these short-term events need to be seen in a positive light (i.e., flu-like withdrawal symptoms or sugar-shakes once on a Perfect Whole Foods Diet does not mean the diet is detrimental). They are not reasons to stop doing what will eventually bring the desired results.

Making even small lifestyle changes is an immense victory for many, and people who are healing need to have their victories validated along the way. The challenge of getting started and continuing the program can be made easier with support and encouragement, especially since there is no way of predicting when they will experience results. Your active role as a supportive coach can make all the difference in their willingness to continue on their path to wellness.

Work with Their Resources: Consider also your patients' available strengths and weaknesses in recommending treatments. I would consciously do my best to give the person healing options requiring the least cost in time, effort, and money. For example, we were renting out GSR machines 25 years ago, as soon as we understood how much money that would save the patient and how much more effective it was for difficult cases. Perhaps it was just an indication of our primary focus: to provide the patients with the least expensive and most effective approaches possible to get results. ■■■

■■■ JAN: To empower my clients, I offer educational handouts, a lending library, books and supplements for sale, a website with self-help articles, and a biannual wellness newsletter. I also spend time teaching them self-help methods like stretching, self-massage, and how to start doing personal growth work. Just listening to some clients talk about what is important in their lives helps them heal. I find it very rewarding to work with individuals who are motivated to assume a large role in their healing process. ■■■

WORKING WITH THE 3LS

Most people must go through a progression to be successful in practicing the 3LS. This is how it goes:

First, they have to fall far enough from good health to be suffering. They want to get better. Next, at least in our culture, they have to exhaust the conventional allopathic symptom-relieving paradigm that our health-care system has become. (This was described in the Afterword.)

Second, they have to begin to look around them, and hopefully see someone who has improved his condition by using holistic approaches.

Third, they have to begin looking for information to help themselves. The Internet has given people who reach this point a lot more options. Our book and holistic practitioners who offer the 3LS also provide information. All this while, most likely the person is getting sicker, but finally when they contact this information, they have an opportunity to learn how to help themselves.

Fourth, they have to learn enough to have a chance to accurately do something (hopefully one part of the Wellness Program) that will bring results in a reasonable length of time.

Fifth, they have to have the discipline to actually do the work.

Sixth, at this point, having gone through the process of accomplishing just one part of the Wellness Program, they have achieved some success. They will most likely want to do more.

Seventh, after practicing the 3LS for a while, they have produced sufficient wellness and energy to learn and study cutting edge research that might give them even more options for healing their particular condition.

This scenario is what we have observed in our own lives, those of our colleagues, and those of our patients who were successful. It was also true of those who were not successful, but we would see them get hung up at one of the above stages.

Usually the hardest part is to motivate the person to begin the first aspect of the Wellness Program. Generally, after people experience just a little bit of wellness, they really move forward with the rest of the 3LS.

3LS Q & A

Q: So, then, how are people best motivated to start the 3LS Wellness Program?

A: In our experience, long-standing pain and suffering (recurrent symptoms) or major health crises are the best motivators. Hearing other people's successful experiences in resolving a similar condition can encourage people. Another good motivator is having already spent thousands of dollars trying to have practitioners or physicians unsuccessfully solve their problems. Read more about beliefs that help people start seeking Wellness in Chapter 6.

Most people will need to start wherever they can. Let them choose something they have enough interest in to actually learn about and that they have the energy to do right. If a patient can do one thing right from the beginning, he or she usually has pretty spectacular results. Few are the patients who will quit after having an eye-opening experience of quick results in health improvement. For the Perfect Whole Foods Diet, it is usually within a week that they will start feeling better. Skilled Relaxation will give some early benefits, but it takes six months to make significant changes. For aerobics, most people will feel changes fairly quickly, but it takes six weeks for the greatest benefit.

As your patients start feeling more energy and health, they become capable of adding the second practice, the one that they would not have been willing or able to do in the beginning. Each practice increases their horsepower, so they have more energy and an easier time doing the other aspects of the Wellness Program. Their success encourages this.

Those who can start with an attitude that wellness practice is positive will get well faster, since this good attitude makes them more open and able to be involved. Yet the most effective way to guide a patient to wellness using a positive attitude is the spiritual way.

By positive attitude and spiritual way, we are talking about the patient welcoming the practice as a good and meaningful part of life and approaching the changes with a positive outlook. Truthfully, a patient's sincere desire to get well is probably more important than any specific protocol. People who already have a view of illness, disease, and health as a meaningful part of the world we live in have the easiest time accepting and implementing these practices.

■■■ WALT: Most people who are sick usually find it a monumental task to learn how to use all three parts right and see practicing wellness as a drudge. I found that when I started talking with them about attitude, spiritual commitment, and so on, their eyes glazed over. I reached a lot more people by starting where I could perceive they were ready to start—very simply. Once the health of their bodymind was strong enough, it took very little for them to change this attitude from drudgery to enthusiasm. Before that, it was impossible.

To encourage their positive attitude, I frequently tell people to make a hobby of wellness. Rather than seeing wellness as a drudge, and being focused on the negative, guide them to see it as an adventure trip with newness and surprise. (The same is true for work, family, and finance.)

Here are a few more tips on how to interest patients:

First, practitioners need to vary their approach to their patients based on a shrewd evaluation of the patients' personalities. If they do not, they run a great risk that the patients will not follow instructions. (Of course, it is not really the practitioner's risk, but the patients', since it is their illness.) For example, some patients who wish to deny their illness cannot tolerate being involved in the management of their problem and so will not listen to explanations. Others cannot bring themselves to follow instructions without a good understanding of what is occurring. With some patients, the authoritarian approach is most effective; with others, it is the least productive. (Authoritarian medicine generally works fine for acute problems but tends not to work for chronic conditions anyway.) Consequently, varying your approach can be helpful.

Second, to interest your patients, be aware that there exists the teachable moment: a moment in time, quite fleeting, in which the transfer of patient education is possible. It often occurs at just that moment when the patient feels at gut level the importance of his condition and before his psychological defenses begin to protect him through denial, anger, or indifference, with thoughts like, "It can't happen to me!" If the physician or practitioner misses this moment of receptivity (it takes skill to catch it), the time when a little effort can transfer a lot of information is lost, possibly forever. Another type of teachable moment is simply when a patient is having an exacerbation of the most painful or bothersome symptoms and is desperate to find a way out.

Since I have always been interested in living up to the meaning of the word doctor (as teacher), I learned early on to recognize the teachable moment, mainly since I was always looking for it. When I had a hospital practice, I began to realize that there were more teachable moments for patients in hospitals than there were while they had more control over their lives. It seems that desperation brings out these moments. As I got healthier myself from practicing Wellness, I also became much more aware of what is now called intuitive medicine. In an intuitive state, recognizing the teachable moment is a lot easier. Then after my center gained an international reputation for helping complex problems, people came to me already carrying the teachable moment with them.

Third, sometimes a dose of direct communication of what is called "tough love" can bring about a gut level response. For example, when faced with a reluctant patient who is likely to have a coronary, try explaining exactly what life is likely to be like (if the coronary does not kill him or her) in graphic details if it is not prevented. By recording this description on cassette and then transcribing it for the patients, many formerly resistant to helping themselves were finally stimulated to change. Of course, you must use your judgment to choose this method carefully for using with certain patients. This means that the physician really has to understand this patient and know he will actually be spurred to change.

That gut-level response is necessary to get some patients' attention, but it must be used carefully to direct them to the educational material. If practitioners become aware they have scored their attention punch, they must immediately actively involve patients in the knowledge transfer. If patients are not immediately and actively involved, their gut-level response will get all the attention, and the factual information presented over the next few minutes will not register (just as though it had never been presented). The way I had them become actively involved was by having them feed back to me exactly what I had asked them to do. In addition, our session was tape recorded for their benefit.

If the person is on the fence and hasn't yet made a decision to try Wellness, that gut level communication I mentioned has to happen. I have found that at times, unless one gets under the individual's skin and they get a bit angry, no action takes place. So perhaps, if you can make a patient angry, they will find the energy at least to try to prove you wrong, and thus start taking steps to help themselves. However, this approach needs to be comfortable as well for you as the practitioner. Do whatever works for you as the practitioner.

Fourth, if you guide most patients to look at their history (hopefully they will bring in a detailed health account), they will notice a definite gradual increase in problems over the years. If they do not believe that they are worsening, tell them to start noting their symptoms on their calendar for the next year or so. Seeing documented evidence that their condition is changing for the worse can motivate them to begin caring for themselves. ■■■

■■■

All we can really do is share what we know at the time and not be attached to anyone taking in any of the information we offer. You can give them "water," but everyone has to "drink" on their own. Simply do not be attached to anyone using anything you lovingly hold out there. If they choose to dither and look elsewhere for options, you have no control over that. There will always be a percentage that will not follow your recommendations, no matter how well you present it.

We are just door openers, and the people who choose to walk through get better. The further they get through the door, the more goodies they will find as they walk down the path. Help as much as you can and do not be discouraged when individuals cannot (or will not) pay any attention or take heed. Perhaps when their problem bothers them enough or recurs in spite of what they have chosen, they will notice that the door is still open. Each person has to find one's own way. The best we can do for some is get them looking in a rewarding direction.

It is not so challenging with every patient. Some people will come to you absolutely eager and ready to begin the program. There is a point when a person is ready to hear what they need to do (and there are different degrees of readiness). Much of this readiness depends in great measure on how much they trust and appreciate you as a practitioner. Without readiness, the time spent trying to educate the reluctant patient can be worthless. Thus, the most effective use of your time is to determine who is ready and willing to do the practices and spend quality time with them. Give them your support. The others who are reluctant to go with the program can just work with the allopathic system until they are ready to consider more promising options. Those patients at least deserve to be told about the 3LS, even if it is clear that they will likely not believe it or do it initially.

Q: How do we know which aspect of the Wellness Program the patient needs to do first?

A: This is part of the skill of the professional, to help your patient choose. Because everyone is so different, sometimes it is hard to know what would be most beneficial to do first. At other times, the most important thing a patient needs to do is obvious to the practitioner from the beginning.

■■■ WALT: I always insisted that my new patients create the kind of health history described on page 271 of Chapter 7 before coming for the first visit. With that information, I could spend my time analyzing the best and most effective first step of the 3LS. Sometimes a practitioner will not choose correctly, any more than a patient. That is why I reiterate that what a patient will actually do is usually the most important determinant (since any aspect of the Wellness Program will help at least some). Anything that helps patients see benefits turns them into believers, and then they have more energy to take the next step.

A good test of patients' determination to help themselves is whether they will bother to learn. The more they are willing to learn before trying, the better chance they have of getting quick results without too much effort. After having an undeniable positive experience, they are more likely to learn more in order to have more of this experience.

Just find a way to get them on track. Once they have started correctly enough to see results begin, their Program typically takes on a life of its own. ■■■

Q: Why are some people reluctant to do the practices?

A: It is amazing at times how much people are willing to suffer rather than even try, for example, a two-week trial of the diet, something very simple for such a short time. They can come up with the most convoluted rationalizations as to why they cannot give it a try to learn if it is beneficial for them. Some would sooner spend thousands of dollars on multiple doctors and various tests and gradually get worse, rather than try something that takes some effort and costs nothing. Never mind that it might help their total health. Although we do not always comprehend this behavior, we do understand a few of the reasons that slow some people down. Here is why some are reluctant to begin practicing the 3LS:

First, one type of resistance comes from people having already been so victimized for years by the health care system that they refuse to believe in anything. When patients discover that allopathic doctors do not have a clue why certain symptoms are present or what to do about them, they often extend this to "nothing any doctor or practitioner does has any value." Of course, this is not true.

Second, dealing with the causes of chronic conditions means learning and doing. The last thing some people want to hear is that they have to educate themselves and make changes based on what they learn. For some, making an effort is much more difficult than just swallowing a pill. For those who really wish to avoid making a significant effort, they will find any reason or excuse not to try. When I was still in practice, there were patients we used to call the "Yes, but" patients. No matter what we told them, if it required the smallest lifestyle change from the one that had gotten them in the predicament they had come to us to "fix," they would always say "Yes, but." And then they would tell us why they couldn't change.

Third, sometimes people have not succeeded at previous attempts to help themselves through similar but different approaches. For example, patients would come into my office telling how they tried (perhaps poorly or half-heartedly) several other dietary approaches to their illnesses (or perhaps they selected inappropriate approaches, and so of course, they didn't have any success). Consequently, now they were suspicious of any dietary approach.

Fourth, people normally do not do anything preventive until they are in a crisis. It is a human tendency to wait until things are desperate before doing anything about them.

Again I refer you to the section about choice in Chapter 6 describing thoughts that slow people down in choosing healthy activities, and new ways to think. This can help you, as a practitioner, work with some of the above situations.

Q: What if people will only do one aspect of the Wellness Program, such as aerobics, and want to stop with that?

A: Just let them do aerobics. After a year of aerobic exercise, rare is the person who does not become interested in the other parts of the Wellness Program. Let them figure that out for themselves. The excitement of discovery is a powerful incentive for more Wellness, and the program takes on a life of its own.

Q: Many of my patients are not disciplined enough to do any of the parts of the 3LS. Perhaps there could be a modified or beginner's plan in some way, something easier?

A: ■■■ WALT: In hundreds of cases of people doing the 3LS, the only failures I have seen were those who thought they could cut corners with the directions. It is true that some people will get benefits with less than accurate practice.

However, I am talking about 100% effectiveness, not partial effectiveness. If people are going to cut down the frequency or perfection of doing these practices, they must be satisfied with very moderate benefits or no benefits at all for a period of time. They must adjust their expectations accordingly. Besides, if people think doing it a little bit less is going to do wonderful things, many will then do a lot less.

If the practices are not done as recommended, and the benefits do not happen, people may give up doing what may likely be the most important single thing for them to accomplish. Consequently, they might not go back to it for years (if ever) because they've "been there and done that," when they have not really done that correctly at all. Any method of practice that is really effective in healing a chronic condition takes energy and dedication. One must at least give it a long enough trial period to find out if it truly helps or not. This has to be their choice, though.

All that being said, I have always tried to tell people what would first and foremost help as many people as possible, as close to a 100% success rate as possible. To make sure this works for everyone is why I may seem strict about how to do the practices. However, a significant percentage of patients will see improvement with doing less than what is recommended, because everyone is unique. Thus the principles I give are just guidelines.

Advanced health thinkers and workers have to tread a tightrope: how to get quick results without driving the patient to distraction with what it takes to get those quick results, and the slower approach that is easier but risks the patient getting impatient for results and giving up prematurely. Practitioners have asked me for statistics about patient compliance with the 3LS and the treatment outcome. First let me tell you that repeated independent studies indicate that after all the time and money spent in doctors' offices, less than 40% of patients follow the advice they were given. This is just with conventional medicine where the instructions are usually something very easy like just taking some pills.

With my patients, the compliance for practicing the 3LS Program was about 5% immediately and double that a year later. This was over 10 years ago, in the days before the holistic approach was at all known. By 5% and 10%, I mean they start doing one leg of the Program. Getting started is the hardest and most important aspect. Once they see results from doing one part, the percentage of those who go on to do a second practice is more than 75% of those who did the first. The percentage of people who practice all three is about 5% of those who do two. These figures are empirical estimates, based on my clinical experience.

I observed that people who were not ready to listen frequently went to a number of doctors again over the next couple of years (the same thing they had been doing before they came to me) and came back worse than they were in the first place. Their first statements were always something like, "Well, here I am—worse. What were you telling me before?" or "You know, I was not ready to hear what you said back then, but now I am. Say it again." Even then, about 50% were still not ready to actually do the work required to deal with their chronic problem. Many went away to repeat what they had been doing all along, which had not helped them. Humans are incredibly stubborn and frequently will do anything but change their minds and habits, even when it's advantageous.

Considering that typically there is only 40% compliance with something as simple as just taking a pill, 10% is not bad. Anyway, my philosophy is that if only 1% of people see the light, it is worth my time. For those people, what is offered here is a godsend. By implementing it, they then serve as examples to their family, friends, and neighbors. I hope in your practice, you can see a much greater percentage of patients starting the 3LS, since you will now have our book and other resources available to teach and inspire them.

Usually only a few people are disciplined, compulsive, or desperate enough to start all three parts of the Wellness Program at once. Depending on what they have and how long they have had it, *all* people who use all three practices consistently and faithfully see improvement in their general health. So treatment outcomes kind of depend upon what you mean by "well." I hesitate to give a definition of wellness because no one really knows what the truly healthy human is capable of in our world.

Some get well with only one part. A larger percentage get well with two and the highest percentage of success occurs with those who follow all three aspects of the protocol. ■■■

Q: How can I as a practitioner become more effective working with my patients with the 3LS?
A: We have stated this before, but it is worth repeating. Practice the 3LS yourself before and while you are recommending it to your patients. "Healer, heal thyself" is always the best example and motivator for the patient. Even if you are already feeling pretty good and don't have a debilitating chronic condition, you may be amazed at how much better you feel doing these practices. Your own experience and testimonial will help others with what might be called

"hopeless conditions" believe in the healing power of the bodymind. Sharing your own personal experience will help the fence sitters begin the program. Personal experience is always inspiring: *"At least it worked for somebody!"*

Also, any healer is more effective the healthier he or she is. This is an especially important reason for health care practitioners to use the 3LS protocol themselves. The healthier you become, the better you can serve others.

■■■ JAN: One advantage of offering the 3LS in a massage office is even if clients don't choose to start the 3LS right away, they may still come for regular massages, and I can continue to gently reinforce the concepts of the Wellness Program. A good time is when their symptoms recur (the teachable moments). Also, several posters on my office wall continually remind clients of principles of holistic healing and the 3LS.

Some people are resistant to the idea of starting the 3LS, but other circumstances may lead them into beginning one practice. When they tell me about it, I reflect back, "Ah, so you started one of the legs of the 3LS Wellness Program." They will usually accept that evaluation with delight and look like a light bulb has been turned on. They have finally caught the concept. This is a great teachable moment.

Others won't start the Program, but are happy to tell me about small improvements they have made such as eating fruit instead of sugary desserts, drinking less caffeine, or taking more time for rest and fun. I always validate their efforts. These are important steps for many people. I am glad to see improvement of any kind, especially when made by their own choice and effort.

I find that after presenting the 3LS Wellness Program, patience is important. Many people start Practicing Serious Wellness eventually, but sometimes it takes years. ■■■

WORKING WITH PATIENTS TO IMPROVE MIND AND EMOTIONS

Here is some guidance for practitioners who assist in healing mind and emotions. Many practitioners approach healing mental-emotional difficulties by offering one method such as psychotherapy or medications. It is our hope through this book that more practitioners will be inspired to take a holistic approach and let patients know that a full range of options are available.

Knowing which part of the 3LS the patient will actually do successfully is a judgment call on the part of the professional. As mentioned, starting where a patient feels most comfortable can be the most effective approach, since the patient is most likely to actually follow through. However, most people already understand exercise, and this is often a good place to start for people with mental or emotional difficulties. By the time it would take them to accept the idea that sitting still in a chair for 20 minutes twice a day would pay dramatic dividends, they could already be getting results from exercise. Thus for many individuals with mental or emotional concerns, start with exercise and do not even mention the other legs of the Program until they have seen benefits from that. Once they begin to become mentally and emotionally more responsive, then suggest nutritional supplements and diet, and lastly, Skilled Relaxation. Approaches for growth of spirit usually need to be personally selected by the patient as he or she gets better.

■■■ WALT: In treating patients with mental-emotional or psychological disorders, the severity of the condition determines the strengths the individual has left to work with reversing the condition. Since it is the individual who does the real work, one has to accurately assess how much they are presently capable of doing and match what is recommended to that ability. I have had patients who were so far gone that I refused to deal with them until a reliable member of the family, who volunteered to participate in the patient's progress, attended every session. Many gave up, but the few that stuck it out were gratified by seeing a loved one return to them. Once the individual begins to get some results, their horsepower (more physical strength, increased energy, clearer mind, and so forth) improves enough that they can begin to take over from the rescuing family member. Assessing the status of when one is ready to help himself or herself can also be challenging. ■■■

INCLUDING THE 3LS IN YOUR PRACTICE

Q: How can I obtain more information and training for offering the 3LS to patients?

A: Many practitioners have a lot of work to do to begin understanding how so many conditions are caused by the same basic mechanisms and how the 3LS addresses them. Besides our book and your personal practice of the 3LS, there are a number of other resources available:

Practitioner Resources

1. Teaching others is often an aid to learning something new. Practitioners have an opportunity to learn more by volunteering on the bulletin board at askwaltstollmd.com. The interactive bulletin board is for asking questions and sharing information and experience.

Everybody learns by publicly sharing their personal experiences and watching the exchange among participants. Patients learn by seeing others with similar problems get well with a holistic approach. Practitioners learn from discussions about application of the 3LS, the perspective of practitioners of other disciplines, reading about a wide variety of diseases and symptoms, and more.

Your expertise can be helpful and you can learn from sharing it with others. All help is welcome. We hope that no one will hold back because they think their knowledge might not help.

Besides the bulletin board, the website has other resources for learning about the 3LS and becoming a holistic practitioner. Reading through the archives may answer questions you didn't know you had. You may do a search of the website to find information about specific conditions or issues. There is also a glossary of terms and concepts on the website, which is worthy of study in itself.

This website differs from many other medical help websites. This website is not-for-profit. All contributors to the website and bulletin board donate their time for no compensation other than the pleasure of helping others learn to help themselves.

2. Walt's first book, *Saving Yourself From the Disease Care Crisis,* provides further information about the 3LS protocol and holistic healing. Watch for the updated and expanded edition written with coauthor Kathleen M. Diehl to be entitled *Beyond Disease Care.*

3. The Resources and Notes for every chapter of our book provide many tools and opportunities for learning more deeply about the background of the three parts of the Wellness Program and other holistic approaches.

4. Visit Jan's website at http://lifespringarts.com. Jan will post information on her website relating to the 3LS Wellness Program, including links to other helpful sites and success stories sent in by practitioners with tips for implementing the program.

5. For additional books and information, plus opportunities for health care practitioners to resell books, check with Sunrise Health Publications at http://www.sunrisehealthcoach.com.

6. Read *Ninety Days to Self-Health,* by C. Norman Shealy, M.D. (Ariel Press, 1988) and *The Textbook of Functional Medicine* by 47 authors, available at www.functionalmedicine.org.

7. Look for schools that teach holistic medicine. Books are available on the topic. The American Holistic Health Association (AHHA) can also help you locate schools and classes (See Chapter 7 resources). Check for magazines at your local health food store.

8. Holistic associations offer benefits such as networking, educational information, and referrals. See Chapter 7 Resources for a list of holistic organizations and visit the AHHA website for a longer list.

Q: I'm a holistic practitioner. I've been using the 3LS Wellness Program for six months myself, and have also spent quite a bit of time studying Walt's books and learning from the Bulletin Board and archives on his website. Now I feel like I'm quite knowledgeable about the 3LS. How can patients seeking assistance with the Wellness Program find me, and how can I find practitioners of other disciplines who use and work with the 3LS also, for mutual referrals?

A: Patients and practitioners working with the 3LS may use the practitioner network of the American Holistic Health Association (AHHA) at www.ahha.org to connect with each other. Practitioners will use the keyword "3LS" or "3LS Wellness Program" in their professional description on the AHHA website to identify themselves, and patients should type in that phrase (or simply "3LS") when looking for a practitioner.

■ ■ ■

To conclude this Appendix, some practitioners who offer the 3LS have shared some of their thoughts. Their writing tells a story and emphasizes the excitement and commitment they bring to what they do. We had asked them to keep their comments short and to the point, but got so many long, enthusiastic responses that we wanted to include everything they said. Personal information and experience is some of the most interesting reading in any book like this, and if you are seeking to enhance your practice, you will appreciate the thinking of these practitioners. The respect we have for those who work with our bodies makes reading about their inner thoughts doubly interesting.

We hope you will become and continue to be a student and teacher of wellness and holistic healing, and wish you success in your practice.

COMMENTS FROM PRACTITIONERS

When I decided 30 years ago that my medical practice was going to emphasize a natural approach and true prevention of illness, the first step I took was to put diet, exercise, and stress-coping measures at the top of my list for every patient. Nothing I could have done would have been more productive. Many patients with severe problems have improved dramatically with this basic approach. The ones who return after not seeing me for a while reporting that they have relapsed often say, "I went off my diet," or "I stopped exercising," or "I just let stress get the better of me." These three core concepts are essential not only for getting well, but also for staying well.

— Terry Chappell, M.D., Bluffton, Ohio

The first client for which I ever tested out the theory that diet, exercise, and regular relaxation-style techniques matter was myself. The proof that the 3LS Wellness Program worked was seen in my initial physical evaluation by Dr. Stoll, which showed no conventional evidence of stress physically or emotionally. Yet the written questionnaire of stress factors in living circumstances (Holmes-Rahe test) revealed that my stress load was almost off the scale. For him as well as for me, this was testimony enough of the power of these three factors in daily wellness and the prevention of stress-related disorders since I had already been doing the diet, exercise, and regular relaxation-style techniques before I came to the center.

After having worked with hundreds of clients and training hundreds of therapists (in the daily health practices of Ayurvedic medicine), my wife Melanie and I know from personal experience and observation that without these three factors in place as the core and foundation, wellness is not possible. In adopting such health-giving practices into one's life, clients also demonstrate their willingness to participate in and be responsible for their own wellness. Diet, exercise, and relaxation, when combined with such intention, is the most powerful of all cures.   *—Robert Sachs, L.I.S.W., L.M.T.*
[Licensed Independent Social Worker, Licensed Massage Therapist]
—Melanie Sachs, O.T. [Occupational Therapist],
Certified Ayurvedic Lifestyle Counselor
Diamond Way Ayurveda
P.O. Box 13753, San Luis Obispo, CA 93406
tel/FAX: (805)-543-9291
Web: www.DiamondWayAyurveda.com

Prescription drugs have helped many of my patients during these past 35 years. At the same time, the most profound and lasting changes in their health and well-being have occurred when they begin to use good nutrition, regular exercise, and skilled relaxation techniques. It seems that these basic human endeavors go to the root causes of problems and begin a profound healing for my patients.

—*Bill Manahan, M.D.*
Assistant Professor of Family Practice and Community Health
University of Minnesota Medical School
Author of Eat for Health
Past President of the American Holistic Medical Association (AHMA)

I have been in the practice of medicine for 55 years in Ohio and Arizona. Family Medicine, as I have practiced it, has included the emphasis on adequate exercise, balanced diet including the consumption of adequate amounts of water; and a diet associated with dietary supplements including vitamins, minerals and enzymes. Through the years I have found and used the help of professionals who are skilled in the use of relaxation techniques such as biofeedback and meditation. The importance of mind, emotions, and spirit as they are actively involved in the process of healing has been a part of this work.

—*Gladys Taylor McGarey, M.D., M.D.(H.)*
Founding Member of the Board of Directors of the AHMA
Former President of the AHMA
Founder of the "Baby Buggy Program"
President of the Arizona Board of Homeopathic Medical Examiners
Adjunct Faculty of Greenwich University, Hilo, Hawaii
Recipient of Lifetime Distinguished Service Award—Muskingum College in Ohio

I have seen thousands of patients who had not responded adequately to conventional medical therapy or who had experienced intolerable side effects. In the majority of these people, a program that emphasized dietary changes and nutritional supplements resulted in considerable and long-lasting improvement.

—*Alan R. Gaby, M.D.*
Past-President, American Holistic Medical Association (AHMA)

I have been offering Skilled Relaxation to my clients for 20 years in a medical clinic, a mental health clinic, and in my private practice. It has been very rewarding to observe that many of those clients have used it. For some, it has meant the relief of physical and emotional pain. For others, it has provided a tool to get centered in their heart and discover an inner peace from which to live their lives. It has helped countless people who suffered from panic and anxiety disorders to find the internal resources to interrupt their symptoms and find they have the power to make another choice. It has helped couples learn that they can connect from their individual centers and experience a deeper love. The list could go on … For all people who have the commitment and motivation to improve the quality of their lives, Skilled Relaxation offers a variety of ways to contribute to that overall goal.   —*Banks Hudson*

Banks Hudson is a 1963 graduate of the US Military Academy at West Point. He has two masters degrees in theology and an accumulation of two years additional formal training in psychology, organization development, and psychotherapy. He is currently licensed in the state of Kentucky as a marriage and family therapist, and his specialty in addition to MFT is treating generalized anxiety disorders, include panic disorder, acute stress disorder, phobias, obsessive-compulsive disorder, and post-traumatic stress disorder. During the past ten years he has researched and developed a sports training system designed to maximize the power of the mind in reaching selected goals and objectives.

The vast majority of Americans are unaware that they live a life that is extraordinarily distanced from that which is optimally natural and healthy. Our lifestyles are directly responsible for most of what ails us. The good news is that we therefore have many opportunities to improve the way we feel. I have found that proper exercise, nutrition and skilled relaxation can help improve health. Therapeutic interventions such as acupuncture, homeopathy, spiritual counseling, manipulative medicine, nutritional supplements, fasting and chelation therapy, when properly applied, can help as well. Everyone who reads this book will find a means to live a more full, healthy and productive life. For some, their very lives will be saved.   —*Scott T. Stoll, D.O., Ph.D.*

Scott T. Stoll, D.O. Ph.D., is a board-certified physiatrist who is Associate Professor and Chairman in the Department of Osteopathic Manipulative Medicine at the University of North Texas Health Science Center. He is Medical Director of the Rehab Center at the Osteopathic Medical Center of Texas and the S.M.A.R.T. Institute, he is Executive Director for the Physical Medicine Institute and Adjunct Faculty in the Department of Integrative Physiology at UNTHSC-FW. He was recently selected as the Executive Director of the Osteopathic Research Center at UNTHSC-FW. He also is the recipient and Principal Investigator of a $1.4 million, 5-year NIH K-30 Research Curriculum Development Award from the National Center for Complementary and Alternative Medicine (NCCAM) designed to train clinicians to conduct OMM research. Dr. Scott Stoll teaches, practices, and lives in Fort Worth with his wife, Myra, and three sons. [This is Walt's son!]

Health care professionals are coming to the realization that what we eat truly affects how we feel, look, think, act, and of course, our health status. As a registered dietitian, I have witnessed dramatic changes in some or all of these areas in everyone I know who has changed to the Perfect Whole Foods Diet (PWFD) as described in my book, *The Healing Power of Whole Foods*. I can honestly say that I have never known anyone who has followed the diet in detail to be disappointed with the results.

—*Beth Loiselle, R.D., L.D. [Registered Dietitian, Licensed Dietitian], Nicholasville, KY*

I ask about diet and patterns of eating with all my patients and espouse organic foods and encourage all who can to learn to raise some of their own food, even if just in a window box. And if testing indicates they will do better (have more normal cholesterol and blood sugars, etc.) if they follow something more akin to the Atkins diet, I do not hesitate to recommend same.

Exercise is wonderful and keeps us all younger longer. Sports, walking, working out in a gym—whatever fits that individual is appropriate. Just doing a bit every day or a bit more every other day can lift the spirits and decrease the bothersomeness of many symptoms in my patients.

Finally, relaxation techniques, meditation, qi gong, biofeedback training, yoga and massage all have their place, and my patients are exposed to or encouraged to incorporate one or more of them in their personal wellness program. Not only do they stay or get healthier doing these things, but the quality of their life and perhaps the length of their life, too, is positively affected.

I wanted to share with you one more thing that I have done over the years, and that was to open a school of medical massage in Lebanon, Ohio 22 years ago. Our goal was to create a learning environment that encouraged the students to explore their own growth and self-care while they were learning how to help others with massage. This is done in the shamanistic style where we, the faculty, continue in our own growth while modeling and encouraging the continued growth of each student. This has been very rewarding for me and for others associated with the school. Massage is a medical license in Ohio, as you might already know. —*Heather Morgan, M.D., F.A.A.I.M.*
[Fellow of the American Association of Integrative Medicine]
Adjunct faculty at Wright State University School of Medicine
in the Family Practice Department for the past 25+ years
Founding Member of the American Holistic Medical Association (AHMA)
Past President of the American Holistic Medical Institute (AHMI)
Founder of School of Medical Massage in Lebanon, OH; Former member of the Board of
Trustees of the AHMA; Faculty at Sinclair College, Dayton, OH
Co-author of Air Streams; *Still makes house calls*

My inner knowing tells me I will live a healthy life void of disease if I follow your "3LS" health approach. I also know that it was no accident I am learning this holistic approach to healing oneself as I embark on a career in natural healing. A big incentive for me to naturally and holistically attain and maintain wellness is to be the example for my future clients who are looking to do the same. Thank you, Jan and Walt, for the leg-up on my journey to wellness and my new career in natural healing.

—*Julia M. Schloesser, Licensed Massage Therapist, Colorado Springs, CO*

■
■
■

Quick References for the Perfect Whole Foods Diet

(excerpted and updated from *The Healing Power of Whole Foods* by Beth Loiselle, R.D., L.D.)

Use these convenient guides to help you determine which foods, ingredients, and additives you may use on the Perfect Whole Foods Diet. Although I have not attempted to investigate all foods, the list is complete enough so that you'll be able to make decisions concerning foods not included.

If you're looking for a specific item in question, refer to either the Quick Reference for Foods or the Quick Reference for Additives. In general, foods containing additives should be consumed less often than those without additives.

My decisions for determining what is acceptable and what is not are based on the guidelines of the Perfect Whole Foods Diet as listed below.

Totally Eliminate	**Avoid**
All sugars	Excessive fat
All refined complex carbohydrates	Hydrogenated fats including margarine
All alcohol	
All fruit—for a while	Refined oils
All dried fruit and fruit juice	Most canned foods
All caffeine	Dry cereals
	Most additives
	Tap water

Totally Eliminate means that you should not eat these while on the perfect diet.

Avoid means that you should try to refrain from using them or use them only in very small amounts.

Occasionally a food or additive is derived from sugar, starch, or alcohol but has been changed chemically and is no longer a sugar, starch, or alcohol. In this case, the resulting food or additive may be used on the perfect diet. For example, the refined sugar in apple juice (the fruit sugar became refined when the fiber was removed in the juicing process) is converted into an acid when apple cider vinegar is produced. Vinegar is, therefore, appropriate for the Perfect Whole Foods Diet since it is not a source of refined carbohydrates.

Explanation of quick references

Yes: You may use this item on the Perfect Whole Foods Diet.

No: Totally eliminate this item while on Perfect Whole Foods.

Avoid: Use occasionally, only if absolutely necessary. These foods will not interfere with the Perfect Whole Foods Diet but should not be used regularly for one reason or other. In most cases, they include an ingredient that is not health-promoting. In small amounts occasionally, they should not be a problem. But regular use is not wise.

Maybe (1): Before using this product, determine what is in it by very carefully reading the ingredient list, and in a few cases you may need to find out from the manufacturer how an ingredient is made. For example, natural lemon flavor might be lemon juice, lemon peel, or lemon oil. Only the manufacturer knows which it is when the term *natural lemon flavor* is used on the ingredient list.

Maybe (2): Not if you are avoiding fruit.

Maybe (3): This item may contain trace amounts of refined carbohydrates, which causes some people to react, while other people can tolerate it well. If you notice adverse reactions from its use, then avoid while on the Perfect Whole Foods Diet.

QUICK REFERENCE FOR FOODS

Since there are so many fruits and vegetables available, it is unlikely that this list will cover them all. If you don't find something listed, you may have it on the perfect diet, as long as it is fresh or frozen with no added sugar or starch. It may be eaten raw or lightly cooked.

Food or Ingredient   Used on Perfect Diet

Acidophilus (bacteria culture as well as others) ....yes
Acorn squash ....yes
Aduki beans, fresh or dried...yes
Agar or agar-agar..yes
Alfalfa sprouts ....yes
All-purpose flour...no
Almond butter ....yes
Almonds, raw or toasted...yes
Aloe vera juice ....yes
Amaranth flour..yes
Amaranth grain...yes
Amasake ....no
Anasazi beans, fresh or dried.......................................yes
Apple, canned ....no
Apple cider ....no
Apple cider vinegar (preferably raw)................maybe (3)
Apple, dried...no
Apple, fresh ....maybe (3)
Apple juice, fresh or canned ....no
Applesauce, canned ....no
Applesauce, homemade ....maybe (2)
Apricot, canned ....no
Apricot, fresh ....maybe (2)
Apricot, dried...no
Arame...yes
Arrowroot...no
Arrowroot flour..no
Arrowroot starch ....no
Artichokes, globe (canned)...no
Artichokes, globe (fresh or frozen) ....yes
Artichokes, Jerusalem ....yes
Artichoke flour, Jerusalem ....yes
Artificial sweeteners, granulated or powdered ....no
Asparagus, canned ....no
Asparagus, fresh..yes
Asparagus, frozen..yes
Avocado, fresh ....yes

Bacon (if sugar is added) ....no
Baking powder...no
Baking soda..yes
Baking yeast...yes
Banana, dried ....no
Banana, fresh..maybe (2)
Balsamic vinegar...maybe (3)
Bancha tea (caffeine)...no
Barley flakes (refined)...no
Barley flour (from pearled barley) ....no
Barley flour (from hulled barley) ....yes
Barley grits (if whole)...yes
Barley, hulled (whole)...yes
Barley malt (sweetener) ....no
Barley, pearled (refined) ....no
Barley, pot (lightly refined)..no
Barley, scotch (lightly refined) ....no
Barley syrup...no
Basmati brown rice..yes
Basmati white rice...no
Basil, fresh or dried...yes
Beans, dried (canned)..no
Beans, dried (cooked or sprouted) ....yes
Beans, green (canned)...no
Beans, green (fresh) ....yes
Beans, green (frozen) ....yes
Bee pollen..maybe (3)

Bee propolis (if no honey is added) ....maybe (3)
Beef, deli-style sliced (sugar)..no
Beef-flavored broth powder (starch) ....no
Beef, fresh or frozen (grass fed is preferable)..............yes
Bell pepper ....yes
Beer ....no
Beer, non-alcoholic..no
Beet, canned ....no
Beet, fresh..yes
Beet sugar..no
Black beans, canned ....no
Black beans, dried (cooked or sprouted) ....yes
Black olives...maybe (3)
Black tea (caffeine) ....no
Blackstrap molasses ....no
Blackstrap molasses, fermented ....no
Bleached wheat flour ....no
Blue corn (if whole grain)..yes
Blue corn, treated with lime, lye,
   or wood ash (if whole grain) ....yes
Blueberry, canned ....no
Blueberry, fresh ....maybe (2)
Blueberry, frozen...maybe (2)
Bologna ....no
Bolted cornmeal (refined)..no
Bouillon cubes (sugar) ....no
Bran (wheat, corn, oat, or rice).....................................yes
Bread crumbs (refined) ....no
Bread, 100% whole grain, unsweetened ....yes
Bread, sourdough, 100% whole grain, unsweetened ..yes
Brewer's yeast ....yes
Broccoli, fresh..yes
Broccoli, frozen (plain, no sauce) ....yes
Broth powders (contains starch or sugar) ....no
Brown rice ....yes
Brown rice, partially milled ....no
Brown rice syrup ....no
Brown sugar ....no
Brussels sprouts, fresh ....yes
Brussels sprouts, frozen..yes
Buckwheat..yes
Buckwheat flour ....yes
Buckwheat groats ....yes
Bulgur ....yes
Bulgur wheat..yes
Butter Buds..no
Butter, salted ....yes
Butter, unsalted or sweet ....yes
Buttermilk, commercial..maybe (1)
Buttermilk, homemade ....yes
Buttermilk powder (added whey) ....no

Cabbage, fresh ....yes
Cake flour ....no
Cane juice, granulated ....no
Cane sugar...no
Candy, sugar-free (contains sorbitol) ....no
Canola oil, expeller-pressed ....yes
Cantaloupe, fresh..maybe (2)
Capers, canned ....yes
Caramel ....no
Caramel coloring..no
Caramel flavoring ....no
Carob candy..no
Carob candy, unsweetened (contains malt) ....no
Carob chips, unsweetened (contains malt) ....no

Carob flour ....yes
Carob powder ....yes
Carrot, canned ....no
Carrot, fresh ....yes
Carrot juice, fresh (1 cup only per day) ....yes
Carrot juice, canned ....no
Cashew butter ....yes
Cashews, raw or toasted ....yes
Cauliflower, fresh or frozen ....yes
Celery, fresh ....yes
Chamomile tea ....yes
Chapattis, 100% whole wheat (if no baking powder
    or sweetener added) ....yes
Cheese, natural ....yes
Cheese, low-fat ....maybe (1)
Cheese, shredded artificial (contains starch) ....no
Cherries, canned ....no
Cherries, dried ....no
Cherries, fresh ....maybe (2)
Chestnuts, water, canned ....yes
Chewing gum ....no
Chewing gum, sugar-free (contains "ol" ingredients) .no
Chicken-flavored broth powder (contains starch) ....no
Chicken, fresh or frozen ....yes
Chicken eggs, preferably farm, not factory ....yes
Chicory ....yes
Chickpeas, canned ....no
Chickpeas, dried (cooked or sprouted) ....yes
Chickpea or garbanzo flour ....yes
Chile peppers, dried ....yes
Chocolate ....no
Chocolate chips ....no
Cider ....no
Cocoa ....no
Coconut (sweetened) ....no
Coconut, dried ....no
Coconut, fresh (unsweetened) ....maybe (2)
Coconut milk (fresh) ....maybe (2)
Coconut oil (non-hydrogenated) ....yes
Coffee (contains caffeine) ....no
Communion bread or wafers ....no
Confectioner's sugar ....no
Converted rice ....no
Corn, canned ....no
Corn chips, whole grain baked—
    (check ingredients) ....maybe (1)
Corn chips, whole grain, no hydrogenated oil,
    sugar, or starch added ....yes
Corn, cracked & degerminated ....no
Corn flour (refined) ....no
Corn, fresh ....yes
Corn, frozen (whole kernel, not cream-style) ....yes
Corn fructose ....no
Corn oil, expeller-pressed ....avoid
Corn oil, refined ....avoid
Corn oil, unrefined ....yes
Corn pasta (refined) ....no
Corn sugar ....no
Corn sweetener ....no
Corn syrup (sugar) ....no
Corn tortillas (if whole grain) ....yes
Corn, treated with lime, lye,
    or wood ash (if whole grain) ....yes
Cornmeal (check with manufacturer) ....maybe (1)
Cornmeal, bolted (refined) ....no
Cornmeal, degerminated (refined) ....no

Cornmeal, enriched ....no
Cornmeal, stone ground (only if whole grain) ....yes
Cornmeal, unbolted (only if germ is present) ....yes
Cornmeal, whole grain ....yes
Cornstarch ....no
Cottage cheese ....maybe (1)
Couscous (most is refined) ....no
Couscous, whole wheat ....yes
Cracked wheat ....yes
Cranberry juice ....no
Cranberries, canned ....no
Cranberries, fresh ....maybe (2)
Cranberries, frozen (if sugar-free) ....maybe (2)
Cream, whipping, half & half ....yes
Cream of tartar ....yes
Cucumbers ....yes
Currants, dried ....no

Dark rye flour (whole grain) ....yes
Date sugar ....no
Dates, dried ....no
Dates, fresh ....maybe (2)
Decaffeinated coffee ....no
Decaffeinated tea ....no
Degerminated corn ....no
Demerar sugar ....no
Dextrin ....no
Dextran ....no
Dextrose (sugar) ....no
Diastatic malt, homemade
    (sprouted, dried, & ground grain) ....yes
Diastatic malt, most commercial ....no
Diet soft drinks, decaffeinated .... avoid/maybe (1)
Dried beans, canned ....no
Dried beans, cooked ....yes
Dried beans, sprouted & cooked ....yes
Dried fruit ....no
Durum ....no
Durum flour ....no
Durum pasta ....no
Durum, whole ....yes

Egg white powder (if no other ingredients) ....yes
Eggs, preferably farm, not factory ....yes
Enriched cornmeal (denotes refined) ....no
Enriched flour (refined) ....no
Enriched pasta ....no
Enriched rice ....no

Farina (refined wheat) ....no
Fish, fresh ....yes
Fish, frozen (no breading) ....yes
Fish oil ....yes
Flax seeds ....yes
Flaxseed oil ....yes
Flour (denotes refined) ....no
Fortified grain ....no
FOS (fructo-oligosaccharides) ....no
Fructose ....no
Fruit, canned ....no
Fruit, cooked from fresh ....maybe (2)
Fruit, dried ....no
Fruit, fresh or frozen (unsweetened) ....maybe (2)
Fruit juice concentrate ....no
Fruit juice, fresh or canned ....no
Fruit sugar ....no

Galactose .... no
Garbanzo beans, dried .... yes
Garbanzo or chickpea flour .... yes
Garlic, fresh .... yes
Garlic oil .... yes
Garlic powdered or granulated .... yes
Garlic salt (powder is preferred) .... yes
Gelatin .... yes
Germinated barley .... yes
Glaze, food (if sugar or starch) .... no
Glue on envelopes & stamps .... no
Gluten (contains some starch) .... no
Gluten flour (contains some starch) .... no
Glycerin .... maybe (3)
Granulated artificial sweeteners
    (contain sugars) .... no
Granulated cane juice .... no
Granulated garlic .... yes
Granulated onion .... yes
Granulated rice .... no
Grapes, canned .... no
Grapes, fresh .... maybe (2)
Grape juice .... no
Grape sugar .... no
Grape sweetener .... no
Grapefruit, fresh .... maybe (2)
Green olives .... yes
Green tea (contains caffeine) .... no
Green tea, decaffeinated (caffeine in trace amount) ..no
Greens, fresh or frozen .... yes
Grits, corn, most commercial (if refined) .... no
Grits, corn, whole grain .... yes
Grits, wheat .... no
Grits, whole wheat .... yes
Ground beef (grass fed is preferred) .... yes

Ham (contains sugar or honey) .... no
Hard whole wheat berries .... yes
Hard whole wheat flour .... yes
Herb tea, caffeine-free (read ingredient list to avoid
    those with malt or other sweeteners) .... maybe (1)
Herb blends (read ingredient list) .... maybe (1)
Herbs, fresh or dried .... yes
High-fructose corn syrup .... no
High gluten flour .... no
Hominy (refined) .... no
Hominy grits (refined) .... no
Hominy, whole (refined) .... no
Honey .... no
Honey, raw .... no
Hulled barley .... yes
Hulled oats (hull is not edible) .... yes
Hydrolyzed cereal solids .... no
Hydrogenated starch hydrolysate (sweetener) .... no

Instant brown rice .... yes
Instant rice (refined) .... no
Instantized flour .... no
Invert sugar .... no

Jam, no sugar added (made with juice) .... no
Jelly, no sugar added (made with juice) .... no
Job's tears .... yes

Kale, canned .... no
Kale, fresh .... yes

Kale, frozen .... yes
Kamut flour (whole grain) .... yes
Kamut whole grain .... yes
Kanten .... yes
Kefir, flavored .... no
Kefir, plain (check ingredients) .... maybe (1)
Kelp .... yes
Koji .... maybe (3)
Kombu .... yes
Kraut .... maybe (3)
Kudzu (starch) .... no
Kukicha tea (caffeine) .... no
Kuzu (starch) .... no

Lamb .... yes
Lactose (as an added ingredient) .... no
Lactose (only as naturally present
    in dairy products) .... yes
Lecithin, liquid .... yes
Lecithin, granules .... yes
Leeks, fresh .... yes
Legumes, all dried .... yes
Lemon flavor .... maybe (1)
Lemon, fresh (only if pulp is included) ...... maybe (2)
Lemon juice, canned in bottle .... no
Lemon juice, fresh or frozen .... no
Lemon oil (read ingredient list) .... maybe (1)
Lemon peel, dried or fresh .... yes
Lemon powder (contains added sugar) .... no
Lentils, green or red .... yes
Lettuce .... yes
Lime, fresh (pulp included) .... maybe (2)
Lime juice, canned .... no
Lime juice, fresh .... no
Lime oil (read ingredient list) .... maybe (1)
Lime peel .... yes
Lime, used to treat corn (not a fruit) .... yes
Light rye flour (is refined) .... no
Long grain brown rice .... yes
Long grain rice (is refined) .... no
Luncheon meat .... no

Macaroni (is refined) .... no
Macaroni, enriched .... no
Macaroni, 100% whole grain .... yes
Macaroni, semolina .... no
Malt (unless you know it is pure diastatic malt or
    sprouted grains, dried & ground) .... no
Malt extract .... no
Malted barley syrup .... no
Malted grain syrup .... no
Maltodextrin .... no
Maltol .... no
Maltose .... no
Mango, fresh .... maybe (2)
Mannitol (sweetener) .... no
Maple sugar .... no
Maple syrup .... no
Margarine .... avoid
Masa (refined) .... no
Masa corn flour (refined) .... no
Masa harina (refined) .... no
Mayonnaise, most commercial .... no
Mayonnaise, sugar and starch-free .... maybe (1), (3)
Medium grain brown rice .... yes
Medium grain rice (is refined) .... no

Medium rye flour (is refined) ....no
Melon, fresh or frozen ....maybe (2)
Milk, chocolate ....no
Milk sugar ....no
Milk, whole, 2%, 1%, 1/2%, skim ....yes
Milled corn (is refined) ....no
Miller's bran ....yes
Millet ....yes
Millet flour ....yes
Milo (sorghum grain) ....yes
Mirin (alcohol) ....no
Miso, white (contains refined rice) ....no
Miso, (if made without grains or with
    whole grains) ....maybe (3)
Mixed vegetables, canned ....no
Mixed vegetables, frozen (if no potatoes added) ....yes
Mochi (read ingredient list) ....maybe (1)
Mochi rice flour (sweet brown rice flour) ....yes
Modified food starch ....no
Molasses ....no
Molasses, fermented ....no
Mouthwash (check ingredients carefully
    since most contain alcohol) ....maybe (1)
Mustard (if no sweetener, starch or wine). maybe (1), (3)
Mustard, dried ....yes
Mustard flour ....yes
Mustard powder ....yes
Mustard seeds ....yes

Natural flavor ....maybe (1)
Natural sweetener ....no
Nightingale flour (refined wheat) ....no
Nigari ....yes
Noodles (term denotes refined noodles) ....no
Nonfat milk solids ....yes
Nonstick cooking sprays containing alcohol ....no
Nutritional yeast ....yes
Nut milk (if no sugar or starch added) ....yes
Nuts, fresh, raw ....yes
Nuts, roasted (if no sugar or starch added) ....yes

Oat bran ....yes
Oat flour (if bran is removed) ....no
Oat flour (if whole) ....yes
Oat groats ....yes
Oats, hulled ....yes
Oatmeal, instant, containing sugar,
    starch or dried fruit ....no
Oatmeal, quick ....yes
Oats, rolled ....yes
Oats, steel cut ....yes
"ol," words ending in (are sugars or alcohols) ....yes
Olives, black and green ....yes
Oolong tea ....no
Orange flavor (if pure oil or peel, not juice) ....maybe (1)
Orange, fresh ....maybe (2)
Orange juice ....no
Orange oil (read ingredients) ....yes
Orange peel ....yes
Orange Pekoe tea ....no
Orange powder (contains sugar) ....no
Oregano, fresh or dried ....yes
Orzo (refined rice-shaped pasta) ....no
"ose," words ending in (except for cellulose) ....no

Palm kernel oil ....yes

Palm shortening ....yes
Pancakes, commercial ....no
Pancakes, homemade, allowed ingredients ....yes
Panocha (flour from sprouted wheat) ....yes
Paprika ....yes
Parboiled rice ....no
Partially hydrogenated oil ....avoid
Partially milled brown rice ....no
Partially polished brown rice ....no
Pasta (term denotes that it is refined) ....no
Pasta, 100% whole grain ....yes
Pastry flour ....no
Patent flour ....no
Peach, canned ....no
Peach, dried ....no
Peach, fresh ....maybe (2)
Peach, frozen unsweetened ....maybe (2)
Peanut butter, most commercial brands ....no
Peanut butter, natural style, no sugar added ....yes
Peanuts (with no sugar or starch added) ....yes
Pearled barley ....no
Pearled wheat ....no
Peas, split & dried ....yes
Pecan meal ....yes
Pecans ....yes
Pectin (fiber) ....yes
Peeled potatoes ....no
Pentose ....no
Peppercorns ....yes
Peppermint oil (flavoring) ....yes
Peppers, fresh, assorted kinds ....yes
Peppers, dried ....yes
Pickles, dill or sour (if no sugar added) ....maybe (3)
Pickles, sweet ....no
Pimento ....yes
Pineapple, canned ....no
Pineapple, dried (with or without added sugar) ....no
Pineapple, fresh ....maybe (2)
Pineapple juice, fresh or canned ....no
Plum, fresh ....maybe (2)
Poi (from starchy taro root) ....no
Polished rice ....no
Polydextrose ....no
Popcorn, commercial ....no
Popcorn, home popped with allowed ingredients ......yes
Pork, cured (if sugar is an ingredient) ....no
Pork, fresh ....yes
Pot barley (lightly refined) ....no
Potato chips ....no
Potato, dried (peeled) ....no
Potato flour ....no
Potato, mashed (if peeled) ....no
Potato, mashed (if not peeled) ....yes
Potato, peeled ....no
Potato, small and with skin ....yes
Potato starch ....no
Potato, sweet (peeled) ....no
Potato, sweet (with skin) ....yes
Powdered sugar ....no
Processed cornmeal ....no
Protein powder, rice (contains trace of starch) ....no
Protein powder, soy (if no refined ingredient added) .yes
Protein powder, whey (contains trace lactose) ....no
Prune (dried plum) ....no
Prune juice ....no
Psyllium seeds & their husks ....yes

Puffed cereal, refined grains ....no
Puffed cereal, whole grain ....avoid
Pumpkin, canned..no
Pumpkin, fresh cooked ....yes

Quinoa flour...yes
Quinoa grain..yes
Quinoa pasta (contains partially refined corn)............no

Raisins ....no
Raw honey ....no
Raw sugar ....no
Reduced lactose whey ....no
Refined sugar ....no
Ribitol...no
Rice (term for refined rice)..no
Rice, Basmati, brown...yes
Rice, Basmati, white ....no
Rice, brown, short, medium, or long grain..................yes
Rice, brown, partially milled...no
Rice cakes with degerminated corn ....no
Rice cakes without refined grains such as
    Degerminated corn added ....avoid
Rice flour (is refined) ....no
Rice flour, brown ....yes
Rice, long grain ....no
Rice pasta (if 100% whole grain) ....yes
Rice syrup ....no
Rice, white ....no
Rice, white Basmati..no
Rice, wild, pure...yes
Rice, wild, blend of white & wild rice,
    labeled wild rice ....no
Roast beef (cooked at home, not from deli) ....yes
Roasted malt ....no
Rolled oats ....yes
Rose hips..yes
Rusk flour (refined) ....no
Rye (term for refined rye)...no
Rye berries (whole grain) ....yes
Rye flour (term for refined rye flour) ....no
Rye flour, dark (if whole grain) ....yes
Rye flour, light (refined) ....no
Rye flour, medium (partially refined) ....no
Rye flour, pumpernickel..yes
Rye flour, sifted (refined) ....no
Rye flour, stone ground ....yes
Rye flour, whole or whole grain ....yes
Rye, light (refined) ....no
Rye meal (refined) ....no
Rye meal, whole..yes
Rye, sprouted ....yes
Rye, whole grain...yes
Rye, whole ....yes

Saccharin, liquid ....avoid
Saccharin, powdered & tablets .... avoid/maybe (1)
Safflower oil, expeller-pressed ....avoid
Safflower oil, refined ....avoid
Safflower oil, unrefined...yes
Salt, Celtic or Real Salt..yes
Salt, iodized (contains dextrose) ....no
Salt, rock .... maybe (1)
Salt, sea (iodized) ....no
Salt, sea (non-iodized)...yes
Salt, table (if not iodized)..yes

Salt, unrefined mineral ....yes
Salted processed foods with no sugar, starch,
    alcohol, or caffeine (processors use the least
    expensive, non-iodized salt) ....yes
Samp (coarse hominy grits) ....no
Sausage containing sugar or starch ....no
Scotch barley (lightly refined)..no
Sea vegetables..yes
Seitan (contains some starch)..no
Self-rising flour...no
Semolina (refined flour used in pasta)..........................no
Semolina flour ....no
Sesame butter ....yes
Sesame oil, refined ....avoid
Sesame oil, unrefined ....yes
Sesame seeds, hulled ....yes
Sesame seeds, whole...yes
Sesame tahini ....yes
Shortening...avoid
Shoyu soy sauce (if no wheat or
    alcohol added)..maybe (3)
Shrimp, no breading...yes
Sifted rye flour (refined) ....no
Sifted whole rye flour (refined) ....no
Soba (only if 100% buckwheat) ....yes
Soft whole wheat berries ....yes
Soft whole wheat flour ....yes
Sorbo (sweetener) ....no
Sorbitol (sweetener)..no
Sorghum (sweetener) ....no
Sorghum, whole grain ....yes
Soup, canned...no
Soup, homemade with allowed ingredients ....yes
Soup, dehydrated mix with allow ingredients.............yes
Soy milk, with sweetener added ....no
Soy milk powder ....yes
Soy oil, refined...avoid
Soy protein isolate (check ingredient list) ....yes
Soy protein powder (check ingredient list) ....yes
Soy sauce powder (contains dextrin) ....no
Spaghetti (refined grain)...no
Spaghetti sauce, most commercial brands ....no
Spaghetti sauce, no sugar or starch added...................yes
Spaghetti, whole wheat ....yes
Spelt berries ....yes
Spelt flakes ....yes
Spelt flour ....no
Spelt flour, whole...yes
Spelt pasta (if from whole spelt flour) ....yes
Spelt, whole grain...yes
Spices, pure (ingredient lists must name them
    specifically, not just say "spices"............................yes
Spinach, canned..no
Spinach, fresh or frozen ....yes
Split peas, dried ....yes
Squash, fresh or frozen..yes
Steel-cut oats ....yes
Stevia product (herbal sweetener),
    check ingredients....................................... maybe (1)
Stevia pure (herbal sweetener) ....yes
Stone ground rye flour (is refined)................................no
Stone ground wheat flour (is refined)...........................no
Stone ground whole wheat flour ....yes
Strawberry, fresh...maybe (2)
Strawberry, frozen, no sugar added ....maybe (2)
Sucanat (evaporated cane juice)....................................no

Sugar, any kind ....no
Sugar cane ....no
Sunflower seeds, raw or roasted ....yes
Sweet brown rice (a variety of brown rice) ....yes
Sweetleaf (herbal sweetener, if pure) .... maybe (1)
Syrup ....no

Tahini ....yes
Tamari soy sauce (if no wheat or
   alcohol added) ....maybe (3)
Tap water ....avoid
Tapioca (thickener) ....no
Tapioca grits ....no
Taro root (starch) ....no
Tea, black, green, or white ....no
Tea, pure red Rooibos ....yes
Tea, decaffeinated ....no
Tea, herb with no caffeine (read ingredient
   list carefully to avoid malt and
   dried fruit) ....maybe (1)
Teff ....yes
Teff flour ....yes
Textured vegetable protein (TVP) ....yes
Tofu, fresh ....yes
Tofu, silken ....yes
Tomato juice, canned, for cooking, not drinking ....yes
Tomato juice, fresh ....yes
Tomato paste ....yes
Tomato puree ....yes
Tomato sauce, canned, if no sugar or starch added ....yes
Tomatoes, canned ....yes
Tomatoes, dried ....yes
Tomatoes, fresh ....yes
Tortillas, corn, treated with lime, lye,
   or wood ash (if whole grain) ....yes
Tortillas, corn (if from whole grain corn) ....yes
Triticale flour (if whole grain) ....yes
Triticale kernels (whole grain) ....yes
Tuna, canned in water ....yes
Turbinado sugar ....no
Turkey, deli-style (if it contains sugar or starch) ....no
Turkey, fresh ....yes
Turkey, frozen (if without sugar or starch) ....yes
Turkey, ground ....yes
Turmeric ....yes

Unbleached flour (refined) ....no
Unbleached whole wheat flour ....yes

Vanilla bean ....yes
Vanilla extract, containing alcohol ....no
Vanilla extract, containing glycerin ....maybe (3)
Vanilla flavor ....maybe (1)
Vanilla oleoresin (contains alcohol) ....no
Vegetables, canned, commercial or home canned
   (Tomatoes used in cooking are an exception) ....no
Vegetable food starch ....no
Vegetable shortening ....avoid
Vegetables, most fresh (see potatoes) ....yes
Venison ....yes

Vermicelli (a refined grain) ....no
Vinegar, Balsamic ....maybe (3)
Vinegar, distilled ....avoid
Vinegar, pasteurized .... avoid/maybe (3)
Vinegar, raw cider ....maybe (3)
Vinegar, raw wine ....maybe (3)

Walnuts ....yes
Water chestnuts ....yes
Water, distilled ....yes
Water, purified ....yes
Water, tap ....avoid
Wheat (term for refined product) ....no
Wheat bran ....yes
Wheat, cracked ....yes
Wheat, farina ....no
Wheat flour ....no
Wheat flour, enriched ....no
Wheat germ, defatted ....yes
Wheat germ flour (white flour + wheat germ) ....no
Wheat germ, fresh & refrigerated ....yes
Wheat germ, sold in jar
   (read ingredients) ....maybe (1)
Wheat malt (if sprouted wheat, dried & ground) ....yes
Wheat, pearled ....no
Whey (contains lactose) ....no
Whey protein concentrate (source of lactose) ....no
Whey protein powder (contains lactose) ....no
Whey, reduced lactose ....no
White flour ....no
White sugar ....no
White rice ....no
White rice flour ....no
White rye flour ....no
White spelt flour ....no
White whole wheat berries ....yes
White whole wheat flour ....yes
Whole durum flour ....yes
Whole durum wheat flour ....yes
Whole meal flour ....yes
Whole rye flour ....yes
Whole rye meal ....yes
Whole wheat berries ....yes
Whole wheat pastry flour ....yes
Whole wheat flour ....yes
Wild rice blend with white rice ....no
Wild rice, pure ....yes
Wine ....no
Winter squash ....yes

Xylitol (sweetener) ....no

Yeast, baking ....yes
Yeast, brewer's or nutritional ....yes
Yogurt, fruit-flavored (contains sweetener) ....no
Yogurt, plain (read ingredients to
   avoid starches) ....maybe (1)
Yogurt, vanilla-flavored (contains sugar) ....no

Zest, citrus (peel) ....yes

QUICK REFERENCE FOR ADDITIVES

Since most foods on the Perfect Whole Foods Diet are simple and minimally processed, your intake of additives will automatically be restricted. Although many additives are allowed in the chart that follows, I do not encourage you to use them often. I'm listing them only because I have been asked about many specific additives in the past and want to help you as much as possible with questions I can anticipate.

I would urge you to avoid whenever possible additives such as artificial coloring, artificial flavoring, phosphates, sulfites, MSG, nitrites, nitrates, and aluminum-containing products. These additives are associated with health problems I have mentioned elsewhere in the book.

You may use artificial sweeteners like aspartame (the brand name is NutraSweet) and saccharin but I don't encourage them since most have not been shown to be 100 percent safe. Also, some people continue craving sweets as long as they continue to eat anything sweet-tasting including artificial sweeteners. And finally, there are some who respond to aspartame with such reactions as rashes, headaches, stomachaches, and even seizures. Before using any such products, pay close attention to the ingredient list to avoid those products with added ingredients such as lactose, dextrose, sorbitol, maltodextrin, dextrin, and other ingredients not allowed on the Perfect Diet. Liquid saccharin and tablets are more likely to be acceptable than powdered artificial sweeteners.

The success of the Perfect Diet is not dependent on the total elimination of many additives. If you happen to be sensitive to any, then eliminate them from your diet.

The chemical structure determines whether or not an additive may be included on the Perfect Whole Foods Diet. If an additive is a sugar, starch, alcohol, or caffeine or if an additive contains one of these, that additive should be eliminated from the perfect diet.

Explanation of quick references

Yes: You may use this item on the Perfect Whole Foods Diet.

No: Totally eliminate this item while on Perfect Whole Foods.

Avoid: Use occasionally, if absolutely necessary, but not regularly or in large amounts.

Maybe (1): Before using this product, determine what is in it by very carefully reading the ingredient list, and in a few cases you may need to find out from the manufacturer how an ingredient is made. For example, natural lemon flavor might be lemon juice, lemon peel, or lemon oil. Only the manufacturer knows which it is when the term natural lemon flavor is used on the ingredient list.

Maybe (2): Not if you are avoiding fruit.

Maybe (3): This item may contain trace amounts of refined carbohydrate, which cause some people to react, while other people can tolerate it well. If you notice adverse reactions from its use, then avoid while on the Perfect Whole Foods Diet.

Additive	Used on Perfect Diet
Acacia (gum Arabic)	yes
Acetates	yes
Acetic acid	yes
Acid modified starch	no
Agar-agar (seaweed extract)	yes
Alcohol	no
Alum or kasal (firming agent)	yes
Algin (thickener, from seaweed)	yes
Algin gum	yes
Ammonium salts	yes
Annatto extract (coloring)	yes
Ascorbic acid (nutrition, curing meats)	yes
Artificial color	avoid
Artificial flavor	avoid
Aspartame (if no sugar or starch added)	avoid
Autolyzed yeast (flavoring)	yes
Baking powder (contains starch)	no
Baking soda (leavening)	yes
Barley malt (sweetener)	no
Benzoate of soda	yes
Benzoic acid	yes
Benzoyl peroxide	yes
Beta carotene (coloring, nutrition)	yes
Beet powder	yes
BHA (antioxidant)	yes
BHT (antioxidant)	yes
Bicarbonate of soda (leavening)	yes
Bran (nutrition)	yes
Bromines	yes
Butyl paraben (preservative)	yes
Caffeine	no
Calcium acid phosphate (baking acid)	yes
Calcium bromate (oxidizing agent)	yes
Calcium carbonate	yes
Calcium caseinate (nutrition and flavoring)	yes
Calcium chloride (firming agent)	yes
Calcium citrate	yes
Calcium disodium EDTA	yes
Calcium iodate (oxidizing agent in bread)	yes
Calcium lactate (batter conditioner)	yes
Calcium oxide (acidity regulator)	yes
Calcium peroxide (dough conditioner)	yes
Calcium propionate (preservative)	yes
Calcium salts (firming agent)	yes
Calcium stearoyl-2-lactylate (dough conditioner)	yes
Calcium sulfate (firming agent, conditioner)	yes
Caramel (coloring or flavoring from sugar)	no
Carob bean gum (thickener)	yes
Carotene (color)	yes
Carrageenan (thickener)	yes

Additive	Used on Perfect Diet
Casein (thickener, whitening agent)	yes
Cellulose (fiber)	yes
Cellulose gum (thickener)	yes
Char-smoke flavor	yes
Cinnamaldehyde (flavor)	yes
Citric acid (acidifier)	yes
Corn polysaccharides	no
Cornstarch	no
Cream of tartar	yes
Dextran (sweetener)	no
Dextrin (product of starch)	no
Dicalcium phosphate (dough conditioner)	yes
Diethyl pyrocarbonate	yes
Diglycerides (emulsifier)	yes
Disodium guanylate (flavor enhancer)	yes
Disodium inosinate (flavor enhancer)	yes
EDTA (preservative)	yes
Enzymes	yes
Equal (contains dextrose and maltodextrose)	no
Erythorbic acid (antioxidant)	yes
Essence of fruit (flavor)	yes
Essential oils (flavor)	yes
Ester gum (thickener)	yes
Ethyl alcohol (solvent)	no
Ethyl maltol (flavor enhancer)	no
Ethyl vanillin (contains alcohol)	no
Ethylene dibromide	yes
Ethylene oxide	yes
Ferrous gluconate (coloring, nutrient)	yes
Ferrous sulfate (nutrition)	yes
Fig pep (sweetener made from fig extract)	no
Food glaze	no
Fumaric acid (acid and antioxidant)	yes
Gelatin (jelling agent)	yes
Gelatinized wheat starch (thickener)	no
Gluconolactone (acid)	yes
Gluten (protein of wheat containing starch)	no
Gluten flour (contains starch)	no
Glycerin	maybe (3)
Green tea extract (contains caffeine)	no
Guar gum (fiber thickener)	yes
Gum gluten	no
Gums (arabic, cellulose, ghatti, karaya, tragacanth, xanthan)	yes
Gypsum	yes
Heptyl paraben (preservative)	yes
Hydrochloric acid (acidifier)	yes
Hydrogen peroxide (bleaching agent)	yes

Hydrogenated starch hydrolysates.................................no
Hydrolyzed plant protein or HPP (seasoning).............yes
Hydrolyzed vegetable protein or HVP ....yes
Hydroxylated lecithin (emulsifier) ....yes

Imitation flavoring (if not alcohol-based)...............avoid
Irish moss ....yes
Irish moss extract...yes

Lactic acid (acidifier) ....yes
Lactalbumin (protein from milk) ....yes
Lecithin (emulsifier) ....yes
Lime used to soften corn hull (not a fruit)...................yes
Liquid smoke..yes
Locust bean...yes
Locust bean gum...yes
Lye used to soften corn hull...yes

Magnesium silicate...yes
Magnesium stearate ....yes
Malic acid (acidifier from apples) ....yes
Malt ....no
Malt, diastatic (most commercial brands)...................no
Malt, diastatic (sprouted, dried, & ground grain) ....yes
Malt extract...no
Malt, wheat (if diastatic malt) ....yes
Maltodextrin...no
Maltol ....no
Menthol ....no
Methyl paraben (preservative) ....yes
Milk serum (contains lactose) ....no
Modified food starch (thickener) ....no
Modified starch ....no
Monocalcium phosphate (dough conditioner) ....yes
Monoglycerides (emulsifier) ....yes
Monosodium glutamate or MSG (flavor enhancer) ....yes
Monostearate..yes

Natural flavor...maybe (1)
Natural smoke flavors (flavoring) ....yes
Niacin (enrichment) ....yes
Nigari ....yes
Nitrates ....yes
Nitrites...yes
NutraSweet .... avoid/maybe (1)
Nutritional yeast ....yes

Oleic acid ....yes
Oleoresin paprika (coloring) ....yes
Oleoresin turmeric (coloring) ....yes
Orange powder (contains sugar) ....no
Oxystearin (prevents fat crystallization) ....yes

Palmitic acid ....yes
Papain (enzyme) ....yes
Paprika...yes
Pectin (fiber which sets fruit jelly)...............................yes
Peppermint oil (flavor) ....yes
Phosphoric acid (acidifier)..yes
Polysorbate 60, 65, 80 (emulsifier) ....yes
Potassium alum (firming agent) ....yes
Potassium bicarbonate (leavening) ....yes
Potassium bromate (oxidizing agent) ....yes
Potassium citrate (acidity control) ....yes
Potassium iodate (oxidizing agent) ....yes
Potassium sorbate (preservative) ....yes

Potassium sulfite (preservative) ....yes
Propyl gallate (antioxidant)...yes
Propyl paraben (preservative) ....yes

Propylene glycol (flavor solvent)..................................yes
Propylene glycol alginate (thickener) ....yes
Propylene glycol monostearate......................................yes
Propylene oxide...yes

Quinine (flavoring) ....yes

Reduced iron (nutrition) ....yes
Rennet (enzyme that causes milk curdling)................yes
Rennin (enzyme that causes milk curdling) ....yes
Riboflavin (nutrition) ....yes
Rye-sour flavor..no

Saccharin, liquid...avoid
Saccharin, tablets or powder.....................................avoid
Salicylic acid ....yes
Salt (if not iodized)..yes
Salt, Celtic or Real Salt..yes
Salt, iodized ....no
Salt, mineral..yes
Saltpeter (curing agent) ....yes
Sea salt, iodized ....no
Silicon dioxide (anticaking agent)...............................yes
Smoke flavoring...yes
Smoked yeast ....yes
Sodium alginate (thickener)..yes
Sodium aluminum phosphate (leavening)...................yes
Sodium ascorbate (nutrition, curing of meats) ....yes
Sodium benzoate (preservative)....................................yes
Sodium bicarbonate (leavening) ....yes
Sodium bisulfite (preservative) ....yes
Sodium carboxymethyl cellulose (thickener) ....yes
Sodium caseinate (thickener, whitening agent)..........yes
Sodium citrate (controls acidity)..................................yes
Sodium chloride (table salt) ....yes
Sodium chloride, if iodized ....no
Sodium diacetate (preservative)...................................yes
Sodium erythorbate (curing agent)..............................yes
Sodium hexametaphosphate (texture modifier).........yes
Sodium metabisulfite (preservative) ....yes
Sodium nitrate (curing agent)......................................yes
Sodium nitrite (curing agent) ....yes
Sodium phosphate (consistency regulator).................yes
Sodium propionate (preservative) ....yes
Sodium pyrophosphate
    (firms meat when water is added) ....yes
Sodium saccharin...avoid
Sodium stearoyl-2-lactylate (dough conditioner).......yes
Sodium sulfite, sodium bisulfite...................................yes
Sorbic acid (mold inhibitor) ....yes
Sorbitol (sweetener)...no
Soy lecithin ....yes
Soy-protein concentrate (seasoning)...........................yes
Soy protein isolate (check ingredient list) .... maybe (1)
Splenda Sugar Blend (contains sugar) ....no
Splenda Sweetener (contains dextrose
    & maltodextrin)..no
Starch ....no
Stearic acid..yes
Stevia, herbal sweeteners
    (check ingredient list) ....maybe (1)
Sucanat (granulated cane juice) ....no

Succinic acid..yes
Sucrose (sugar) ....no
Sugar, any kind ....no
Sulfur dioxide (preservative) ....yes
Sweetleaf (herbal sweetener) ....maybe (1)
Sweet One packet (artificial sweetener
    contains dextrose) ....no
Sweet'n Low (contains dextrose).................................no

Talc (filler in tablets and capsules)..............................yes
Tannin (tannic acid)...yes
Tapioca (thickener)...no
Tartaric acid (baking acid, from grapes) ....yes
TBHQ or tertiary butylhydroquinone (antioxidant) ..yes
Textured vegetable protein (TVP)................................yes
Thiamine/mononitrate (nutrition)..............................yes
Titanium dioxide (coloring) ....yes
Torula yeast..yes
Tricalcium phosphate (prevents lumping) ....yes
Turmeric (coloring) ....yes

Ultramarine blue (coloring)..yes
Unmodified starch..no

Vanilla bean ....yes
Vanilla extract, with alcohol ....no
Vanilla extract, with glycerine ....maybe (3)
Vitamin C (if tablets are sugar and starch-free) ....yes

Whey (milk component, includes lactose)...................no
Whey protein concentrate (includes lactose) ....no

Xanthan gum (thickener) ....yes
Xylitol ....no
Xylose (wood sugar) ....no

Yeast, baker's (leavening) ....yes
Yeast, brewer's or nutritional (nutrition) ....yes
Yeast, torula ....yes

Preface

1. Jan DeCourtney has two certifications in massage therapy. One is from the Boulder College of Massage Therapy and the other is from the National Certification Board for Massage Therapists and Bodyworkers (NCBMTB).

Chapter 1: How to be Healthy

1. Walt: This is a generous estimate. I was taught 40 years ago in medical school that 95% of health problems will get better on their own unless our allopathic treatment makes them worse. Since then, I have read this information in many sources as being around 90%. The national statistics provided by the Family Practice organization says the same: 90% of conditions seen in the Family Practice office will get well on their own. Even in Hippocrates' time, this understanding that treatment can worsen conditions was the basis for the first tenet of the Hippocratic Oath: "First, do no harm."

2. Functional Medicine Update, 1980-2003. This was specifically discussed in the January, 2000 edition with references from:
U.A. Meyer, Pharmagenetics and adverse drug reactions. *Lancet.* 2000; 356 (9242): 1667-1671.
C.K. Lee, R.G. Klopp, R. Weindruch, T.A. Prolla. Gene expression profile of aging and its retardation by caloric restriction. *Science.* 1999; 285: 1390-1393.
J.J. Ramsey, M.E. Harper, R. Weindruch. Restriction of energy intake, energy expenditure, and aging. *Free Radical Biology & Medicine.* 2000; 29(10): 946-968.
And in the March 2001 edition from:
J.F. Fries. Aging, natural death, and the compression of morbidity. *New England Journal of Medicine.* 1980; 303: 130-135.
A.J. Vita, R.B. Terry, H.B. Hubert, J.F. Fries. Aging, health risks, and cumulative disability. *New England Journal of Medicine.* 1998; 338: 1035-1041.
For a discussion of the differences between genome and phenome, see Richard Lewontin, "The Genotype/Phenotype Distinction," *The Stanford Encyclopedia of Philosophy (Spring 2004 Edition)*, Edward N. Zalta (ed.), http://plato.stanford.edu/archives/spr2004/entries/genotype-phenotype (accessed August 21, 2005).

Chapter 2: Skilled Relaxation

1. For more information, see *The Stress of Life*, by Hans Selye (McGraw Hill, second edition 1978); *Mind as Healer, Mind as Slayer*, by Kenneth R. Pelletier (Delta, 1977); and *90 Days to Self-Health*, by C. Norman Shealy, M.D. (Dial Press, 1977), pages 2-12. Selye did the basic

research, and his book is considered to be a classic work in the field of stress research. Others came later and added to his knowledge, but it can all be understood in terms of Selye's basic research and model. See also http://www.majon.com/articles/New_Age/stress_management_new_age_104.html. (accessed February 25, 2006).

2. Here is a reference for learning more about how the stress effect may be stored—*Functional Medicine Update*, August 2003, from:

   K.B. Schmaling, D.H. Lewis, J.I. Friedelak, R. Mahurin, D.S. Buchwald. Single-photon emission computerized tomography and neurocognitive function in patients with chronic fatigue syndrome. *Psychosomatic Medicine*. 2003; 65(1):129-136.

   D.J. Torpy, D.A. Papanicolaou, A.J. Lotsikas, R.L. Wilder, G.P. Chrousos, S.R. Pillemer. Responses of the sympathetic nervous system and the hypothalamus-pituitary-adrenal axis to interleukin-6. *Arthritis & Rheumatism*. 2000; 43(4): 872-880.

3. Hans Selye, *The Stress of Life*, Chapters 5, 6, and 7; and Kenneth Pelletier, *Mind as Healer, Mind as Slayer*. See also *Sound Mind, Sound Body*, by Kenneth Pelletier (Simon & Schuster, 1994), pages 84-86.

4. Walt: The standard percentage was taught to us in medical school 40-plus years ago. At that time, the percentage was considered 85% and the curve showed that the percent was increasing every year. I am assuming that it is far past 90% by now. The one thing certain is that it will continue to increase with our current medical model. This is common knowledge in the profession. Some references to this information can be found in: *Mind as Healer, Mind as Slayer*, by Kenneth Pelletier, page 7, and *Prescription for Nutritional Healing*, by James F. Balch and Phyllis A. Balch (Avery, 1997), page 496.

5. The term "bracing" has been implemented by Dr. Walt Stoll to describe chronic full-body muscle tension. In other literature, the phenomenon is also referred to as armoring, engrams, or chronic full-body muscle tension. For more information about bracing, read *Mind as Healer, Mind as Slayer*, pages 4, 17-18, 93, 122, 270, 271.

6. Walt remembers reading this statistic in medical journals many years ago. There are hundreds of references to Leaky Gut Syndrome, including: *Optimal Digestion*, edited by Trent Nichols, M.D. (Avon, 1999).

   Also F. Guarner, J.R. Malagelada. Gut flora in health and disease. *Lancet*. 2003; 360: 512-519; X Hebuterne. Gut changes attributed to aging: effects on intestinal microflora. *Current Opinion in Clinical Nutrition & Metabolic Care*. 2003; 6:49-54; and J.A. Spanier, C.W. Howden, M.P. Jones. A systematic review of alternative therapies in the irritable bowel syndrome. *Archives of Internal Medicine*. 2003; 163(3):265-274.

7. *Mind as Healer, Mind as Slayer*, pages 197 and 207, and Herbert Benson, *The Relaxation Response*.

8. *Mind as Healer, Mind as Slayer*, pages 198-199 and 289-290, and *The Relaxation Response* (Avon, Reissue edition 1990).

9. This list has been compiled through Dr. Walt Stoll's professional and personal experiences.

10. Walt: Some of my most effective Skilled Relaxation was done with eyes open, although that was not the case when I was just learning. But soon I was able to get up and walk around while in this state. I could see and hear more clearly. Colors were brighter and sounds were clearer. Sometimes people's energetic qualities became visible. At first this effect only lasted a few minutes after my Skilled Relaxation session was over, but the duration gradually lasted longer until it was all the time.

    I found I had the time because I only needed a couple of hours to lie down to rest my body. I never actually went to sleep. This went on for years. My entire life was spent in the alpha rhythm, and I felt better than I had ever felt in my life.

    There were many gradual effects that I received from doing Skilled Relaxation, but they would not necessarily be what anyone else would notice. Now, I have no serious conditions amenable to conventional diagnostics, and I attribute much of that to following the 3LS for 15 years.

Chapter 3: The Whole Foods Diet

1. List compiled from the clinical experience of Dr. Walt Stoll and from *The Healing Power of Whole Foods*, by Beth Loiselle, R.D., L.D. (Healthways Nutrition, 1993), page 384.

2. For information about refined foods, diet, and nutrition see: *Food for Nought: The Decline in Nutrition*, by Ross Hume Hall (Vintage Books, 1976); *Human Life Styling: Keeping Whole in the 20th Century*, by John C. McCamy, M.D., and James Presley (Harper Colophon, 1977); *How You Can Beat the Killer Diseases*, by Harold W. Harper, M.D., and Michael L. Culbert

(Arlington House, 1978); and *Staying Healthy with Nutrition,* by Elson M. Haas, M.D. (Celestial Arts, 1992), pages 375-376. Also just note the large percentage of refined and processed food in the typical grocery store.

3. E. Cheraskin and W.M. Ringsdorf. *American Laboratory.* 1974; 6: 31.

4. This may have been published in the USDA literature in the late 1800s. An interesting article describing research in the 1800s may be found at http://4optimallife.com/ Dangers-Of-SUGAR-To-Your-MENTAL-HEALTH.html (accessed February 25, 2006), which references McCollum, Elmer Verner, *A History of Nutrition: The Sequence of Ideas in Nutritional Investigation,* Houghton Mifflin Co., Boston, 1957, p. 87 and 88.

5. Gleaned through Dr. Walt Stoll's personal and professional experience. See also *Orthomolecular Nutrition: New Lifestyle for Super Good Health,* by Abram Hoffer, Ph.D., M.D., and Morton Walker, D.P.M. (Keats, 1978), page 78; and *Fighting Depression,* by H. Ross (Larchmont Books, 1975).

6. Walt: People with food allergies (sometimes called food hypersensitivities) tend to crave and eat the very foods to which they are allergic. It is interesting that this is similar to what happens in an addiction. Addicts always crave their addictive substance. So is a habit of eating refined carbohydrates an addiction or an allergy? One day perhaps researchers will discover that allergy and addition are two properties of one phenomenon, just like researchers in physics finally defined the properties of light as including the characteristics of both particles and waves rather than insisting upon an either/or situation.

   At present, what we can say is refined carbohydrates cause both an immune system problem *and* an addiction. This description explains the observed phenomena that occur during the initial months of following a Perfect Whole Foods Diet and is what we have to work with until a better explanation comes along.

   Some experts suggest that these reactions originate from a genetic trait or a hypoglycemic response (see note 5). Another theory postulates that the ratio between micronutrients needed for the Krebs cycle and calories eaten causes the allergic/ withdrawal reaction. Refined carbohydrates have low micronutrients and high calories, and this greatly imbalanced ratio might cause the reactions.

   At this time, all we have are theories about how and why the allergic/withdrawal response happens. Even if we were to list all of the theories and possibilities for the cause of these reactions, it is likely that within the year (or at least within the next five years), they will become outdated. Research moves that quickly in the medical world.

7. The ratio of fructose (fruit sugar) to the micronutrients in fruit is so great that a person with an already damaged Krebs cycle responds to the fruit as pure fructose (pure sugar). Any food containing a substance that ends with –ol or –ose reacts the same with the Krebs cycle. In contrast, whole milk, although it contains naturally occurring lactose (remember on the list that anything ending in –ose is a sugar), is much more slowly absorbed, and the protein, fat and micronutrients necessary to run the lactose through the Krebs cycle are sufficient to prevent an allergic/addiction response in nearly all people (unless you have a food allergy or sensitivity to it).

8. See Note 6 for Chapter 2.

9. Although the terms food hypersensitivity, food allergy, and food intolerance are sometimes used interchangeably, the term "allergy" is typically used in medicine to refer to reactions to an environmental antigen or to drugs. In this book, we use the terms "hypersensitivity" or "allergy" interchangeably, since certainly foods are environmental antigens. The vast majority of hypersensitivities are due to the leakage of Leaky Gut Syndrome, whereas traditional allergies are mostly serum of unknown cause.

Chapter 4: The Right Exercise for You

1. *Aerobics,* by Kenneth Cooper, M.D. (Bantam, 1988); *The Wellness Guide to Lifelong Fitness,* by Timothy P. White, Ph.D. (Rebus, 1993), pages 19-25; and *IFA Fitness Manual,* by Chuck Krautblatt, International Fitness Association, http://ifafitness.com/book1/index.html (accessed August 22, 2005). See also *Healing Moves: How to Cure, Relieve, and Prevent Common Ailments with Exercise,* by Carol Krucoff and Mitchell Krucoff, M.D. (Harmony Books, 2000), pages 18-19; and *Saving Your Brain,* by Jeff Victoroff, M.D. (Bantam, 2002), pages 344-347.

2. *Fitness Training Manual* by International Fitness Association, (www.ifafitness.com, 1995-2004).

3. See the original works of Kenneth Cooper, M.D., in particular his initial book on the topic, *Aerobics.*

4. Ibid. See also *Saving Your Brain,* by Jeff Victoroff, M.D.
5. See *The Wellness Guide to Lifelong Fitness,* by Timothy P. White, Ph.D. (Rebus, 1993); *Active Isolated Stretching,* by Aaron Mattes (Aaron L. Mattes, 2000); and *Fitness for Dummies,* by Suzanne Schlosberg and Liz Neporent (Hungry Minds, 2000) for more information about stretching. In these books, there is some disagreement about the best way and time to stretch. Through personal and clients' experiences, I have found the guidelines I have given to be very helpful.
6. *Mind as Healer, Mind as Slayer,* page 307.

Chapter 6: How Did This Happen?—Causes of Illness

1. See note 1 for Chapter 2.
2. For further information, see the classic book on stress by Hans Selye, *The Stress of Life* (McGraw-Hill, 1956).
3. See note 4 for Chapter 2.
4. You may find information about this in the books *Mind as Healer, Mind as Slayer,* by Kenneth R. Pelletier, Ph.D., (Delta, 1977). *Human Life Styling,* by John McCamy, M.D. (Harper-Colophon 1975). *The Global 2000 Report to the President,* Volumes I & II, (Blue Angel, Inc., July 1981). See Pages 97-98 of *The Stress of Life,* by Hans Selye. Many other references are available. Just one representative sample is: P. Liechtenstein, N.V. Holm, P.K. Verkasalo, et al. Environmental and heritable factors in the causation of cancer. *New England Journal of Medicine.* 2000; 343:78-85. See also note 1 for Chapter 2.
5. For more information on biophysical effects of stress, see *Mind as Healer, Mind as Slayer,* by Kenneth R. Pelletier, and *The Stress of Life,* by Hans Selye. Just the possibility that about 75% of people have at least some clinically significant LGS contributes to being close to the cliff edge.
6. This was announced at one of their annual meetings in the early 1990s. See also note 1 for Chapter 2 and http://pubs.acs.org/hotartcl/cenear/960916/software.html. (accessed February 25, 2006)
7. For more information, see *Nuclear Evolution: Discovery of the Rainbow Body,* by Dr. Christopher Hills (University of the Trees Press, 1977). See also note 1 for Chapter 2.
8. *The Stress of Life,* by Hans Selye. See the entire book, especially chapters 5, 6, and 7.
9. Stress-effect is described in *The Stress of Life* and *Mind as Healer, Mind as Slayer.* It is related to what they called the General Adaptation Syndrome (GAS). The negative effects of stress-effect start when you reach the down slope of the GAS, after you have already accumulated a certain amount of stress-effect storage. In *The Stress of Life,* see Chapters 3, 6 and 8 for a description of GAS and its consequences.
10. See note 2 for Chapter 1.
11. See note 6 for Chapter 2 and note 5 for Chapter 6.

Chapter 7: Adjunct Approaches to the 3LS

1. *The Relaxation Response,* by Herbert Benson, M.D. *Time Magazine,* Special Issue, August 4, 2003 (various articles). *Time Magazine,* Special Issue, January 20, 2003 (various articles).
2. People interested in this can experience a session at one of the many tank farms that have sprung up all over the country. If you're interested, look in the Yellow Pages under Stress Management or Isolation Tanks.
3. Thousands of nutrients are already known. Reference: M. Muller, S. Kersten. Nutrigenomics: goals and strategies. *Nature Review.* 2003; 4: 315-322.
4. See *Fats That Heal, Fats that Kill: The Complete Guide to Fats, Oils, Cholesterol, and Human Health,* by Udo Erasmus (Alive Books, 1999) for more information.
5. Opening statement from the founding meeting of the American Holistic Medical Association, 1977.
6. Excerpt quoted from "Holistic Health: What Is It?" and "The Holistic Health Practitioner: What Standards Set Him Apart?" by JoAnn Louk Axton, presented at the first holistic health conference of the Association for Holistic Health in 1975.
7. This is like saying, "If we took a car apart into its smallest parts, we would finally understand the essence of a car." A human bodymind is infinitely more complex than a car, and it is ultimately absurd to think anything but seeing it function as a whole will allow us to understand it. Think about it.

8. Walt remembers many years ago seeing the effectiveness statistic in the FDA literature and the side effects statistic in double-blind studies. We searched but were unable to find the exact references for these statistics. However, we found that the FDA does not even use a standard 66% effectiveness rate. If it is a condition without effective treatment, and if initial studies show even the littlest bit of efficacy, the treatment is approved. Studies are continued while the general population is receiving the drug and if the drug is found to be dangerous, it is pulled from the market then. The average length of time for the studies for certain diseases such as cancers without effective treatment before the drug is put on the market is 6 months. For more information on how the FDA accepts drugs, see *http://www.fda.gov/cder/reports/rtn/2001/rtn2001-1.htm#NewDrugReview.* See also the *Physicians Desk Reference* for information on side effects on individual drugs.
9. January issue of the *New England Journal of Medicine,* 1993. See also *The Complete Encyclopedia of Natural Healing,* by Gary Null, Ph.D. (Bottom Line, 2002), page ix.

Chapter 8: Health for the Complete You: Mind, Emotions, and Spirit, Too

1. For more information on this topic, read *The Second Brain: A Groundbreaking New Understanding of Nervous Disorders of the Stomach and Intestine,* by Michael Gershon, M.D. (Perennial, 2000). This book describes how the digestive tract produces brain hormones. It is the first book we know of that documents this relationship between brain and body chemistry. This is also mentioned in *Patient Heal Thyself,* by Jordan S. Rubin (Freedom Press, 2003), pages 31-34.
2. Linus Pauling and Abram Hoffer, among many other world-class researchers, showed this 40 to 50 years ago and repeatedly showed it ever since. It has taken all this time for the conventional medical establishment (whose power is centralized in the national organizations) to catch on.
3. From Dr. Stoll's clinical experience.
4. For further information on this topic, see *Putting It All Together: The New Orthomolecular Nutrition,* by Abram Hoffer and Morton Walker (Keats, 1978). Some individuals need supplementation with other nutrients in addition to niacin. See also *The Natural Medicine Guide to Schizophrenia,* by Stephanie Marohn (Hampton Roads, 2003), pages 67-74; and *Natural Healing for Schizophrenia and Other Mental Illnesses,* by Eva Edelman (Borage, 2001).
5. For more information, see *Physicians Handbook on Orthomolecular Medicine,* edited by Roger Williams, Swight Kalita and Abram Hoffer, M.D. (Keats, 1977). See additional references inside first page. Also see *Natural Healing for Schizophrenia and Other Mental Illnesses,* by Eva Edelman. For further information on balancing brain chemistry, see *Saving Your Brain: A Revolutionary Plan to Boost Brain Power, Improve Memory, and Protect Yourself Against Aging and Alzheimers,* by Jeff Victoroff M.D. (Bantam, 2002).
6. From Dr. Stoll's clinical experience. For more information, see Philpott's book, *Brain Allergies,* (Keats, 1980); *Mental and Elemental Nutrients,* by Carl Pfeiffer, Ph.D., M.D., (Keats, 1975); Alexander Schauss' book, *Diet, Crime and Delinquency* (Parker House, 1981); and *Nutritional Influences on Illness,* by Melvyn Werbach, M.D. (Keats, 1987). See also note 5.
7. For more information on prayer and healing, see *Healing Words,* by Larry Dossey M.D. (Harper, 1993).

Conclusion

1. See *Voluntary Controls: Exercises for Creative Meditation and for Activating the Potential of the Chakras,* by Jack Schwartz (EP Dutton, 1978). Also, see the Menninger Clinic archives.

Afterword

1. There are many, many references that document the policy of the American Medical Association to suppress or discount any other form of medicine from being practiced. Furthermore, it is commonplace for them to revoke the licenses of holistic M.D.s. To understand this, read *The Assault on Medical Freedom,* by P. Joseph Lisa (Hampton Roads, 1994). Other references include *The Great Medical Monopoly Wars,* by P. Joseph Lisa (International Institute of Natural Health Sciences, Inc., 1986); *Racketeering in Medicine: The Suppression of Alternatives,* by James P. Carter (Hampton Roads, 1992); *Dirty Medicine: Science, Big Business, and the Assault on Natural Health Care,* by Martin Walker (Slingshot Publications, 1993); *Reclaiming Our Health: Exploding the Medical Myth and Embracing the Source of True Healing,* by John Robbins (HJ Kramer, 1996). See also Note 3.

2. Ibid.
3. Documented and broadcast in, "From Simple Beginnings," with Jack Perkins on CNBC at noon CST, March 10, 1996. Copies available through the American Chiropractic Association. The court case lasted 10 years, from 1980 to 1990. See also *Reclaiming Our Health: Exploding the Medical Myth and Embracing the Source of True Healing,* by John Robbins for a description of this and similar accounts about the AMA.
4. *Planet Medicine: From Stone Age Shamanism to Post-Industrial Healing,* by Richard Grossinger (Anchor Books, 1980), pages 161, 239-240.
5. Ibid. For more information, see also *Divided Legacy: The Conflict Between Homeopathy and the AMA, Science and Ethics in American Medicine* (North Atlantic Books, 1973); and the World Health Organization. Current statistics comparing health care in different countries may be found online at *The Commonwealth Fund's* website at http://www.cmwf. org/topics/topics.htm?attrib_id=9121&portal=yes (accessed August 30, 2005).

Appendix A

1. From the American Holistic Health Association Website at www.ahha.org.

If you don't find the term you are looking for here, check with a dictionary, do an Internet search, or call your reference librarian.

3LS Wellness Program (also called Serious Wellness, 3LS, or Wellness): A healing protocol consisting of Relaxation, Diet, and Exercise. Dr. Stoll's version includes Skilled Relaxation, Whole Foods Diet, and Aerobic Exercise. Your own version will be whatever works best for you.

Acute: Occurring over a short period of time, or lasting a short time. Having a sudden onset, sharp rise, and short course. Acute can also mean severe, but is used in this book to describe the duration of a symptom.

Acute stress: Acute stress comes and goes quickly, in contrast to chronic stress, which is long-term. A certain amount of acute stress is good for people, because the bodymind is benefited by responding and acting on a stressor through fighting or fleeing. (Chapter 6)

Aerobic exercise (AE): Any extended physical activity that makes you breathe hard while using the large muscle groups at a regular, even pace. Aerobic activities help make your heart stronger and more efficient. Specific heart rates for different ages are part of the definition. (Chapter 4)

Alexander technique: A simple method developed around 1900 by E. M. Alexander for learning to be more aware of how we move as we go about our everyday activities. The aim is to regain the natural grace and balance of a child and to discover easier and more efficient ways of movement, thus reducing the everyday tensions that have built up over the years. It is particularly helpful for correcting bad posture and the stress that may result from it.

Allergy (also known as hypersensitivity): In this book, we expand the definition of allergy past the classical limited definition (of having immunological reactions to environmental or drug allergens) to defining allergy as an abnormal response to a food, drug, or something in our environment that usually does not cause symptoms. Also, we can view an allergy as anything that weakens the body's energy system. (Chapter 3)

Allopathic medicine: The kind of medicine taught in medical schools and practiced by M.D.s and D.O.s for the past 100 years in the US. The term allopathic medicine (in Greek, "allo" means other) was coined by Samuel Hahnemann, M.D., in the late eighteenth century in reference to using therapeutic modalities to treat (i.e., oppose) symptoms. Allopathy claims its basis as scientific and the focus on treating symptoms seems to have developed as one of the guiding treatment principles. Allopathic medicine primarily uses medication and surgery. (Chapter 7)

Alpha: A brainwave ranging from 8 to 12 hertz. Alpha is a state of light relaxation. (Chapter 2)

American Medical Association (AMA): A professional association of physicians and medical students. Its stated goals are to protect the interests of American physicians, advance public health, and support the growth of medical science.

Amino acids: A class of organic compounds known as the building blocks of protein molecules. (Chapter 7)

Atomism: Atomism holds that the human bodymind is nothing more than tiny particles that get combined and recombined. That means eventually, if we broke things down into small enough pieces, we would be able to explain and control everything in terms of manipulating those small pieces. (Chapter 7)

Autogenic training: A set of techniques designed to generate a state of psychophysiological relaxation to relieve stress. Originally developed in 1930 by Johannas Schultz as a method of psychotherapy, it is used by the trainee to affect his/her autonomic nervous system and inner state by repeating a series of phrases that suggest relaxation while focusing on different parts of the body.

Autonomic nervous system: The part of the nervous system that regulates involuntary action of organs and glands, etc. The ANS is divided into two parts: sympathetic nervous system and parasympathetic nervous system. The ANS performs the most basic human functions more or less automatically, without conscious intervention from higher brain centers.

Beta: A brainwave ranging from 14 to 20 hertz. Beta is the state of usual, wakeful consciousness with ordinary or fast thinking. (Chapter 2)

Bioenergetics: A system of body-oriented psychotherapy developed by Alexander Lowen, M.D. Bioenergetics emphasizes the use of physical postures to energize chronically tense parts of the body and ultimately facilitate muscular relaxation. (Chapter 8)

Biofeedback: A therapeutic method that enables an individual to learn to consciously control internal physiological processes. Biofeedback machines monitor internal activity and display sensory signals to patients so that they can recognize what they are doing that changes certain physiological activities. (Chapter 2)

Biophysical environment: Our physical world, including gravity, radiation, atmosphere, and every other factor known to impinge upon us. (Chapter 6)

Biophysical stressors: Biophysical stressors include anything that causes physical or biological stress to the body. The body's response to biophysical stressors is the FOF response. Biophysical stressors include physical stressors, nutritional stressors, biochemical stressors, and electromagnetic smog stressors. Smaller stressors, like chemical additives in the food you eat, all create the same effect, but usually in a less dramatic way. (Chapter 6)

Bodymind: Research in the past 50 years has shown that there is no separation between body and mind. This term demonstrates the connection between the two. For example, the mind leads the body, so by changing what you believe, you can often change what your body is capable of doing. Also, the body leads the mind, so, for example, stand up straight and walk tall, and you will both think and feel better. (Chapter 5)

Bodymind laboratory: This refers to the process of trial and error (i.e., testing) and paying attention to the physical results of a particular course of treatment. Your body is by far the most sensitive laboratory ever developed, and the better you can listen to it, and the clearer it is, the more your body can help you know what is right for you. (Chapter 5)

Bodywork: This term is used to describe methods of manipulating the body, such as massage or Rolfing. These methods are different from physical therapy. (Chapter 8)

Bracing: Chronic tension in muscles due to storage of chronic stress (unexpressed FOF). Bracing is unrelenting, constant chronic muscle tension throughout the entire body. Bracing is usually below conscious awareness, meaning a person cannot usually feel it. (Chapter 2)

Bulletin board: The bulletin board on Dr. Stoll's website www.askwaltstollmd .com is a place where participants post messages to ask questions, share healing information, and discuss health topics. (Chapter 5, Appendix A)

Candida-related syndrome: Candida is a common fungal parasite that is normally part of the gastrointestinal flora. It becomes a harmful syndrome when the ordinary yeast (or seed form) sprouts into the fungal form, creating problems in any system of the body. (Chapter 3)

Carbohydrate: A food produced by plants that includes sugars, starches, celluloses, and related compounds. (Chapter 3)

Chiropractic: A healing art that considers the nervous system to be the crucial element in proper bodily functioning. Chiropractic's primary form of therapy, spinal manipulation, relieves pressure in the nerves as they emerge from the spinal column.

Chronic: Persisting over a long period of time, or recurring (repeating). Chronic has nothing to do with severity, just with the duration of symptoms.

Chronic illness: An illness or symptoms that persist over a long period of time or recur (repeat). Most chronic conditions appear suddenly but have been building over a length of time. The natural progression of chronic conditions is to become more severe.

Chronic stress: Long-term, continuous, or recurrent stress. (Chapter 6)

Clinical ecology: The study and treatment of aberrant psycho-physiological responses to foods, chemicals, and other environmental factors. Clinical ecologists are broadly concerned with all allergies, hypersensitivities, and a wide range of environmental stresses.

Complementary and alternative medicine (CAM): A commonly used term that describes all other healing methods and modalities besides allopathy (drugs and surgery). (Chapter 7)

Conditioning exercises: Exercises designed to prepare an individual for a certain activity or sport.

Conventional medicine: See allopathic medicine.

Cure: A permanent reversal or remission of symptoms in a disease or health condition with no further treatments. For chronic conditions, the concept of cure is applied a little differently: a cure from chronic illness may require a lifetime of attention to lifestyle. (Chapter 5)

Deficiency: The lack of a specific nutrient or nutrients.

Degenerative diseases: Diseases that cause permanent deterioration of tissues, such as osteoarthritis, cancer, and arteriosclerosis.

Delta: A brainwave ranging from two to four Hertz. Delta is a state of deep sleep or trance-like consciousness. (Chapter 2)

Dysbiosis: An imbalance of the bacteria in the gastrointestinal tract. (Chapter 3)

Edge of the cliff: The point at which symptoms begin to appear. The genetic limit for any functional body system to cope with or tolerate stress. (Introduction and Chapter 6)

Electro-Encephalo Gram (EEG): A diagnostic test that measures activity of the brain (brain waves) using a highly sensitive machine or equipment. An EEG biofeedback machine uses a tone or signal to indicate changes in brainwave activity for the purpose of self-awareness and change. (Chapter 2)

Electromagnetic medicine: Healing approaches that work with the electromagnetic, energetic, or vibrational fields of the body. (Chapter 8)

Electromagnetic smog: An accumulation of radiation from electronic and magnetic sources that exists in the environment, particularly in the modern home and urban areas. It is also called electropollution and includes both non-ionizing electromagnetic radiation and magnetic fields. (Chapter 6)

Energy medicine: Healing approaches that involve balancing and enhancing the energy field or vibrational frequency of the bodymind. Also called vibrational or electromagnetic medicine. Energy medicine's approaches to healing range from bodywork methods to magnets to the use of substances like essential oils.

Engrams: A lasting mark or trace. The term is applied to the definite and permanent trace left by a stimulus in the protoplasm of a tissue. In psychology it is the lasting trace left in the psyche by anything that has been experienced psychosocially. (Chapter 8)

Enzyme: A substance, usually protein in nature and formed in living cells, which brings about chemical changes.

Essential amino acid: An amino acid that cannot be made in the body by the human organism. (Chapter 7)

Essential fatty acids (EFA): Certain oils necessary for the healthy function of many areas of metabolism. They are slightly acidic. (Chapter 7)

Exacerbation: Aggravation of symptoms (or an increase in the severity of a disease). After you start feeling better, a temporary period of time when your symptoms return. The opposite of remission. (Chapter 5)

Feldenkrais: The Feldenkrais Method is an approach to working with people that expands their repertoire of movements, enhances their awareness, and improves function. This is done by using movement sequences that bring attention to the parts of the self that are out of awareness and uninvolved in functional action. The movements attempt to improve the individual's relationship with gravity and re-establish connection between the motor cortex and the muscular and nervous system, which have been short-circuited or rerouted by bad habits, chronic tension, and/or physical trauma.

Fight or flight (FOF): The body's response to an emergency (in order to be prepared to either flee or fight) which includes intense stimulation of the sympathetic nervous system and the adrenal glands. The heart and respiratory rates, blood pressure, and blood flow to muscles are increased. This is also called sympathetic nervous system activation. (Chapter 2)

Functional disease: Some part of the body does not work as well as it should, but does not show any measurable structural changes, such as changes on a blood test.

Galvanic Skin Response (GSR): A change in electrical resistance of the skin, occurring in emotion and certain other conditions. A GSR biofeedback machine uses a tone or signal to indicate a change in electrical resistance for the purpose of self-awareness and change. (Chapter 2)

Gastro Esophageal Reflux Disorder (GERD): (also called acid reflux or hiatal hernia). A disorder characterized by recurrent return of stomach contents into the esophagus (throat), causing pain (heartburn) and sometimes causing tissue damage. It often feels worse when lying down. (Chapter 3)

Genetics: The study of the physical inheritance of our bodies and personality. (Chapter 6)

Genome: The combination of all of a person's genes or the entire DNA structure of an individual. (Chapter 6, see also Human Genome Project and Phenome)

Guided imagery: A diagnostic and therapeutic method in which a therapist asks a patient to visualize particular images or scenes. May be done with a recorded cassette or CD. (Chapter 7)

Healing: The use of inner power and resources of our mind and body to restore our own unique balance and harmony. It is this balance and harmony that results in full health and gives us the ability to live lives of vitality and joy. (Chapters 5 and 7)

Healing crisis: The healing crisis is a return to experiencing symptoms of the past with less intensity, or times during healing characterized by reorganization and integration in the bodymind. Healing crisis symptoms are positive in that they herald a good outcome. They are temporary and are a normal part of the healing process. (Chapter 5)

Hellerwork: A series of one-hour sessions of deep tissue bodywork and movement education designed to realign the body and release chronic tension and stress. Verbal dialogue is also used to assist the client in becoming aware of emotional stress that may be related to physical tension.

Holistic health: A state of health in which body, mind, and spirit function in an integrated way in a supportive environment. Holistic healing is used to denote a type of health care responsive to all aspects of a person that incorporates a wide variety of therapeutic modalities into the traditional medical model. (Chapter 7)

Homeodynamic: A dynamic, moving state of equilibrium in the living body. This term replaces the term homeostasis since it is a more accurate description that the body's balance is dynamic and moving rather than still or static. Now it is known that body systems are in a constant state of homeodynamics that can be established in a sick mode as well as in a well mode and every setting between. An individual's state of homeodynamics may become reset to greater wellness by practicing the 3LS. (See also Homeostasis.)

Homeostasis: A state of equilibrium in the living body in which various physiological functions maintain balance. This state of balance (considered static) was taught in medical school 40+ years ago. Homeodynamic is a more accurate description of the body's equilibrium. (See Homeodynamic.)

Holistic medicine: Holistic medicine, in its broadest sense, could include practically every type of healing philosophy and modality in the world. Holistic medicine encompasses all safe methods of diagnosis and treatment (including drugs and surgery), and searches for the root cause of illness. It emphasizes the necessity of looking at the whole person, including analysis of physical, nutritional, environmental, emotional, spiritual, and lifestyle values. Holistic medicine particularly focuses upon patient education and patient responsibility for personal efforts to achieve balance. (See also Wholeness, Holistic health, and Chapter 7.)

Hormone: A chemical substance that is secreted into body fluids and transported to another organ, where it produces a special effect on metabolism (chemical function of the body).

Human Genome Project: Begun in 1990, the US Human Genome Project is a project coordinated by the Department of Energy and the National Institutes of Health. Project goals are to identify all of the approximately 30,000 genes in human DNA and determine the sequence of the 3 billion chemical base pairs that make up human DNA. (Chapter 6)

Human species: The term "human race" is incorrectly used in common speech. If you look up the biological tree of life, you will see how living things are categorized. First is "kingdom" (plants vs. animals), next is "phylum," which includes mammals. Then there is "species" (anything that can interbreed). Following that is "breed," which for humans is called race. So there is a human species and four different races: white, black, yellow, and red. In dogs, this level would be spaniels, poodles, beagles, etc.

Hypersensitivity: See Allergy.

Hypothalamic overload: A change in function of the hypothalamus and output of hypothalamic hormones due to chronic stress-effect. (Chapter 2)

Hypothalamus: A portion of the brain that lies beneath the thalamus and secretes substances (hormones), which control metabolism by exerting an influence on pituitary gland function. The hypothalamus is also involved in the regulation of body temperature, water balance, blood sugar, and fat metabolism. Additionally, the hypothalamus regulates the nervous system and other glands such as the ovaries, parathyroids, and thyroid. (Chapter 2)

Iceberg, Treating the Tip of the: Treating symptoms instead of addressing the underlying causes.

Integrated exercises: Exercises combining more than one philosophy, technique, or method. (Chapter 4)

Krebs cycle: A metabolic (chemical) process in the body that accomplishes the production of energy (ATP) from carbohydrates. (Chapter 3)

Leaky Gut Syndrome (LGS): A weakening of the intestinal lining that enables poorly digested proteins to leak into the blood supply causing the immune system to make antibodies to them. (Chapter 3)

Locus of control: In this book, locus of control is a concept that explains how people's viewpoint about the origins of health and illness contributes to what actions they are likely to take to improve their health. *Internal locus of control* describes a basic understanding that health originates inside the body, and thus decisions, changes, beliefs, and the discipline to change all come from inside you. *External locus of control* describes the belief that outside influences determine your health (and destiny) and you are helpless to control your fate. (Introduction, Chapter 6)

Massage: The practice of kneading or rubbing various parts of the body, usually with the hands, for the purpose of stimulating circulation, relieving muscle tension, and enhancing joint flexibility. (Chapter 2, Chapter 7)

Maximal heart rate: Take the number 220 and subtract your age from it. The number that you get is your maximum or highest heart rate recommended for your heart. Never exercise even near the maximum heart rate but only at a percentage of it. (See Target heart rate and Chapter 4.)

Megadose: A large dose of a nutritional supplement, used therapeutically, which is often 100 to 1,000 times as much as that required to prevent deficiency diseases. (Chapters 7 and 8)

Metabolism: Chemical changes in living cells by which energy is produced and new material is assimilated for the repair and replacement of tissues. (Chapter 4)

Middle of the field: Refers to the concept of the edge of the cliff (the point at which symptoms begin). If a person is operating in the middle of the field, it means they are not close to the edge of the cliff and do not have symptoms. (Introduction, Chapter 6)

Macronutrients: The major nutrients derived from food, including fats, carbohydrates, protein, and water. These nutrients provide calories, fatty acids, glucose, fiber, and amino acids. (Chapter 3)

Micronutrients: The minor nutrients derived from food, including minerals, vitamins, and all the co-factors needed for assimilation of nutrients and proper function of the body, such as enzymes, phytochemicals, and antioxidants. These nutrients are generally needed in small amounts, compared to the macronutrients. (Chapters 3 and 7)

Nutrient: A substance needed by a living thing to maintain life, health, and reproduction. (Chapters 3 and 7)

Nutrition: The science that deals with the relationship between food and our needs for all the nutrients required to nourish the cells of the body.

Nutritional dose: A standard dose of a dietary supplement used to prevent or slowly correct chronic conditions or enhance health. The nutritional dose of a particular nutrient might be obtainable from whole foods, but is often taken through dietary supplementation. (Chapter 7)

Orthomolecular medicine: Curing disease by means of nutritional therapy. The prevention and treatment of disease by varying the molecular concentrations of substances normally present in the human body. (Chapters 7 and 8)

Orthomolecular nutrition: Nutrition that recognizes the individuality of each person and notes that some people require very large amounts of specific nutrients. It takes into account that nutrients are often synergistic and work in harmony together. (Chapters 7 and 8)

Parasympathetic nervous system: The part of the autonomic nervous system originating in the brain stem and the lower part of the spinal cord that, in general, inhibits or opposes the effects of the sympathetic nervous system. The parasympathetic nervous system tends to stimulate digestive secretions, slow the heart, constrict the pupils, and dilate blood vessels. The keywords for the parasympathetic nervous system are "rest and relax" in contrast to the sympathetic nervous system, which are "fight or flight."

Pathological mechanism: The mode and means by which a disease process originates and progresses in an organism.

Perfect Whole Foods Diet (PWFD): A healing diet that calls for total avoidance of refined carbohydrates, sugars, and nicotine. (Chapter 3)

Personal Growth Work: Personal growth work is learning ways to improve your character, personality, skills, mind, emotions, and relationships. This may be accomplished through self-help methods such as books or groups, or with the assistance of a therapist or counselor. (Chapter 8)

Pharmacological dose: The pharmacological (or therapeutic) dose of a nutritional supplement is a dose meant to produce certain therapeutic effects. Therapeutic doses are generally large doses (megadoses) prescribed or supervised by an orthomolecular specialist or other qualified health care practitioner. (Chapters 7 and 8)

Phenome: The expression of a person's genes. The health possibility or potential for that person. (Chapter 6, see also Genome.)

Physiology: All of the functions of a living organism or any of its parts.

Phytochemicals: A non-nutritive bioactive plant substance, such as a flavenoid or carotenoid, considered to have a beneficial effect on human health.

Polarity Therapy: A health care system developed by Dr. Randolph Stone, D.O., that uses energy medicine, awareness training, exercise, and diet to rebalance the body.

Practicing Serious Wellness: Practicing the 3LS Wellness Program, plus doing whatever else it takes to become healthy, including learning and study. (Introduction)

Probiotics: Live microbial food supplements that beneficially affect the gastrointestinal tract by improving the intestinal microbial balance.

Protocol: The plan for a course of medical treatment.

Psychosocial environment: All psychological and social factors that impinge upon every individual including culture, education, training, family, and experience with disease and health. (Chapters 6 and 8)

Psychosocial stress: The type of physical and emotional stress that arises from a person's personal situation and interaction with others. Psychosocial stress is typically produced by conflicts, unreasonable expectations, and frequent or rapid changes in workplace, family, personal, and social situations. (Chapters 6 and 8)

Refined foods: Previously whole or natural foods that humans have processed, changed, or fragmented. (Chapter 3)

Reflexology: A diagnostic and therapeutic massage technique based on the premise that each of our organs has corresponding reflex points on other parts of the body. Practitioners of the technique believe that the presence of sensitivity at a particular reflex point is indicative of disorder in the associated organ or zone of the body and that stimulation or sedation of this point will facilitate the body's natural healing process. (Chapter 7)

Relaxation response: A unique state of physical and mental relaxation that reverses stress-effect storage at an accelerated rate. (Chapter 2)

Remission: A complete or partial disappearance of the signs or symptoms of disease in response to treatment. The period during which a disease is under control. A remission is not necessarily a cure. Remission is the opposite of exacerbation. (Chapter 5)

Rolfing: A system of deep tissue massage developed in the 1930s by Ida Rolf, a biochemist, to increase movement and ease in the body. By stretching the fascial (connective) tissue, moving muscles around, and breaking up adhesions between muscle and bone, a Rolfer attempts to release blocks in the body's musculature that occur as a result of physical and emotional traumas and chronic tension. Rolfing also includes movement education.

Self-help: Self-help is about observing yourself, your habits, thoughts, feelings, and actions. It is about examining those aspects of yourself (body, mind, emotions, spirit) that contribute to your health condition and finding ways to make lifestyle changes that will enhance and improve your health and well-being. (Chapter 6)

Serious Wellness: The 3LS Wellness Program, plus doing whatever else it takes to become healthy. (See also Practicing Serious Wellness.)

Skilled Relaxation (SR): Any process (i.e., meditation, guided imagery, etc.) that reliably produces alpha or theta brainwaves and the physical relaxation response. (Chapter 2)

Spiritual healing: A term used to describe incidents of physical healing that cannot be explained in purely medical, physical, or psychological terms. (Chapter 8)

Spirit or spirituality: The meaning of these terms are subject to individual interpretation, but for the purpose of this book and for improving health through the 3LS, we will define spirit as the non-physical aspect of life. Spirit or spirituality may also be considered a sense of connection with life itself or with something greater, wiser, and more powerful than an individual's sense of self. The growth of a person's spirit involves becoming aware of a higher meaning to life and life's experiences and a movement towards a more positive and mature personal expression. (Chapter 8)

Stress: Anything that puts the body in fight-or-flight mode (FOF) causing an increase in the heart, respiratory and blood pressure rates, and moving blood away from the digestive organs and into large muscles in preparation for a fight or flight. There are countless things that can activate the fight or flight response. (See also acute stress, chronic stress, biophysical stress, psychosocial stress, and stress-effect, autonomic nervous system, sympathetic nervous system, parasympathetic nervous system, and Chapter 6.)

Stress-effect: Stress-effect is an internal perception and amplification of stress. It is an individual's interpretation of what is experienced (often a totally unconscious process) and is intensely personal. Stress-effect has the physical manifestations of FOF (sympathetic activation). (Chapters 2 and 6)

Stored stress-effect: When stress occurs, the effect of the stressor (the "stress-effect") that is not discharged becomes stored in the hypothalamus as "stored stress-effect." (Chapter 2)

Supplement: A nutrient taken in addition to regular food in one of many forms, such as pills, powder, or liquid. (Chapter 7)

Sympathetic nervous system: The part of the autonomic nervous system originating in the thoracic and lumbar regions of the spinal cord that in general inhibits or opposes the physiological effects of the parasympathetic nervous system. The sympathetic nervous system tends to reduce digestive secretions, speed up the heart, and contract blood vessels. The keywords for the sympathetic nervous system are "fight or flight," in contrast to the parasympathetic nervous system, which are "rest and relax."

Synergetics: A gentle series of movements for exercise that have no impact or stress, developed by Taylor and Joanna Hay. (Chapter 4)

Synergistic effect (synergy): The interaction of two or more agents or forces so that their combined effect is greater than the sum of their individual effects. Cooperative interaction that creates an enhanced combined effect.

Systemic disorders: Conditions that negatively affect an entire functional body system.

T'ai chi chuan: A traditional Chinese meditative exercise and martial art. T'ai chi consists of a complex series of slow dance-like movements that are intended to harmonize mental and physical functions and enhance energy flow.

Target heart rate: A range of optimum heart rate for safe and effective cardiovascular exercise, based on factors such as an individual's age and fitness level. A target heart rate is usually 60% to 90% of a person's maximal heart rate. (See Maximal heart rate.)

Theta: A brainwave ranging from four to eight Hertz. Theta is a state of deep relaxation, a semi-aware state sometimes characterized by deep, dreamy thoughts. (Chapter 2)

Top of the mountain: The pinnacle of spiritual and physical wellness. Only a few humans have reached this spot over recorded history. The best documentation is in the book, *Cosmic Consciousness,* by Richard Maurice Bucke, M.D., published by E.P. Dalton in 1901 and reprinted many times since. (Introduction, Conclusion)

Trace mineral: An element present in minute quantities that is essential to the life of an organism. (Chapter 3)

Transit time: This is the amount of time needed for the stomach contents to move from the stomach through the intestines, finally being eliminated from the body via the rectum and anus. For most people it is 24 to 48 hours. (Chapter 3)

Vibrational Medicine: See energy medicine.

Vitalistic medicine and philosophies (Vitalism): The healing philosophy which holds that the human bodymind has within it the capacity to protect itself from the ravages of the environment and aging. Vitalistic healers focus on supporting the bodymind to heal itself. Hippocrates was the first recorded vitalist. (Chapter 7)

Vitamin: An organic substance found in food that performs specific and vital functions in the cells and tissues of the body. Most vitamins are not produced by the body but must be obtained from external sources. (Chapter 7)

Website: Dr. Stoll's website: www.askwaltstollmd.com. (See also Jan DeCourtney's website at www.lifespringarts.com and the Sunrise Health Coach Publications website at www.sunrisehealthcoach.com.)

Wellness: Exuberant life, happiness, creativity, and energy; the infinite capacity for forgiveness and loving support of others. There are many degrees of wellness just as there are many degrees of illness. (Conclusion)

Whole Foods: Unrefined foods such as fruit, vegetables, meat, nuts, and everything else grown in nature and consumed in as close to its natural state as possible. Foods that have no parts removed. (Chapter 3)

Whole Foods Diet (WFD): A way of eating that avoids refined foods. (Chapter 3)

Wholeness: High level wellness. Development and integration of all parts of a person to reach wellness, health, or a sense of completion. (Chapter 8, Conclusion).

Workbook: A reference to *The Relaxation and Stress Reduction Workbook.* (Chapter 2)

Yoga: Yoga is a gentle exercise that uses posture and breathing to build strength, endurance, and flexibility. (Chapter 4)

··

Note: Practitioners, products, and companies have not been evaluated and, unless otherwise indicated, are not endorsed by the authors or publishers. This information is included for your convenience and to provide a sample of the many good resources available. All information was correct at publication time. Since websites often change and companies go out of business, to obtain current information, use an Internet search engine or consult your library. Although some of the books listed have older publication dates, we believe the information in them is still valid. Often they were 30 years ahead of their time when published. If these "classics" are no longer in print, your library should be able to provide you a copy through their electronic lending network (Interlibrary Loan).

··

Skilled Relaxation (Chapter 2)

Learning and Practicing Skilled Relaxation—General

Books

Key Resource: *The Relaxation and Stress Reduction Workbook,* by Davis, Eschelman and McKay (Fifth Edition, 2000, New Harbinger Publications, Inc.; published continuously since 1980). This is the most effective self-help book to learn a variety of Skilled Relaxation techniques. Earlier editions are also good. This book contains information on the following Skilled Relaxation methods: breathing, progressive relaxation, meditation, visualization, applied relaxation training, self-hypnosis, autogenics, recording a relaxation tape, combination techniques, and thought stopping. The fifth edition also includes useful information about body awareness, stress management, coping skills, time management, assertiveness training, and exercise. This latest edition is an example of a book that has been exclusively about the one topic of Skilled Relaxation for 25 years. It recognizes the importance of the 3LS by including short information about diet and exercise. This is an excellent self-help book.

Awakening (Ways to Psycho-Spiritual Growth), by C. William Henderson (Spectrum, Prentice-Hall 1975). This book contains the largest number of Skilled Relaxation techniques. The first and biggest part of the book carefully explains different approaches, so the individual can choose which one makes the most sense personally. Then the last part of the book gives resources for each approach, about 150 different organizations and their publications, addresses, branches, programs, courses, and retreats. There are many newer modalities and approaches not listed in this book, though.

The Relaxation Response, by Herbert Benson, M.D. (Avon, reissue edition 1990). A classic book which is based on studies at Boston's Beth Israel Hospital and Harvard Medical School. Dr. Benson showed that relaxation techniques such as meditation have immense physical benefits, from lowered blood pressure to a reduction in heart disease. This book gives a great explanation of the relaxation response and is easy to read. It discusses only one Skilled Relaxation technique, however.

Meditation for Children, by Deborah Rozman (Integral Yoga Distribution, 2002). This resource contains information about what meditation is (useful for anyone to read who is considering starting meditation practice), what works for children at different ages, meditating individually and as a family, yoga exercises for children, and insight about how to bring about deeper contact between parents and children. This is a great self-help book.

Mind as Healer, Mind as Slayer, by Kenneth R. Pelletier (Delta, 1977; reissue edition 1992). Dr. Pelletier helps you identify the sources of your own stress and evaluate if your stress levels are dangerously high. Then he explores proven techniques for reducing stress, giving your immune system a boost, and speeding the healing process. This book is currently not in print, but used copies may be obtained or found in libraries. This book is moderately technical and contains some self-help instructions.

The Stress of Life, by Hans Selye (McGraw Hill, second edition 1978). This is a fairly technical work, written for the public as well as physicians, which describes the progressive effects of chronic stress on the body. Ultimately, the whole of Dr. Selye's work was about how a person's entire metabolism is changed when the hypothalamus is forced to stay in the fight-or-flight mode.

Specifically for Active Skilled Relaxation

Read the *Relaxation and Stress Reduction Workbook* mentioned above to learn active techniques that you can do yourself.

Look for classes in meditation, t'ai chi, yoga, breathing, etc. in your locality. Health food stores often have bulletin boards full of flyers announcing such classes.

Look in the Yellow Pages for specific practices.

Find religious and spiritual groups that teach Skilled Relaxation techniques such as meditation and yoga.

Search for books, CDs, and videotapes giving instruction for active Skilled Relaxation techniques (for example, progressive relaxation and visualization) in local or on-line bookstores.

Specifically for Passive Skilled Relaxation

Audiocassettes or CDs

Amazon.com currently offers the following CDs (recommended by Bulletin Board participants.) Also, you might go to a bookstore or music store and ask a salesperson to show you the relaxation music or CDs. Some Skilled Relaxation practitioners suggest having a few different CDs to rotate for use on different days.

Brainwave Suite—Theta, by Dr. Jeffrey Thompson (sounds)

Spectrum Suite, by Stephen Halpern (musical sounds)

Rainbow Meditation, by Michael Patrick Bovenes (narration with music)

Healing Mantras, by Shri Anandi Ma & Shri Dileeji Pathak

Magical Healing Mantras, by Namaste (East Indian chants with music)

Soma, by Tom Kenyon

Internet Resources

BrainSync, PO Box 3120, Ashland, OR 87520—1-800-984-SYNC, info@brainsync .com and www.brainsync.com. You can download an example to listen to. Try Total Relaxation, Healing Meditation, Guided Relaxation, or Guided Meditation.

Centerpointe Research Institute (Holysync), 4720 SW Washington St., Suite 104, Beaverton, OR 97005, 1-800-945-2741, support@centerpointe.com. Their website at www.centerpointe.com has a free download. Stereo headphones must be used to listen to these CDs.

Jan DeCourtney, C.M.T., has a list of recommended soothing, relaxing, massage-type music on her website at http://lifespringarts.com/products_music.shtml with access to ordering through Amazon.com.

Gaiam, Inc., also called the Relaxation Company, 360 Interlocken Blvd., Suite 300, Broomfield, CO 80021-3440, 877-989-6321, www.gaiam.com (Do a search for "relaxation" on their site.)

Skilled Relaxation machines (entrainment devices): Try doing a search on the web for "mind machines" or "light and sound machines." Bulletin Board participants have recommended the following companies:

Photosonix Product Group, 20206 State Road, Cerritos, CA 90703, 1-800-258-2566, http://www.photosonix.com/

Tools for Wellness, 9755 Independence Avenue, Chatsworth, CA 91311-4318, 1-800-456-9887 http://www.toolsforwellness.com

Transformation Technologies, 4110 Lyceum Avenue, Los Angeles, CA 90066, 1-877-287-0912 http://www.braintuner.com/

Specifically for Biofeedback

Books

The Awakened Mind: Biofeedback and the Development of Higher States of Awareness, by Maxwell Cade and Nona Coxhead, (Harper-Collins UK, reissue edition 1991). If you want to learn more about brainwaves, read this book. This book is written for the layperson and describes the development as well as early discoveries of biofeedback training.

Megabrain: New Tools and Techniques for Brain Growth and Mind Expansion, by Michael Hutchinson (Ballantine Books, reprint edition 1987). This book also has information about brainwaves, brain function, and consciousness technology.

Internet

http://www.holistic-online.com/biofeedback.htm has an informative article on using biofeedback.

http://www.lindaland.com/free.htm contains free books you can download on biofeedback, stress, stress management, positive thinking, and personal development.

Finding a biofeedback technician or practitioner

Look in the Yellow Pages under Biofeedback, Pain Management, Psychologists or Neurologists.

The Biofeedback Network maintains a list of technicians and links to equipment suppliers and biofeedback associations at http://www.biofeedback.net

Also try www.bcia.org for practitioners and articles.

Biofeedback machines (GSRs) are available from:

Web Ideas International—BiofeedbackZone.com, #110, 4335 Pheasant Ridge Drive NE, Suite 224, Blaine, MN 55449, 651-494-3977, www.biofeedbackzone.com

New-Mindmachines.com, 2856 S. Full Moon Drive, Tucson, AZ 85713, 520-405-2842

www.stresseraser.com

www.thoughttechnology.com

See also Tools for Wellness (listed under Skilled Relaxation machines above).

Other Resources

Look in the Chapter 7 Resources for information about locating bodyworkers (massage therapists, Hellerworkers, Rolfers, etc.) mentioned in this chapter.

Whole Foods Diet (Chapter 3)

Books

Key Resource: *The Healing Power of Whole Foods,* by Beth Loiselle, R.D. (with foreword by Walt Stoll, M.D.), (Healthways Nutrition, 1993). Beth's easy-to-understand and inspirational book is an invaluable resource for those wanting to learn every aspect of the basics of eating and healing through whole foods. It contains information about following the Perfect Whole Foods Diet, a liberal Whole Foods Diet, recipes, and adapting your diet to address candida, food allergies/sensitivities, a soft diet, and weight loss. It also has references for determining if specific foods, additives, and brand name products are appropriate for the Perfect Whole Foods Diet. Order from Healthways Nutrition, 93 Summertree Drive, Nicholasville, KY 40356-9190, (859) 223-2270 or (800) 870-5378, or online at www.wholefoodsforlife.com.

Saving Yourself from the Disease Care Crisis, by Walt Stoll, M.D., (Sunrise Health Coach, 1996). Look for the revised, expanded edition of this book entitled *Beyond Disease Care,* co-authored with Kathleen Diehl. You will find a chapter entitled "Leaky Gut Syndrome," which discusses LGS in detail as well as other gastrointestinal problems (including Crohn's and Ulcerative Colitis) mentioned in this chapter. The ginger root juice protocol for symptomatic relief of GERD is outlined in this book as well. Hypersensitivities and elimination diets are also discussed.

Staying Healthy with Nutrition, by Elson M. Haas, M.D. (Celestial Arts, 1992). An important reference guide for nutrition, vitamins and minerals, foods, diet, detox, nutritional therapies, and supplements.

Optimal Digestion, edited by Trent W. Nichols, M.D. and Nancy Faass, M.S.W., M.P.H. (Quill, 1999). This book explores the mechanics of the digestive system as well as the causes and potential remedies for over 30 chronic digestive disorders.

Neanderthin: Eat Like a Caveman to Achieve a Lean, Strong, Healthy Body, by Ray Audette, et al. (St. Martin's Press, 1999). This book can be an adjunct to *The Healing Power of Whole Foods* for those who include meat in their diet.

The Yeast Connection: A Medical Breakthrough, by William G. Crook, M.D. (Vintage Books, 1986). Dr. Crook's work gives the basic information about candida and includes topics on parasites, digestive disorders, and allergies, to name a few.

> Note: Where I differ with his approach is my experience that: 1) It is not necessary to avoid fermented foods. 2) Doing an effective practice of Skilled Relaxation is necessary for a permanent resolution. 3) It should not take two years to resolve the condition with a 40% relapse rate. My success rate in treating candida was an average of three to six months with a 10% relapse rate. —Walt Stoll, M.D.

Allen Carr's Easy Way to Stop Smoking, by Allen Carr (Barnes and Noble Inc., 1999). This easy-to-read, inspiring book offers a unique, simple, and enjoyable approach to giving up a nicotine addiction.

> Note: We were not able to find one book that discusses and compares all the different dietary approaches on the market, although there may be such books available. Check with your local bookstore for current books about individual dietary approaches and digestive disorders.

Other Resources

Beth Loiselle's website at www.wholefoodsforlife.com has additional recipes for the Perfect Whole Foods Diet.

Dr. Stoll's website at www.askwaltstollmd.com has archives with information about following the Perfect Whole Foods Diet.

Orthomolecular Nutrition: We have listed resources for orthomolecular nutrition under Chapter 8 (healing mind, emotions, and spirit).

Perfect Whole Foods Diet Practitioners: At the time this book was written, most nutritionists, dieticians, physicians, and other practitioners are not acquainted with the Perfect Whole Foods Diet. Thus we cannot refer you to conventional sources for additional assistance. However, check with the American Holistic Health Association (AHHA) at www.ahha.org, PO Box 17400, Anaheim, CA 92817-7400, 714-779-6152, mail@ahha.org. We are encouraging professionals acquainted with the 3LS and the Perfect Whole Foods Diet to register with AHHA's practitioner network. Thus, as the 3LS Wellness Program becomes more widely known, the AHHA will be the most likely place to find a practitioner familiar with this nutrition plan. Visit their website at www.ahha.org and click the button for resource and referral lists, then click the button for holistic practitioners, then in the specialty field type in "3LS" or "3LS Wellness Program." (Note that neither the AHHA nor the authors of this book regulate, certify, or endorse practitioners.)

Where to Buy Whole Foods

Health food stores, food co-ops, and farmers' markets are the most likely places to find the widest variety and selection of whole foods and whole foods products. Also look in the fresh and frozen departments, as well as the bulk or health food sections of your regular grocery store.

Just by doing a search on the web, we found three health food stores willing to ship whole foods by mail order. Further searches may turn up more mail-order suppliers.

Down to Earth Whole Foods, 305 Grant Avenue, Endicott, NY 13760, 607-785-2338, 866-811-2338, downtoearth@clarityconnect.com, http://www.dteweb.com

Amazing Grace Whole Foods, 1133 Bardstown Road, Louisville, KY 40204, 502-485-1122, fax 502-485-1144, us@amazinggrace.com, http://www.amazing gracewholefoods.com

Fresh Life, 2300 E. Third St., Williamsport, PA 17701, 570-322-8280, Fax 570-322-4460, freshlife@earthlink.net, http://www.freshlife.com/index.htm

Resources for Whole Food Supplements

Whole Food Supplements: Perfect Food is the best whole food supplement we know. However, recently the manufacturer started adding fermented molasses so it is not suitable for the PWFD. Other brands contain fruit. Check at your local health food store for new products, and be sure to read the labels.

Mineral Salt: RealSalt by Redmond. Redmond RealSalt, PO Box 219, Redmond, UT 84652. 800-367-7258, mail@realsalt.com. www.realsalt.com. Also available in many health food stores.

The Right Exercise For You (Chapter 4)

Books

Key Resource: *Fitness for Dummies*, by Suzanne Schlosberg and Liz Neporent (Wiley, John & Sons, 1999) is the best exercise book we have seen. This is a great reference book that covers a wide variety of exercises and describes them in detail. They cover cardio, strength, and flexibility exercises (including different types of yoga, for example), setting exercise goals, buying equipment, choosing an exercise class, health club, or exercise videos, hiring a trainer, exercising at home, fitness rip-offs, common injuries, and more. Even their foray into nutrition is close enough to the facts to be worthy.

The Aerobics Way, by Kenneth Cooper, M.D. (Bantam, 1989) was one of his first authoritative books on the subject but is out of print, so you might look for a used copy. Your library may have one or be able to obtain one for you by Inter-Library Loan. Dr. Cooper's initial concept is included in the rest of his aerobics books, so any one of them would do. His other books include: *Aerobics, The New Aerobics, Aerobics for Women,* and *The Aerobics Program for Total Well-Being.*

The Relaxation and Stress Reduction Workbook, has a short chapter about exercise, which also highlights the benefits of aerobics. See the Skilled Relaxation chapter resources.

The Health Fitness Handbook by B. Don Franks, Edward T. Howley, and Yuruk Iyriboz (Human Kinetics, 1999). This book is big on exercise and pretty good with that. They recognize a little of the importance of combining nutrition and stress reduction with exercise (a less focused version of the 3LS).

The revised, expanded edition of *Saving Yourself from the Disease Care Crisis,* to be called *Beyond Disease Care,* by Walt Stoll. M.D. and Kathleen M. Diehl, contains a section about rebounding.

Synergetics: Your Whole Life Fitness Plan, by Taylor and Joanna Hay (Synergetics Health Publications, Inc., 1991). Requiring only two non-impact, 12-minute non-aerobic workouts a day, here is a revolutionary new fitness plan that is safe and effective. Nine years of research have created a unique system that activates one's natural synergy and the harmony of mind, body, and spirit. It's a great way to get started if you haven't exercised or have been ill. A book and videotapes are available, we recommend the video. Their website is www.pocketgym.com, and you can also reach them at 1-800-336-1993.

A New Foot Health Solution, by Dennis Denlinger (eBookstand, 2001) teaches a simple way to use the foot muscles naturally to relieve foot pain and foot problems, including plantar fasciitis, foot arch pain, Achilles tendon pain, heel spur pain, etc. This book is great reading for those who have been avoiding exercise due to foot problems.

Vic Braden's Mental Tennis: How to Psyche Yourself to a Winning Game, by Vic Braden and Robert Wool (Little, Brown & Co. 1994) provides instruction on using Skilled Relaxation techniques such as mental imagery to improve one's performance in competitive sports.

Walkaerobics (Walk Away the Pounds) Videotapes, by Leslie Sansone make up a graduated program for slowly and easily building up strength and stamina by walking in place in your own home. A variety of videos are available, including tapes for one to four mile walks. Look for them at your local discount store or online.

The Wellness Guide to Lifelong Fitness (Rebris, 1993) has a whole body stretching routine. So does *Specific Stretching for Everyone* and *Active Isolated Stretching*, both by Aaron Mattes (Aaron L. Mattes, 2000).

Other Resources for Exercise

Aerobics and other exercise and fitness programs and classes are available at health clubs, gymnasiums, fitness clubs, community recreation centers, and YMCA's.

Athletic equipment, heart rate monitors, and exercise videos may be found at sporting goods stores, discount stores, and department stores. There are also many exercise programs on TV. Used sporting equipment may also be available on Internet auctions, yard sales, thrift shops, or in the classified advertising section of your local newspaper.

Fitness information is available online at the International Fitness Association's website at http://www.ifafitness.com. They have several free online manuals including a stretching manual and fitness manual, several online videos, a library with articles, fitness calculators, healthy advice, a gym locator and more.

Personal trainers can be located through health clubs, recreation centers, and YMCA's. There are also many on-line certification programs that offer referrals.

Sports medicine specialists can be located by looking in your phone book yellow pages under physician, specialties, sports medicine, or orthopedics.

Survivors of life-altering illnesses, such as cancer, multiple sclerosis, heart disease, and stroke may contact the Active Survivors Network, a non-profit group based in Baltimore, MD. The Active Survivors Network links those who have been affected by serious illness with the support and resources they need to remain active. Membership is free and open to both men and women. Contact them at (410) 823-0562 or www.activesurvivor.org.

The 3LS and Your Daily Life (Chapter 5)

Key resource: Visit Dr. Stoll's website www.askwaltstollmd.com for help, support, and information about the 3LS and holistic healing. The most effective way to use his website is to first read the articles, archives, and glossary concerning your health conditions and the practice of the 3LS. The website search engine is available for researching particular topics. Then, if after studying existing material on the website, you still have a question, post your message on the website's Bulletin Board. People experienced in practicing the 3LS Wellness Program volunteer their time to answer questions posted by newer participants. Many health care practitioners volunteer their time and expertise, too.

Other Resources for the 3LS and Daily Life

Jan DeCourtney's website http://lifespringarts.com has many resources available for individuals practicing the 3LS.

Read Dr. Stoll's first book, *Saving Yourself from the Disease Care Crisis* (Sunrise Health Coach, 1996). The revised, expanded edition, co-authored with Kathleen Diehl to be entitled *Beyond Disease Care*, contains a section on the 3LS. Whichever book is currently available may be ordered from the publisher at www.sunrise healthcoach.com, amazon.com, and through your local bookstore.

Jan DeCourtney is available for consultations and bodywork sessions at her office in Boulder, Colorado. For more information and to find out if she is accepting new clients, visit her website at http://lifespringarts.com, e-mail her at info@lifespringarts.com, or write her at PO Box 21132, Boulder, CO 80308. Jan is also available for public speaking.

Contact the American Holistic Health Association (AHHA), www.ahha.org, PO Box 17400, Anaheim, CA 92817-7400, 714-779-6152, mail@ahha.org. We are encouraging health care professionals acquainted with the 3LS Wellness Program to register with the AHHA's practitioner network. Thus the AHHA is your best bet for finding a physician or practitioner knowledgeable about the practices that comprise the 3LS. Search the American Holistic Health Association's website at www.ahha.org by first clicking the button for resource and referral lists, then clicking the button for holistic practitioners, then in the specialty field type in "3LS" or the words "3LS Wellness Program." You may also look for practitioners who are knowledgeable about one or more aspects of the Wellness Program (for example, for help with Skilled Relaxation, look for biofeedback practitioners). (Note that neither the AHHA nor the authors of this book regulate, certify, or endorse practitioners.)

Resources for Further Learning and Study

Check first with your health care practitioner who guided you to this book to see if he or she has any additional books or materials that might address your condition.

Do research at your local library. If they don't have the book you need or if it is out of print, ask your librarian to obtain it through Inter-Library Loan. Most books can be obtained that way, and it's usually at no charge or for a small fee. If your home computer has Internet access, use your library's on-line card catalog if they have one. Some libraries will even mail books to you for a small fee, so you may be able to look for and obtain books without even leaving your home.

Most local bookstores have a health section and/or an alternative health section. Health food stores often sell books on a wide variety of healing topics, especially nutrition and alternative healing modalities. Used bookstores sometimes have helpful titles at low cost.

On the Internet, find books through sites such as www.amazon.com and www .bn.com (Barnes and Noble). Each site sells most books still in print, has reader reviews for you to peruse, and can show you lists of other books related to your topic. Both sites can also help you find used books and out-of-print books.

Use a search engine to find a current website on the Internet. It sometimes takes some digging to find appropriate information on the Internet, so expect to spend some time. However, some of the most up-to-date and interesting information can be found there. Websites come and go and are updated regularly, and new information is constantly being added. Consequently, repeating a search several months later may turn up new informational treasures.

Here are a few other specific resources that can be very helpful in your learning and study. Some of this information may also be available on-line at various health websites.

For skin conditions: Go to your medical school library and ask the librarian for the best color dermatology atlas they have available. Look up your skin condition by examining the photographs. You will also find a short explanation about it. Then, if you want, you can look for more written information about your condition in a dermatology text.

If you are taking medications: No one should ever take a prescription medication without reading the entire package insert first. Also, look up your medications in the *Physician's Desk Reference* (PDR), available at your local library. It will tell you nearly everything known about each medication. There are also less technical versions of the PDR at bookstores and libraries. Of necessity, these are less complete, but they are easier to read and understand. These resources help you understand exactly what you are taking, what the side effects are, and if the medications you take react with each other.

If you are taking herbs or vitamins: These substances may have side effects too and sometimes react or interact with drugs or other natural medicines. It is wise to know something about what you are taking. Most health food stores and holistic pharmacies make available current reference books for looking up herb and vitamin interactions and usage. This information is also available on some health websites.

For chronic musculo-skeletal disorders: Go to a library or medical school library and look at a good picture anatomy book. Knowing the names and locations of muscles and bones can be helpful when consulting with practitioners or doing self-massage.

For toenail problems: Go to a medical school library and have the reference librarian help you find a good color atlas of toenail problems.

For understanding medical terminology: Use medical encyclopedias or medical dictionaries. There are also easier textbooks about medical terminology for beginners.

For learning about specific healing methods or modalities: There are books that give short descriptions of a wide variety of modalities so you can compare and select them. There are also primers on most individual healing methods.

For understanding your specific condition: Read books about your specific illness or condition written by people who have had and resolved the same condition. These books can be inspirational and full of useful ideas. Sometimes, workbooks related to healing specific conditions are available, too.

Also study the Glossary of this book for further general learning about health.

For additional enlightenment, take advantage of free wellness and health education programs as well as lectures offered by health food stores, some physicians or practitioners, and hospitals. Watch health education programs on TV, and check your local talk radio or National Public Radio station for holistic health programs. Look for printed information on health issues in literature racks at practitioners' offices, health food stores, and public health agencies. Attend community health fairs. Classes or weekend seminars for laypeople are also offered in many communities at massage schools and other learning institutions.

Causes of Illness (Chapter 6)

Genetics

The cutting edge of genetics is the Human Genome Project. The map of the entire genome has been completed, but to my knowledge the understanding is still being explored, and no books written for the layperson are yet available. Keep watching for them.

Biophysical Stress

Books

Home Safe Home: Protecting Yourself and Your Family from Everyday Toxics and Harmful Household Products in the Home, by Debra Lynn Dadd (JP Tarcher, 1997)

Toxics A to Z: A Guide to Everyday Pollution Hazards, by John Harte, et al. (University of California Press, 1999)

Food Additives: A Shopper's Guide to What's Safe and What's Not, by Christine H. Farlow (Kiss for Health Publishing, 2001)

Psychosocial Stress

The Relaxation and Stress Reduction Workbook, by Davis, Eschelman and McKay. (New Harbinger Publications, Inc., Fifth Edition, 2000) The fifth edition includes useful information about stress management, coping skills, time management, and assertiveness training.

See also our Chapter 8 Resources.

Stress-Effect

See *Mind as Healer, Mind as Slayer* and *The Stress of Life* as described in the Chapter 2 Resources and read about the General Adaptation Syndrome.

Choice

The Mind of the Soul: Responsible Choice, by Gary Zukav, (Free Press, 2003). This is a clear, practical workbook for understanding choice and taking the steps to making beneficial choices in your life.

Adjunct Approaches (Chapter 7)

Resources for Finding Self-Help Materials

There are so many good books on the market and in libraries these days, and with new books always becoming available, any list we could make would be too long and soon out of date. Also, we do not want to list so many other books that you will get lost in all those options and bypass doing the 3LS Wellness Program. After all, the 3LS will probably benefit you the most. So instead of listing titles, we recommend several options for you:

Use the learning and study resources in Chapter 5 of this Resource List for guidelines about where to look for books and other materials for self-help.

Look for websites that specialize in self-help books. Jan found three:

1. wellnessbooks.com primarily offers books for physical health and specific conditions, and

2. www.solveyourproblem.com mostly offers books for mental and emotional wellness.

3. www.newharbinger.com

For self-help support groups: *Self-Help Sourcebook: Your Guide to Community and Online Support Groups* (7th edition), by the American Self-Help Group Clearinghouse, 100 East Hanover Ave., Suite 202, Cedar Knolls, NJ 07927-2020, phone (973)-326-6789. This entire book is also available online at www.selfhelp groups.org.

See the list that Jan DeCourtney maintains of selected self-help books and other resources on her website: http://lifespringarts.com/self_help.shtml.

See also Dr. Stoll's first book, *Saving Yourself from the Disease-Care Crisis* (Sunrise Health Coach, 1996), for self-help information. The revised, updated edition co-authored with Kathleen Diehl, entitled *Beyond Disease Care,* contains how-to information about essential fatty acids, not compresses, preventing body odor, influenza and the common cold, stool withholding in children, GERD (hiatal hernia), headaches, fungal infections of the feet, and also includes a section about being your own best advocate for health care.

If you don't have health insurance, see Jan DeCourtney's website at www .lifespring.netfirms.com/selfhelp_no_health_insurance.shtml for self-help ideas and resources.

Nutritional Supplementation Resources

Always read the ingredient list to ascertain that a product is safe for the Perfect Whole Foods Diet. Also be aware that since no standards have been set for supplements, there is a wide variety of quality variations in nutritional products. Research the reputation of companies before selecting their products. Better quality products are usually found in health food stores.

Esterified vitamin C, vitamin E (mixed tocopherols, with selenium) and magnesium: Metagenics brand (same as Ethical Nutrients, which is available in health food stores) is good, but there are other suitable ones out there. Metagenics products are available only through health care practitioners. To find a practitioner, try www.metagenics.com.au or e-mail order@healthworld .com.au, Health World Ltd., PO Box 830, Hamilton QLD 4007 Australia.

Amino Acids: SeaCure by Proper Nutrition Inc., PO Box 13905, Reading, PA 19612, 800-247-5656, info@propernutrition.com or http://propernutrition.com. However, by reading the label very carefully, we see that many of the amino acids have a casein base. That means that anyone hypersensitive to cow's milk would not be able to use it.

EFAs and B Complex 100s: NOW brand is available in many health food stores, but these are standard so nearly any reputable company can be used.

How to find local allopathic and holistic physicians and other practitioners in your area

Look in the Yellow Pages under physicians, chiropractors, acupuncturists, etc.

Your own health care practitioners may be able to give you referrals to practitioners of other healing modalities.

The American Holistic Health Association (AHHA) has a list of almost 100 professional organizations that provide referrals to various types of health care practitioners or to a variety of modalities. Most sources are national organizations, educational institutions, or marketing services for practitioners. (See below for the AHHA contact information.)

Ask your library to find you a copy of the *Alternative Medicine Yellow Pages*, published by Future Medicine Publishing, Inc.; complied and edited by Melinda Bonk.

Health food stores often have bulletin boards or free publications describing local resources for healing and practitioner advertising.

The resources section of Chapter 8 has information about practitioners who work with healing the mind and emotions.

Ask your friends, family, and colleagues for recommendations.

Also, contact any of the following holistic organizations:

American Holistic Medical Association, 12101 Menaul Blvd. NE, Suite C, Albuquerque, NM 87112, (505)-292-7788, info@holisticmedicine.org; both holistic M.D.s and D.O.s are in this organization, and these are the only ones who can combine both conventional and holistic medicine. Practitioners of other healing therapies can be associate members in this organization. Their website at http://www.holisticmedicine.org has a doctor finder by state and locality.

American Holistic Health Association (AHHA), www.ahha.org, P.O. Box 17400, Anaheim, CA 92817-7400, (714)-779-6152, mail@ahha.org. The AHHA website contains access to their network of holistic practitioners, healing centers, and practitioner referral sources for a wide variety of healing modalities. The AHHA also offers a free booklet entitled "Wellness From Within," which explains the basics of holistic healing. To receive a copy, e-mail or mail your request, and include your name and address.

American Holistic Nursing Association, PO Box 2130, Flagstaff, AZ 86003-2130, (800)-278-AHNA, www.AHNA.com. Their website has an online resource directory, a listing of practitioners by state, and descriptions of healing modalities.

Holistic Dental Association, PO Box 5007, Durango, CO 8130, hda@frontier.net

The Pain and Stress Treatment Center is a holistic chronic pain center based upon the originator (Norman Shealy, M.D., Ph.D.), and dedicated to service rather than economic goals. Call 417-865-5940 and ask for a recommendation to a center near you.

Some bodywork associations include:

Massage: American Massage Therapy Association, 820 Davis St., Suite 100, Evanston, IL 60201-4444, 888-843-2682, www.amtamassage.org or Associated Bodywork and Massage Professionals, 1271 Sugarbush Dr., Evergreen, CO 80439-9766, 800-458-2267, expectmore@abmp.com. To find a qualified therapist, look in the Yellow Pages under Massage Therapy. Not all states have competency laws, so look for a therapist who is nationally certified or licensed.

Rolfing: To locate a Rolfer, try the Yellow Pages under Massage Therapy or call 800 530-8875 for information and the names of the closest Certified Rolfers. www.rolf.org

Hellerwork: To find a Hellerwork practitioner, try www.AlternativeMedicine. com. For more information, www.josephheller.com

Alexander Technique: www.alexandertechnique.com This site maintains links to professional organizations worldwide who register teachers of the Alexander Technique method.

Feldenkrais: Feldenkrais Guild of North America, 3611 SW Hood Avenue, Suite 100, Portland, OR 97239, 800-775-2118, www.feldenkrais.com

For our readers outside the United States searching for professional help, look for holistic medical associations in your country.

The American Holistic Health Association (AHHA) accepts as members professional health care providers in any country. While all practitioners are on the online list of AHHA Practitioner Members, only those in the U.S are on the printed version of the list. The AHHA also includes in their membership holistic healing centers in North America. AHHA has a Practitioner Referral Sources list that includes about 100 other organizations offering referrals to health care professionals. Many of these organizations are international professional associations.

Any other organization mentioned in this book may also have international chapters.

Resources for Healing Mind, Emotions, and Spirit (Chapter 8)

Crisis and Suicide Hotlines and Websites for Emergency Situations

Crisis Intervention: Dial 9-1-1

Crisis Helpline (for any kind of crisis): 800-233-4357. They will refer you to local agencies in your area.

Girls and Boys Town National Crisis Line: 800-448-3000. Children and parents can call with any problem, any time. Staffed by caring professionals.

National Hope Line Network (Crisis): 800-suicide or 800-784-2433. The Hope Line connects people in immediate distress to a local crisis center. Calls are answered by certified counselors 24/7.

www.metanoia.org/suicide contains conversations and writings for suicidal persons to read.

1-800-therapist or call 800-843-7274: A free referral service during normal business hours. After an initial telephone evaluation, they can refer you to the full range of mental clinicians including a psychiatrist, psychologist, marriage or family therapist, clinical social worker, licensed professional counselor, or psychiatric nurse when available in your area. A website is also available at http://www.1-800-therapist.com/find_a_therapist.htm (offering guidance about how to select and evaluate an appropriate therapist for you).

Orthomolecular Nutrition and Therapy

Books

Saving Yourself from the Disease Care Crisis, by Walt Stoll, M.D. (Sunrise Health Coach, 1996). Read the entire book for wellness concepts and then focus on the chapter about "Mood, Mind, Memory, and Behavior." The revised, expanded edition of this book, *Beyond Disease Care,* co-authored with Kathleen Diehl, contains a chapter entitled, "Disorders of Brain Chemistry."

The Edge Effect, by Eric R. Braverman (Sterling, 2005). Dr. Braverman reveals the dramatic impact that proper brain nourishment can have on the quality of life. His key to longevity and well-being is balancing the brain's four important neurotransmitters.

Nutrition and the Mind: Dietary Approaches to Mental Illness from Alcoholism to Migraines, by Dr. Gary Null (Four Walls, Eight Windows, 1995). This book describes basic mechanisms for known, approachable brain chemistry influences upon mood, mind, memory, and behavior that the reader can try without risk. The updated version of this book is called *The Food-Mood-Body Connection: Nutrition Based and Environmental Approaches to Mental Health and Physical Well-Being,* by Dr. Gary Null. (SevenStories Press, 2002).

Brain Allergies: The Psychonutrient and Magnetic Connections, by William Philpott, M.D. (McGraw Hill, 2000). In this book, Dr. Philpott shares his research and clinical experience that has proven how hypersensitivities to things in the environment can profoundly influence behavior.

Natural Healing For Schizophrenia and Other Mental Illnesses, by Eva Engleman (Borage Books, 2001). This book gives an overview of orthomolecular nutritional therapy and brain chemistry, and what they accomplish. It discusses and gives details about using specific vitamins and minerals, as well as offers extensive resources. A very informative book!

Orthomolecular Nutrition: New Lifestyle for Super Good Health, by Abram Hoffer Ph.D., M.D. and Morton Walker, D.P.M. (Keats, 1978). This easy-to-read book explains what orthomolecular nutrition is, how it works, why it is necessary, and gives suggestions for supplementation as well as case studies. It also has an extensive list for further reading. Dr. Hoffer is the first world-class practitioner to be knowledgeable in this area. Because of his age, there may be some younger clinicians who have followed his teachings that have gone beyond the teacher. Dr. Perlmutter in Florida is one of them.

The Brain Chemistry Diet, by Michael Lesser, M.D. (G. P. Putnam's Sons, 2002). Renamed *The Brain Chemistry Plan* in subsequent printings. This user-friendly book about orthomolecular nutrition discusses diet, supplements, and lifestyle choices designed to keep a person in balance. Take a short quiz to determine which of the six personality types you are based upon brain chemistry. This is a great self-help book. It is basically an updated and more reader-friendly form of *Mental and Elemental Nutrients,* by Carl Pfeiffer (Keats, 1976).

Mental and Elemental Nutrients: A Physician's Guide to Nutrition and Health Care, by Carl Curt Pfeiffer (Keats, 1976). One of the pioneers in the field of brain chemistry brings that state-of-the-art information to the lay person.

Nutrigenetics: New Concepts for Relieving Hypoglycemia, by R.O. Brennan (New American Library, 1977). This book describes mechanisms for management of the symptoms of hypoglycemia and discusses conventional and unconventional approaches to this stress-related condition.

Diet, Crime, and Delinquency, by Alexander Schauss with an introduction by Michael Lesser, M.D., another pioneer in this area (Parker House, revised 1981). It is a classic in the field! In this short book, an internationally known criminologist presents the first clear guide to correcting behavior through diet. He clearly and concisely documents how food allergies can foster violence, how nutrition and vitamin therapy help alcoholism and drug addiction, and how junk foods and environmental pollutants favor the development of crime.

The Second Brain: A Groundbreaking New Understanding of Nervous Disorders of the Stomach and Intestine, by Dr. Michael Gershon (Perennial, 2000). Dr. Gershon has proved that the intestinal tract creates a much higher dosage of all the brain hormones we've discovered so far than the brain does. We used to think people had intestinal symptoms because of their mental attitude. It turns out that it is probably the other way around, that we have a mental attitude because of the malfunction of the intestinal tract. This book is fairly technical, but so far it is the only book we know of available on the subject.

Is This Your Child: Discovering and Treating Unrecognized Allergies in Children and Adults, by Doris Rapp, M.D. (William Morrow & Co., 1992). Dr. Rapp reveals that common allergies may be the cause of many health and behavioral problems.

The Advancement of Nutrition, by Roger J. Williams, Ph.D. D.Sc. (International Academy of Preventive Medicine, 1982). He gives a concise overview and explanation of the nutritional principles summarized in this chapter and in Chapter 3 (about diet).

Feed Your Body Right: Understanding Your Individual Body Chemistry for Proper Nutrition without Guesswork, by Lendon H. Smith, M.D. (M. Evans, 1994). Includes information on nutritional research, body chemistry, how to read and interpret blood tests, and the chemistry of mental and emotional dysfunction, immune system (allergies and sensitivities), and more.

Staying Healthy with Nutrition, by Elson M. Haas, M.D. (Celestial Arts, 1992). In addition to thorough information about foods and diets, this book contains a detailed discussion of vitamins and minerals, including uses and dosages.

Some of the cutting edge research that ties together brain chemistry, function, and self-directed immunity has come from the work of Carl Simonton. If you would like to learn more about the research and health benefits, read Michael Murphy's book, *The Future of the Body: Explorations into the Further Evolution of Human Nature* (J.P. Tarcher, 1993) or search for Simonton's work for the scientific background.

Orthomolecular Practitioners

Orthomolecular practitioners may be hard to find. The AHMA (see Chapter 7 resources) may be able to help you find a practitioner. Many of the books listed above on the topic have further resources for contacting practitioners.

Huxley Institute for Biosocial Research, 86B Dorchester Dr., Lakewood, NJ 08701, www.schizophrenia.org

International Society for Orthomolecular Medicine (replaced the Academy of Orthomolecular Psychiatry), 16 Florence Avenue, Toronto, Ontario, Canada M2N 1E9, (416)-733-2117, www.orthomed.org. or centre@orthomed.org. Has an online list of orthomolecular societies throughout the world and a list of orthomolecular treatment and research institutes. They also provide referrals for local practitioners.

Society for Orthomolecular Health Medicine, 2698 Pacific Avenue, San Francisco, CA 94115, (415)-922-6462, Sohm@aol.com

www.restoreunity.org/list_of_ortho_doctors.htm

Safe Harbor, at www.alternativementalhealth.com, provides practitioner references and resources for drug-free healing of mental health problems.

Psychosocial and Personal Growth Resources

Books

You can find many good personal growth self-help books on a wide range of topics, and new ones are available all the time, so we won't even attempt to list them. It would be better to go to your local library or bookstore and browse the shelves, or check Amazon.com for the latest titles.

The Relaxation and Stress Reduction Workbook (described in Chapter 2 Resources) includes chapters on goal-setting, time management, and assertiveness skills. Other chapters, including job stress management, goal setting and time management, and assertiveness training, focus on daily scenarios people often find distressing. Lessons in identifying key elements that trigger unpleasant responses and ways to react differently to these stressors are designed to defuse perceived conflicts. The fifth edition has added topics on worry control, anger management, and eye-movement therapy. This is a valuable tool for therapists, their patients, and the stressed-at-large.

Jan DeCourtney maintains a list of selected self-help books and links to other self-help resources on her website: http://lifespringarts.com.

Psychosocial Practitioners/Psychotherapists

If you are looking for a practitioner, ask for referrals from other health care practitioners, people you know, or check the Yellow Pages. Therapists have different areas of expertise and specialization. To find a practitioner with whom you are comfortable, it's a good idea to interview several of them before making a choice. Ask them questions regarding their training, experience and approach to therapy, as well as their fees and payment methods. It is important that you feel comfortable and safe with a therapist during the time you spend in a healing relationship.

Bodywork, Vibrational Medicine, Combination Approaches

Books

Discovering the Body's Wisdom, by Mirka Knaster (Bantam, 1996.) This book presents an overview of many bodywork techniques, energy medicine and combination approaches and how to make use of them.

Vibrational Medicine: The #1 Handbook of Subtle-Energy Therapies, by Richard Gerber M.D. (Inner Traditions International, Revised Edition 2001). A standard reference book that provides an encyclopedic treatment of energetic healing.

A Practical Guide to Vibrational Medicine: Energy Healing and Spiritual Transformation, by Richard Gerber, M.D. (Quill, 2001). This book provides a new way of thinking about healing and explains the benefits of energetic therapy and how it works.

Vibrational Medicine for the 21st Century, by Richard Gerber, M.D. (Bear & Company, 1988). A self-help work that combines scientific evidence with case studies of real patients.

Resources for Spirit and for Non-Physical Approaches to Healing

Books

Awakening: Ways to Psycho-Spiritual Growth, by C. William Henderson (Spectrum, 1975). The first and primary part of the book carefully explains different approaches, so the individual can choose which one makes the most sense personally. The last part of the book gives resources that go deeply into those approaches. Basically, it describes about 150 different organizations that accomplish this, their publications, addresses, branches, programs, courses and retreats. There are many newer modalities and approaches not listed in this book, nonetheless.

Cosmic Consciousness, by Richard Maurice Bucke, M.D. (E.P. Dutton, 1969). In this book, Dr. Bucke relates his own experience and then discusses 50 people whose experience of cosmic consciousness is evidenced in their writing or life.

The Awakened Mind: Biofeedback and the Development of Higher States of Awareness, by C. Maxwell Cade and Nona Coxhead (Delacorte Press, 1979). C. Maxwell Cade is unique among researchers and clinicians in his field because of his enormous wealth of experience in each of three distinct fields. He is not only a psychologist, but also a Zazen meditator and teacher of Raja Yoga, as well as a research scientist and distinguished physicist.

Healing Words, by Larry Dossey, M.D. (Harper San Francisco, 1993) or any of the other books by Dr. Dossey. His books probe links between medicine and spirituality, such as the healing power of prayer. This is not news to the religious world, but to the scientific world, it is a revelation. His work links the two.

Joy's Way: A Map for the Transformational Journey, by W. Brugh Joy, M.D. (J.P. Tarcher Inc., 1979). In this book, Dr. Joy describes his own personal spiritual transformation.

Websites

How to cope: www.coping.org is a public service website that offers tools for coping with a variety of life's psychosocial stressors. This award-winning website has much self-help information and articles including:

Tools for Raising Responsible Children

Tools for Handling Loss

Tools for Personal Growth

Tools for Relationships

Tools for Communication

Tools for Anger Work-Out

Tools for Handling Control Issues

Tools for Healing the Inner Child

Tools for a Balanced Lifestyle

Program for Recovery

Online Courses

Trauma information pages: www.trauma-pages.com/index.phtml. This website has much information, resources, links, and an extensive book list for those wishing to heal traumatic life events.

Peer Counseling: www.rc.org. Re-evaluation Counseling Communities, 719 Second Avenue North, Seattle, WA 98109, 206-284-0311, www.rc.org, ircc@rc.org. Re-evaluation Co-counseling is a low-cost way to do personal growth work in groups and with other individuals who are also working on themselves. You take a class (low cost) to learn simple, basic listening and counseling skills. Following completion of the class, you become a member of the co-counseling community and can trade sessions with other co-counselors. Re-Evaluation Co-Counseling is a large organization with communities in many areas of the US and abroad. There may be other similar organizations.

Groups

Self-Help Groups: See the Clearinghouse information in the resources section of Chapter 7.

Twelve Step Groups: Do an Internet search or check your phone book or Yellow Pages for AA (Alcoholics Anonymous). AA can usually help you find other local twelve-step groups addressing different conditions.

Yahoo Groups: At yahoo.com, go to the link for groups and type in your interest to locate an online discussion group about your topic, health issue, or concern.

Index

A

acid reflux, 38, 43, 116, 373
acne, 42, 125, 126, 209
Active Isolated Stretching (Mattes), i, 365–366, 388
active skilled relaxation, 47, 382
Active Survivors Network, 388
acupressure, 245, 264, 276
acupuncture, 245, 276, 300, 326, 332, 349, 393
acute sickness, 15, 117, 217, 225, 262, 318, 336, 369
ADD. *See* attention deficit disorder
addiction, 229, 265. *See also* withdrawal
    to alcohol, 99
    to caffeine, 84–85, 86
    to nicotine, 99, 105, 385, 396
    to refined carbohydrates, 84–86, 92, 98–101, 104, 121, 133–134, 244, 294
addictions counseling, 265
additives, 352–358
adenosine triphosphate (ATP), 83–84
adrenal fatigue/exhaustion, 42
adrenal glands, 373
Aerobic Exercise (AE), 130–132, 134–142, 144–149, 166, 369
    aging and, 135
    Alexander technique in, 130, 150
aerobic metabolic pathway, 142–143

Aerobics (Cooper), 150, 167
affective disorders, 44
affirmations, 47
aging
    aerobic exercise and, 135
    Right Exercise and, 130, 140, 141
    Skilled Relaxation and, 44
agoraphobia, 38, 79, 288
AHHA. *See* American Holistic Health Association
AHMA. *See* American Holistic Medical Association
AHNA. *See* American Holistic Nursing Association
alcohol, 86, 90, 99, 121
    addiction to, 99
alcoholism, 38, 42, 231, 288, 307, 395, 396
Alexander technique, 264, 273, 300, 324, 369
    in Right Exercise, 130, 150, 151
allergic skin reactions, 42
allergies, 385, 396
    to food, 38, 42, 91, 109, 110, 114–115, 117, 126, 241–242, 309, 384–385
allopathic medicine, 369. *See also* modern-day medicine
    adjunct approaches in, 261–262, 266–267, 279, 281
    holistic medicine and, 318, 319, 320–321

in modern-day medicine, 318, 319, 320–321
practitioners/physicians in, 318, 319, 320–321
alpha brainwaves, 40–45, 45, 55, 58, 69, 369
alternative medicine, 310, 317, 326, 393
CAM and, 263, 349, 372
AMA. *See* American Medical Association
American Holistic Health Association (AHHA), 326, 346, 348, 386, 389, 393, 394
American Holistic Medical Association (AHMA), xxiv, 348–350, 397
American Holistic Nursing Association (AHNA), 393–394
American Massage Therapy Association, 394
American Medical Association (AMA), xix, xxiv, 315–318, 370
American Society of Chemical Engineers (ASCE), 222
amino acids, 29, 289, 309, 370, 375, 393. *See also* essential amino acids
anabolism, 143, 144
anaerobic exercise, 66, 150
anaerobic metabolic pathway, 142
anger management, 297, 398
angina pectoris, 42
anorexia athletica, 241
anthroposophic medicine, 264
anxiety, 210, 280, 285, 286, 289, 301, 349
appliances, 108–109, 223, 252
applied kinesiology, 275–276, 325
applied relaxation, 46, 47, 71, 72, 381
arm pain, 42
armoring, 299, 364
aromatherapy, 245, 274, 276
arthritis, 69, 125, 147, 150, 154, 169, 208, 244, 255, 372
rheumatoid, xii, 125, 126–127, 171, 209, 280, 364
ASCE. *See* American Society of Chemical Engineers
assertiveness training, 46, 381, 391, 397
Associated Bodywork and Massage Professionals, 394
asthma, 42, 125
Aston patterning, 264, 273
atherosclerosis, 268
athletes
Perfect Whole Foods Diet and, 88

Right Exercise and, 145, 151, 153, 160, 166, 172
3LS and, 133–134
Atkins diet, 115, 349
atomism, 266, 370
atonic bowel, 116
ATP. *See* adenosine triphosphate
attention deficit disorder (ADD), 42, 79, 288, 309
Skilled Relaxation and, 38
audiotapes/CDs, 48, 60, 71, 72, 373, 382–383
autism, 288
autogenics, 47, 370
autoimmune conditions, 42, 208
autoimmune disease, 208
autonomic nervous system, xxii, 57, 370, 376, 378
avoiding practicing, in 3LS/daily life, 176–177
The Awakened Mind (Cade & Coxhead), 312
Awakening: Ways to Psycho-Spiritual Growth (Henderson), 61, 398
awareness, 184, 264, 332, 383, 399
body, 46–47, 55, 151, 161, 205, 246, 299, 373
conscious, 41, 45, 65, 205, 225, 247, 302, 371
of emotions, 197–198
self, 141, 153, 194–200, 250, 273, 292–293
Ayurvedic medicine, 264, 347
Ayurvedic physicians, 324, 347

B

Bach flower remedies, 274, 300
back pain, 42, 63, 73, 119, 135, 384
Baker's cyst, 42, 147
balance, 263–264
balance beam and, 151–152
balanced B complex, 258
balancing chemistry, 290–291, 305
baldness, 43
beans, 89, 121
behavioral kinesiology, 258, 265, 276, 297
behavioral kinesiologists and, 324
behavioral problems, in children, 289, 309, 396
bell curve, 218–219, 228–230

benefits
  of Perfect Whole Foods Diet, 79–81,
    82–86
  of Right Exercise, 135–136
  of Skilled Relaxation, 39–40, 53
  of Whole Foods Diet, 86
Benson, Herbert, 54
beta brainwaves, 40, 370
beverages, 29, 89, 90, 96, 155
Beyond Disease Care (Stoll & Diehl), 202,
  345, 385, 387, 388, 392, 395
bicycling, 135, 137, 144, 145, 147, 163, 167
biochemical imbalance, 285, 286, 290
bioenergetics, 264, 297, 370
biofeedback, 370, 372, 373, 389, 399
  practitioners, 45, 56–59, 72, 181, 324,
    384
  Skilled Relaxation and, 45, 48, 53,
    56–59, 383–384
biophysical environment, 370
biophysical stressors, 220–224, 226,
  230–231, 238, 285, 370–371, 391.
  See also stressors
bipolar disorder, 42, 79
bleeding gums, 125
blepharospasm, 42
bloating, xi, xii, 127
blood clots, 310
blood lipids, 135
blood pressure, 135, 162, 221, 225, 373,
  377, 382
blood thinners, 310
blood volume/total hemoglobin, 135
body chemistry, 35, 38, 71, 288–291,
  305, 397
body odor, 392
body-centered psychotherapy, 265, 297
bodymind, 371, 394
  healing chronic illness and, 21–22, 194,
    195, 205
  in mind/emotions/spirit, 303–304
  in practicing wellness, 11–12
bodymind laboratory, 195–196, 332, 371
bodywork techniques, 264–265, 299,
  371, 398
bodyworkers, 324, 363, 384
bone density/joint strength, 135, 157
bowel function, 16, 42, 116, 117, 135,
  209, 364
Bowen technique, 264–265

bracing, 371
  Skilled Relaxation and, 35–37, 59–60,
    62–63, 66–67
brain fog, ix, 128, 291
brain function, 294, 295, 384
brain physiologists, 200, 312
brain/body chemistry
  in mind/emotions/spirit, 288–293, 305
  Skilled Relaxation and, 38–39
brainwaves, in Skilled Relaxation, 39–41,
  45, 48–51, 53–65, 71, 72, 248, 370, 377, 383
breathing, 53, 69, 166, 246, 379
  rate, 35, 225
  Skilled Relaxation techniques and, 46,
    47, 71
Breema bodywork, 264
bronchitis, 280
bruxism, 13, 42
bulletin boards, 12, 208, 241, 346, 371, 393
bunions, 281
bursitis, 42

C
caffeine, 90, 100, 105, 121, 294
  addiction to, 84–85, 86
calcium, 157, 360, 362
cancer, 16, 38, 116, 171, 281, 312, 366, 388
Candida, 118, 208–209, 286, 371
  diet, 115
canker sores, 42
carbohydrates, 371
  Perfect Whole Foods Diet and, 84–86,
    98–99, 101–106, 121
  refined, 84–86, 90, 93
cardiac arrhythmias, 42
carpal tunnel syndrome, 42
catabolism, 143–144
celiac disease, 309
centering/prayer, 47
chakras, 300, 367
charlie horse, 309
charts, iv, 174, 207
chelation therapy, 349
chemistry balancing, 290–291, 305
chemistry imbalance, 38, 71, 285, 288, 291
children, Whole Foods Diet and, 127, 182–
  183, 185, 256, 289, 382, 394–395, 397, 399
chiropractic, 63–64, 264, 367, 371
choices, 75–78, 130–131, 137–138, 149–154,
  218, 232–238, 245, 278
cholesterol, 39, 69, 125, 135, 366

chondromalacia, 42, 147, 170
chronic condition reversal, 3, 187–188, 231
chronic conditions, in practicing serious
  wellness, 10–11, 13–14, 15
chronic fatigue, 42, 79, 127, 281, 289, 364
chronic illness, 7, 119, 121, 157, 232, 238,
  244, 262, 266–269, 305, 371
    acute vs., 225–226
    bodymind and, 21–22
    cliff edges and, 21–22, 23
    genetic inheritance and, 22, 24
    healing in, 21–28
    3LS in, 3–4, 7
chronic muscular aches, 42, 79
chronic muscular tension. *See* bracing
chronic pain, 42, 61–62, 250, 394
chronic stress, 33–40, 83, 219–226, 371,
  382. *See also* stress
clinical ecology, 300, 325, 371
coaching, xxiv, 265, 297
cod liver oil, 281
cold hands and feet, 42, 57
colds, xi, xii, 42, 119, 128, 135
colitis, 38, 116, 244, 255, 385
colon, 113, 117–118
colon cancer, 38, 116
combination approaches, 300, 301–302
commitment, to 3LS, 178
common digestive issues, LGS and, 116,
  117, 118
communication, 198, 253, 254, 272, 296,
  337, 399
Complementary and Alternative Medicine
  (CAM), 263, 349, 372
compliance, in 3LS, 341, 342
concentration, 38, 84, 134, 241, 291, 304
conditioning exercises, 372
congestive heart failure, 268
constipation, x, xi, 42, 79, 119
conventional medicine. *See* allopathic
  medicine; modern-day medicine
cool-down time, 31, 50, 139, 140, 146, 194
coordination, 39, 135, 150–152, 241
coping skills, 46, 296, 347, 381, 391, 399
coronary heart disease, 42
cortisol, 35, 225
cortisol levels, 42
Cosmic Consciousness (Bucke), 311, 378, 399
cost
    of Perfect Whole Foods Diet, 94
    of Right Exercise, 160

costochondritis, 42, 73, 74, 210
cough, 16, 42, 101
counseling, 296–299, 301, 305
cramps, 73, 141, 146
craniosacral therapy, 264, 324
cravings, 80, 85, 98, 101, 105, 359
creativity, 19–20, 39, 210, 309, 379
crisis, xxiv, 53, 68, 114, 117, 118–192,
  162, 205
Crohn's disease, 38, 116, 385
cross-training, 114–115
cures, xix, 13, 16, 86, 115, 117, 178, 188,
  231–232

D

dairy products, 89, 93, 121
DeCourtney, Jan, xxi–xxv, 202, 379, 383,
  388, 392
deficiency, 372
degenerative diseases, 224, 372
delta brainwaves, 41
dental problems, 13, 125, 394
dentists, 125, 265, 276, 324
depression, xix, 38, 119, 135, 158, 210, 241,
  282, 308, 365
detoxification, 84, 119, 246, 277, 278, 385
diabetes, 135, 136, 150, 266, 268, 312
diagnosis, 7, 16, 21, 25, 231, 262, 264, 266,
  269, 283, 287, 374
diet, 116
    Candida, 115
    elimination/provocation, 114–115,
      119–120
    food combining, 115
    hereditary/metabolic, 114
    in mind/emotions/spirit, 289
    rotation, 19–120, 114–115
    ten percent fat, 114
    in 3LS Wellness Program, xxi, 9–13
    in Whole Foods Diet choice, 75–78
dietitians, 92, 324, 349
digestive disorders, 27–38, 385
digestive enzymes, 117–118
digestive issues, xxii, 38, 63, 113, 116–118,
  122, 309
digestive weakness, 37–38
digitalis, 268
diverticulitis, 38, 42, 116
dizziness, 38, 42, 101, 102
drug addiction, 64, 288, 396

drugs, xix, xx, 64, 183, 222, 267, 271, 280, 286, 287, 307, 319, 347, 372, 390
dysautonomia, ix, xxii, 42
dysbiosis, 38, 117–118, 294, 372

E

eating out, 109–110
economics, for healthcare practitioners, 326–327
eczema, 84, 255
edge of the cliff, 21, 23, 37, 61, 62, 101, 178, 220, 225–227, 229–230, 372
EEG. *See* electro-encephalograph
EFA. *See* essential fatty acids
eggs, 89, 121
electro-encephalograph (EEG), 372
    Skilled Relaxation and, 57, 58, 59
electromagnetic medicine, 274, 276, 372
electromagnetic smog, 220, 221, 223, 252, 372
electro-myograph (EMG), 57, 59
elimination/provocation
    diet, 114–115, 119–120
    testing, 294
EMG. *See* electro-myograph
emotional disturbances, 135, 250, 284, 291
emotions, 193, 343–344
    awareness of, 197–198
endocrine system, 38, 42, 286
endurance, 174
energy healing, 172, 265, 325, 398
energy medicine, 372. *See also* electro-magnetic medicine
engrams, 299, 364, 372
environmental illness, 79
enzymes, 117–118, 143, 309, 348, 373, 375
essential amino acids, 255, 258, 259–260, 279, 372
essential fatty acids (EFA), 255, 258–259, 279, 294, 372, 392
essential oils, 360, 372
exacerbations, 43, 187, 188, 193, 205, 211, 260–261, 333, 372
exercise, ix, xi, 3, 9–10, 15, 31, 60, 72. *See also* Aerobic Exercise
    flexibility in, 150
    heart rate in, 375
    in mind/emotions/spirit, 295
    in Right Exercise choice, 130–131, 137–138, 149–154
    with Skilled Relaxation, 60

in 3LS Wellness Program, xxi, 3, 9–13
    videos, 133, 155, 387, 388
expectations, in 3LS, 176, 193
expression, 197

F

family, 6, 49, 106–107, 181–185, 205
family therapists, 324, 349, 395
fasting, 246, 349
fatigue, 141, 146–147
fats, 39, 82, 89, 121, 208, 366, 375
Feldenkrais, 62, 264, 273, 373
    practitioners, 324, 394
    in Right Exercise, 151
    Skilled Relaxation and, 62
fight or flight (FOF), 220, 225, 373
    Skilled Relaxation and, 33–34, 35, 39, 71
    Whole Foods Diet and, 77
fitness, 133, 155, 325, 365, 386–388
Fitness for Dummies (Schlosberg & Neporent), 133, 140, 161, 166, 207, 365, 386
flexibility exercise, 150
Flexner report, 317
focusing, 7, 19, 21–24, 27, 29, 47, 198–199, 266–267, 370, 374. *See also* Gestalt therapy
FOF. *See* fight or flight
food(s)
    additives, 91, 221, 257, 261, 351, 359–360, 384–385, 391
    allergies to, x, 38, 42, 76, 91, 109, 110, 114–115, 115, 117, 126, 241–242, 309, 365, 384–385, 396
    combining, 115
    hypersensitivities and, 38, 76, 112, 115–117, 119, 178, 195, 294, 365, 374, 385, 393, 395
    organic, 94, 104, 115, 252, 320, 349
    quick references for, 352–358
    refined, 76, 78, 82, 83, 90, 182, 377
    superfoods, 260
food combining, diet and, 115
foot, x, 248, 281, 387
fructose, 90, 104, 354, 355, 365
fruit
    in mind/emotions/spirit, 291
    in Perfect Whole Foods Diet, 86, 88, 90, 104–106, 115, 121, 291
full stomach, Right Exercise and, 141

functional disease, 12, 35, 373
functional medicine, 263, 346, 363, 364
fungal infections, 118, 308, 371, 392
The Future of the Body (Murphy), 312, 397

G

gall bladder, 43, 191
galvanic skin response, 56–59, 373
gastro esophageal reflux disorder (GERD),
    38, 116–117, 373
gastrointestinal problems, 35, 116, 286,
    294, 372, 385
general adaptation syndrome, 366, 391
genetic inheritance, 22, 24, 218, 227, 231
genetic susceptibility, 157, 178, 228
genetics, 217, 218–219, 223, 227, 238, 285,
    305, 373
genome, 227, 231, 301, 363, 373, 391
GERD. *See* gastro esophageal reflux
    disorder
Gestalt therapy, 297
goals
    healthcare practitioners' guide and,
        323
    in Right Exercise, 131–134, 167
grains
    refined, 90
    whole, 29, 88–90, 123, 194, 310
grief therapy, 297
GSR. *See* galvanic skin response
guided imagery, 48, 72, 133, 200, 248–249,
    278, 373, 387

H

Hahnemann, Samuel, 261–262
Hakomi, 265, 297
headaches, 38, 101, 105, 119, 128, 189, 241,
    253, 359
healing, 21–28, 373
    bodymind and, 21–22
    cliff edge and, 21–22, 23
    crisis, 188–192, 205, 373
    genetic inheritance and, 22, 24
    progression, 187–193
    relationships and, 331
    signs of, 193
    steps to, 243–244
healing tools
    awareness, 193, 194–200, 211–213
    Beyond Disease Care, 201, 343
    body awareness, 201, 343

bodymind, 194, 195, 205
bodymind laboratory, 195–196
emotional awareness, 197–198
expression in, 197
instinct in, 194
knowledge/study, 200–201
mind in, 193, 200–202
practice charts, 211–213
*Saving Yourself from the Disease Care
    Crisis* and, 201
self-awareness and, 196
spirituality and, 199–200, 377
thought awareness and, 198–199
in 3LS/daily life, 193–202, 205
toxins and, 194
websites and, 201, 202
The Healing Power of Whole Foods
    (Loiselle), ii, 30, 91, 94, 104, 109, 113, 121,
    123, 349, 351, 385
health clubs, 158, 387, 388
health food stores, 81, 92, 93, 119, 260–261,
    320, 386, 391, 393
health history, 271, 272, 279, 328, 339
health maintenance, 11, 25, 39, 79, 121
heart attack, 39, 136, 162, 171, 172, 228, 229
heart disease, 42, 114, 130, 131, 136, 169,
    266, 382, 388
heart rate
    maximal, 139, 167, 375, 378
    target, 138–139, 142–143, 160, 167,
        211, 378
Hellerwork, 62, 264–265, 273, 373
hemorrhoids, 43, 69
herbalists, 281, 307, 324
herbology, 265, 276
hereditary/metabolic diets, 114
herpes, 11, 43
hives, 73, 172, 248, 309, 345
Hoffer, Abram, 290
holistic approaches, 287–288, 299–300,
    305, 306
Holistic Dental Association, 394
Holistic Healing Center, 63, 394
holistic health, iv, 202, 263–264, 269, 367,
    373. *See also* American Holistic Health
    Association
holistic medicine
    adjunct approaches to, 262–264,
        269–271, 272, 275–276, 279
    allopathic medicine and, 318, 319,
        320–321

illness causes and, 229–231
in modern-day medicine, 318–321
physicians and, 393–394
in practicing serious wellness, 14, 17
3LS Wellness Program and, xxi–xxii,
4–5, 7, 14, 17
in 3LS/daily life, 203
treatments, 324, 325–326, 326–329
Holmes-Rahe test, 222
homeodynamic, 103, 229, 374
homeopathy, 264, 276, 300, 325, 329, 330,
348, 349, 367
homeostasis, 172, 374
hormones, 35, 84, 222, 288, 374
Human Genome Project, 22, 227, 301,
374, 391
human potential, 311–313
hypertension, x, 43, 69, 172, 182, 266, 268
hypnotherapy, 265, 297, 324
hypoglycemia, x, 30, 43, 88, 123, 126, 242,
365, 396
hypothalamic overload, 35, 39, 244, 374
hypothalamus, 34, 35–38, 44, 56, 57, 71,
148, 172, 225–226, 230, 240–241, 284, 286,
293, 374, 382

I

imagery, guided, 48, 72, 133, 200, 248–249,
278, 373, 387
imagination, 72, 331
immune disorder, xii, 208
immune response, 85–86, 90, 101–103, 121
immune system, 85, 90, 101–103, 116–117,
121, 312, 382, 397
indigestion, 16, 69, 208
informed choice, 245, 278
injuries
Right Exercise and, 140, 147–148, 157,
160–161, 170–171
3LS/daily life and, 13, 16, 133–136, 139,
145–147, 209, 210, 232, 250, 387
insomnia, xxii, 69, 119, 135, 241
instinct, 194
insulin, 30, 88, 114, 123, 135, 268
insurance, medical, xi, 273, 315–317, 320,
321, 329, 392
integrated exercises, 134, 375
integrative medicine, 263, 350
International Fitness Association, iv, 138,
365, 388
interstitial cystitis, 43, 74, 282

irritable bowel syndrome, 43, 364
isolation tanks, 48
isometric exercise, 152

J

Jacobson, Edmond, xix, xx
jogging, 162–163, 169
joint aches, 43, 128, 146

K

key resources, 46, 91, 133, 381, 384–385,
386–388
kinesiology, 258, 265, 275–276, 297,
324–325
knowledge/study, 200–201
Krebs cycle, 374
in Right Exercise, 141
Whole Foods Diet and, 76, 78, 82, 83,
93, 104–105

L

lactose, 90, 93, 355, 357, 359, 365
leaky gut syndrome (LGS), 375. *See also*
digestive weakness
in common digestive issues, 116,
117, 118
mind/emotions/spirit and, 286
3LS/daily life and, 208
learning disabilities, 79, 288, 289, 309
lethargy, 309
LGS. *See* leaky gut syndrome
Liberal Whole Foods Diet
Perfect Whole Foods Diet vs., 86, 91,
111–112, 121
Whole Foods Diet and, 76, 78, 86,
91, 104
lifestyles, 303, 349
mind/emotions/spirit and, 285–287,
305
Perfect Whole Foods Diet and, 106–111
3LS/daily life and, 183–184, 186
light therapy, 245, 300
locus of control, 22–24, 233, 375
Loiselle, Beth
The Healing Power of Whole Foods, ii,
30, 91, 94, 104, 109, 113, 121, 123,
349, 351, 385
Perfect Whole Foods Diet and, 91–92,
104, 349
love, 40, 182, 185–187, 199, 242, 264, 304,
344, 348

lumps, 16, 281
lymph nodes, 43, 171

M

macrobiotic diet, 115, 276
macronutrients, 82, 375
magnesium, 257–258, 268, 279, 280, 294, 307, 309, 392
magnetics, 48, 143, 166, 219–221, 238, 251, 274, 295, 372, 395
malabsorption testing, 294, 309
manic-depression, 38, 43, 79, 288, 307
massage, 36–37, 55, 60, 62–64, 66, 71, 128, 161, 246, 375
    self, 250, 278, 334, 390
    Skilled Relaxation and, 37, 62–64, 66
    sports, 160, 265
        therapists, 37, 59, 62, 64, 128, 146, 149, 160, 210, 250, 324, 328, 347, 350, 394
maximal heart rate, 139, 167, 375, 378
meal preparation, 108–109
meats, 89, 93, 121
medical advice, 15–16
medical conditions, helped by Skilled Relaxation, 42–43
medical insurance, 273, 329
medical records, 271, 279
medication. *See* prescription medications/drugs
medicine systems, 264
meditation, 40–41, 46, 47, 72, 242, 350, 381, 382, 383
megadoses, 256, 305, 375, 376
memory, 207, 288, 291, 312, 367, 395
mental growth, 247
mental health professionals, 68, 324
Mental Tennis (Braden), 133, 387
mental-emotional approaches, 265
mental-emotional problems, 285–293
menus, 87–88, 89
metabolic efficiency, 142–144
metabolic sluggishness, 229, 244
metabolism, 114, 143–144, 223, 375, 382
metal toxicity, 242, 294
micronutrients, 82, 83, 84, 375
middle of the field, 375
migraine, ix, 241, 395
milk, whole, 29, 93, 365
mind, 193, 200–202
Mind as Healer, Mind as Slayer (Peletier), 240, 363, 382, 391

mindfulness, 47, 199
mineral salt, 95, 103
minerals
    trace, 95, 378
    vitamins and, 257
mistakes, common, in 3LS diet, 175–177
modern-day medicine
    in allopathic medicine, 316, 317, 318, 319, 320–321
    holistic medicine in, 318, 319, 320–321
    Saving Yourself from the Disease Care Crisis and, xxiv, 117, 202, 318, 388, 395
    3LS Wellness Program in, 315–318
mood swings, 125, 291
motivation, 158–159
multiple sclerosis, 131, 388
multivitamins, 260, 261
muscular tension, 35–36, 69, 71, 247
myofascial pain, 43, 265

N

naps, 51, 52, 65, 128. *See also* sleep
Native American healing, 234, 264
natural medicine, 263, 367, 390
neck pain, 43, 63, 150
nervousness, 38, 39, 43, 101, 288, 291
neuromuscular therapy, 265, 300
neuropathy, 43, 169
nicotine
    addiction to, 99, 105, 385, 396
    Perfect Whole Foods Diet and, 99, 105, 121
Ninety Days to Self-Health (Shealy), 346
numbness, ix, 53, 169, 193, 225
nutrition, 75–79, 81–84, 86, 91, 94–96, 100, 121, 134, 222–223, 294–302, 325, 364, 367, 375, 395–393. *See also* orthomolecular nutrition
nutritional deficiency, 286, 288–289, 307
nutritional dose, 255, 256, 375
nutritional needs, Whole Foods Diet and, 76
nutritional supplementation, 76, 95, 114, 247, 255–257, 277, 278–279, 292, 294, 344, 392–393
    balanced B complex, 258
    EFAs, 255, 258–259
    essential amino acids, 259–260
    exacerbations, 260–261
    magnesium, i, 257–258

in mind/emotions/spirit, 94
multivitamins, 260
nutritional dose, 255, 256
Omega 3 oils, 259, 261
Omega 6 oils, 259
pharmacological dose, 256–257
superfoods, 260
synergy, 225–256
vitamin C, 258
vitamin E, 258
vitamins/minerals, 257
whole foods concentrates, 257
nutritional supplements
    in adjunct approaches, 247, 255–261,
        278–279
    in Perfect Whole Foods Diet, 95, 114
nutritional therapy, 256, 265, 289, 292, 293,
    385, 395
nutritionists, 114, 257, 324, 386
nuts/seeds, 89, 93, 121

O

older people, 44, 88, 140, 152
Omega 3 oils, 259, 261
Omega 6 oils, 259
organic food, 94, 115, 252, 349
oriental medicine, 324
The Origins of Human Disease (McKeown),
    xix
orthomolecular medicine, i, 290, 292,
    376, 397
orthomolecular nutrition, 376, 395–397
orthomolecular therapy, 256–257, 289, 290,
    294–295, 305, 376, 397
osteoarthritis, 43, 372
osteopathy, 264, 266, 316
overexercising, 145, 241–242
overweight, x, 79, 80, 136, 154, 168
oxygen, 135, 142–144, 246, 295

P

pain, chronic, 61–62
panic attacks, 38, 43, 73, 79, 172, 288, 289,
    291, 307
parasites, 43, 117–118, 185, 371, 385
parasympathetic nervous system, 370,
    376, 378
pasta, 93, 96, 111, 354
pathological mechanisms, 285, 305, 376
patient education, 7, 262, 327, 329,
    331–332, 336, 374

persistence, in Perfect Whole Foods Diet,
    99–101, 112–113
personal growth work, 297–299, 376
personal trainers, 148, 151, 156, 158,
    325, 388
pharmaceutical medication, 262, 278, 279,
    286, 287, 288, 290, 315
pharmacological dose, 256–257, 294, 376
phenome, 227, 230, 301, 363, 373, 376
phobias, 38, 42, 79, 288, 349
physical health, mind/emotions/spirit vs.,
    283–285
physical therapy, 64, 131, 154, 210, 265,
    324, 328
physicians, in allopathic medicine, 318,
    319, 320–321
Physician's Desk Reference, 267
phytochemicals, 82, 255, 257, 375, 376
pilates, 131, 150, 152, 170–171
polarity therapy, xxii, 265, 300, 324,
    328, 376
pollution, 182, 222, 226, 286, 372, 391
poor health, 25, 75, 79, 83, 88, 234
post-traumatic stress disorder (PTSD), 38,
    79, 288, 349
posture, 132, 135, 152, 153, 369, 379
practicing serious wellness, 9–20, 376
    bodymind in, 11–12, 21–22
    chronic conditions in, 10–11, 13–14, 15
    health maintenance in, 10–11, 25
    holistic medicine in, 14, 17
    medical advice in, 15–16
    prescription drugs and, 18–19
    Q&A about, 12–20, 335
    Right Exercise in, xxiii, 9–13, 15, 25, 31
    side effects of, 19–20
    Skilled Relaxation in, xxiii, 9–13, 15, 25,
        27–28
    Whole Foods Diet in, xxiii, 9–13, 15, 25,
        29–30
practitioner-assisted approaches, 243
practitioners, 5, 7, 13, 15, 261, 264, 269,
    272, 274–275, 323–324, 336–337
    effectiveness, 342–343
    health and, 324
    resources for, 324
prayer, 47, 199, 265, 299, 303, 367, 399
pre-menstrual syndrome, 43, 79
prescription medications/drugs, 18–19,
    267–268
probiotics, 117–118, 376

professional help
> for nutrition/digestion, 113–114
> with Perfect Whole Foods Diet,
>> 113–114
> in Right Exercise, 161–162
> for Skilled Relaxation, 68
progress monitoring, 140, 168
progressive resistance, 152
protocols, for wellness, xxi, 3, 11, 25, 115,
> 117, 146, 195, 293, 345, 369, 376, 385
psoriasis, 43, 84, 255
psychiatry, 265, 297, 397
psychological counseling, 236, 287, 290,
> 296–297, 301, 305
psychopathology, 28, 44
psychosocial approaches, 295–299, 306
psychosocial environment, 197, 285, 376
psychosocial stress, 376–377
psychotherapy, 265, 297, 299, 328, 343,
> 349, 370
PTSD. *See* post-traumatic stress disorder
pulse rate, 136–137, 160, 168

Q

Quick-Start Guides, 4–5, 27–31

R

radiation/irradiation, 222, 223, 281, 372
rashes, 191, 253, 359
rebounding, 152–153, 164, 169
refined carbohydrate addiction/allergy,
> 84–86, 98–99, 101–106, 121
refined carbohydrates, 84–86, 90, 93
> addiction to, 84–86, 92, 98–101, 104,
>> 121, 133–134, 244, 294
refined foods, 377
> 3LS/daily life and, 182
> Whole Foods Diet and, 76, 78, 82,
>> 83, 90
refined grains, 90
reflexology, 247–248, 265, 377
relationships, 181–187, 233, 247, 262, 265,
> 269, 293, 296, 331
relaxation, xxi, 3, 9–13
relaxation response, 54–55, 377
*The Relaxation and Stress Reduction
> Workbook* (David, Eschelman & McKay),
> 379
> adjunct approaches and, 249, 255
> illness causes and, 224, 240
> Skilled Relaxation and, 46, 72

relief, immediate, 51, 60, 61–65, 71
religious approaches, 299, 300, 306
remission, 169, 188, 193, 211, 265, 377
restaurants, 81, 94, 106, 109–111, 122, 127,
> 203, 320
rheumatoid arthritis, xii, 125, 126–127, 171,
> 209, 280, 364
Rolfing, 62, 66, 265, 273, 377
rosacea, 43, 73
Rosen method, 265, 300
rotation diet, 114–115, 119–120
running, 146, 162, 163, 194–195

S

salt, mineral, 95, 103
Saving Yourself from the Disease Care Crisis
> (Stoll), xxiv, 95, 103, 201, 317–318, 345
schizophrenia, 285, 288, 290, 307, 367,
> 395, 397
scoliosis, 43, 191, 192
seasonings, 29, 88, 89, 121
secondary/tertiary healthcare providers,
> 325
seizure disorders, 28, 44, 56, 68, 359
self-awareness, 53, 196
self-empowerment, 81
self-esteem, 19, 39, 81, 159, 297
self-help, 6, 8, 10, 15, 17, 25
> devices for, 251
self-help techniques, 243, 245–251, 278
self-hypnosis, 46, 47, 61, 72, 133, 205, 248
self-massage, 249–250, 278, 334, 390
Selye, Hans, 219, 225
sensitivity, 292, 365, 377
serious wellness. *See* practicing serious
> wellness
setbacks, 178, 188, 276
Shealy, C. Norman, xx, 260, 262
> *Ninety Days to Self-Health* and, 346
side effects, of practicing serious wellness,
> 19–20
Silva Mind Training, 47, 69, 72, 202
sinus infections, xi, 69
skin conditions, 310, 390
sleep, 51, 66, 240. *See also* naps
smoking, 99, 100, 136, 252, 385
snacking, 95–97
social influences, on mind/emotions/
> spirit, 296–297
soft diet, 384
somatic approaches, 265, 297, 300, 364

sound/light machines, 48
spasms, 42, 43, 140, 153, 241, 250
spices, 29, 81, 89, 94, 97, 111, 123, 357.
    See also seasonings
spirit, of life, 302–304, 305
spiritual healing, 377
spirituality, 61, 189, 199–200, 299, 303, 377
sports massage, 160, 265
sports medicine specialists, 149, 157, 158,
    161, 162, 325, 388
standard American diet, 83
Stoll, Walt
    Beyond Disease Care and, 202, 345, 385,
        387, 388, 392, 395
    Recapture Your Health and, 202
    *Saving Yourself from the Disease Care
        Crisis* and, xxiv, 95, 103, 201,
        317–318, 345
    3LS Wellness Program and, xxi–xxv,
        315–321
stomach, full, 141
stool withholding, 4, 392
stored stress-effect, 34, 35, 37, 38–39, 51,
    148, 229–230, 286, 378
strengthening exercises, 150, 166
stress, 377–378
    acute, 225–226, 238, 369
    biochemical, 221, 222, 238, 371
    biophysical, 217, 220, 221, 229–231,
        238, 252, 370, 391
    chemical, 220
    chronic, 33–39, 225–226
    decreasing/eliminating, 247, 252–255
    emotional, 220, 373, 376
    management of, 46, 210, 246, 253, 366,
        381, 384, 391, 397
    mind/emotions/spirit and, 285, 305
    nutritional, 222–223
    physical, 220–221, 247, 370–371
    psychosocial, 224, 376, 391
    real, 219–226
    Right Exercise and, 136, 148
    3LS daily/life and, 183
    3LS Wellness Program and, 8
    Whole Foods Diet and, 183
stress-effect, 378
    in illness causes, 217, 220, 224–226,
        229, 238
    mind/emotions/spirit and, 285–286
    Skilled Relaxation and, 34–35, 40, 66
    stored, 150

stressors
    biochemical, 222, 238
    biophysical, 217, 220–224, 238,
        252, 278
    electromagnetic, 222, 238
    interactions, 228–229
    in mind/emotions/spirit, 286
    nutritional, 222–223
    physical, 221, 238
    psychosocial, 217, 224, 238, 253–255
stretching, 130, 140, 145, 146, 152, 163–164
stroke, 131, 186, 388
sugar, 90, 98–99
suicide, 284, 394–395
surgery, 12, 64, 69, 262, 266–268, 279
swimming, 135, 141, 154, 167
The Symbolic Message of Illness (Pop), 255
sympathetic nervous system, 8, 33, 370,
    373, 378
synchronistic treatments, 323–324
Synergetics, 140, 142, 150, 153
synergy, 245, 255–256

T

T'ai chi chuan, 48, 378
T'ai chi/qi gong, 153
target heart rate, 138–139, 142–143, 160,
    167, 211, 378. *See also* maximal heart rate
taste sensitivity, 80–81
teeth, 36, 42, 248. *See also* bruxism
temperature
    body, 52
    skin, 57
ten percent fat diet, 114
The Textbook of Functional Medicine
    (misc), 346
therapeutic dose. *See* pharmacological
    dose
therapeutic touch, 265, 300, 324
therapists, for massage, 37, 59, 62, 64, 128,
    146, 149, 160, 210, 250, 324, 328, 347,
    350, 394
theta brainwaves, 40–41, 44, 45, 50, 54–55,
    72, 377
thought awareness, 198–199
thought stopping, 47
thyroid, 169, 171, 172, 248, 374
time management, 46, 147, 381, 391, 397
timing, in Skilled Relaxation, 50, 60–61
tinnitus, 43, 248
TMJ, 13, 43, 210, 276

toenail problems, 244, 390
top of the mountain, 3, 181, 189, 297, 304, 311, 313, 378
tough love, 337–338
toxins, 195, 222, 246, 286, 289, 302
    healing tools and, 194
    3LS/daily life and, 182
trace minerals, 95, 378
traditional medicine, 373
Tragerwork, 265, 273
transit time, 118, 278
trauma therapy, 265, 297, 324
treatments, in holistic medicine, 324, 325–326, 326–329
treatments, conventional, 287, 305
triggering responses, 86, 90, 101, 103
triglycerides, 79, 135
troubleshooting
    for adjunct approaches, 274–275
    for mind/emotions/spirit, 302
    for Perfect Whole Foods Diet, 112–118
    for Right Exercise, 154–162
    for Skilled Relaxation, 65–68
    for 3LS/daily life, 180–181
tumors, 74, 172
twitching, 52, 241

U

ulcerative colitis, 38, 43, 116, 385
ulcers, 43, 228

V

vegetables, 87–89, 89, 97, 110, 115, 121, 123, 233, 379
vertigo, 43, 73
vibrational energy medicine, 300, 378
violence, 181, 396
viral infections, 135
visualization, 46, 48, 72, 133, 205, 249, 278, 381–382
vitalism, 266, 379
vitamins, 379
    B, 290, 291–292, 294, 307
    C, 258
    E, 258
    minerals and, 257
    multi, 260

W

wakefulness, in Skilled Relaxation, 51–52, 60, 66
Walkaerobics (Sansone), 387
walking, x, 60, 102, 132, 141, 149, 153–154, 157, 164, 167, 170, 210, 387
warm ups, 139–140, 146
warts, 16, 248
water aerobics, 147, 154, 163, 171
websites, xxiv, 8, 98, 136, 184, 201–203, 320, 345, 367, 381, 383–385, 387, 389, 390, 399
weight loss, 144, 209, 384
    Perfect Whole Foods Diet and, 75, 80, 91, 121
weight training, 150, 151, 154
wellness. *See* practicing serious wellness
whole foods concentrates, 134, 257, 279, 294
whole grains, 89, 121
wholeness, 40, 298, 311, 313, 379
withdrawal, 30, 84–85, 97, 98, 101–102, 103–104, 105, 121, 123, 365. *See also* addiction
workbook. *See The Relaxation and Stress Reduction Workbook*

X

xanax, 210, 301

Y

yoga, 71, 72, 133, 151, 246, 265, 379, 399
    Right Exercise and, 153, 164
    Skilled Relaxation and, 48, 68

Z

zero balancing, 265
zoloft, 307

GIVE *RECAPTURE YOUR HEALTH*
TO YOUR FAMILY AND FRIENDS

Postal Mail: Send this completed form with check, money order, or credit card info to: Sunrise Health Coach Publications, PO Box 21132, Boulder, CO 80308.

Internet: Visit www.sunrisehealthcoach.com to place your order and see our other titles. E-books are also available.

Phone: Call toll free 1-877-3LS-WELL (1-877-357-9355) or 303-527-2886 to leave your order on our answering machine. Or, leave your name and phone number, and someone will call back to take your order.

Fax: Call 1-877-3LS-WELL (1-877-359-9355) for faxing instructions.

E-mail: E-mail your order and credit card info to orders@sunrisehealthcoach .com. You may also use Paypal to send your order to this e-mail address.

Please print clearly:

Name:_____

Address: _____

City/State/Zip: _____

Telephone: day_____ evening _____

E-mail address:_____

❏ Send me ____ copy(ies) of *Recapture Your Health* @ $19.95 each. $_____

Sales tax: Add 8.2% for Colorado. $_____

Shipping: $4.00 first copy, $2.00 each additional copy. $_____

For foreign shipping, please order from our website at www.sunrisehealthcoach.com.

Total: .... $_____

Payment: ❏ Check ❏ Money order ❏ Visa ❏ Master Card

Credit card number: __ _____

Name on card: _____

Exp. Date: _____

Signature: _____

Customer service: call toll free 1-877-3LS-WELL
(1-877-357-9355) or 303-527-2886.
E-mail: orders@sunrisehealthcoach.com.

❏ Check here to receive a occasional e-mail newsletter
with health tips and notification of new books and author events.

Thank you for your order!